PULMONARY GAS EXCHANGE

Volume I

Contributors

John W. Evans
Robert A. Klocke
Albert J. Olszowka
Arthur B. Otis
Johannes Piiper
Hermann Rahn
Richard L. Riley
Peter Scheid
Peter D. Wagner
John B. West

PULMONARY GAS EXCHANGE

Volume I

Ventilation, Blood Flow, and Diffusion

Edited by

John B. West

Department of Medicine
School of Medicine
University of California, San Diego
La Jolla, California

ACADEMIC PRESS   1980
A Subsidiary of Harcourt Brace Jovanovich, Publishers
New York   London   Toronto   Sydney   San Francisco

ACADEMIC PRESS, INC.
111 Fifth Avenue, New York, New York 10003

United Kingdom Edition published by
ACADEMIC PRESS, INC. (LONDON) LTD.
24/28 Oval Road, London NW1 7DX

Library of Congress Cataloging in Publication Data
Main entry under title:

Pulmonary gas exchange.

   Includes bibliographies and index.
   CONTENTS: v. 1. Ventilation, blood flow and
diffusion.
   1. Respiration. 2. Blood gases. 3. Respiratory
insufficiency. I. West, John Burnard.
QP121.P78   612'.22   80–12857
ISBN 0–12–744501–3

PRINTED IN THE UNITED STATES OF AMERICA

80 81 82 83   9 8 7 6 5 4 3 2 1

Contents

3 Development of the Three-Compartment Model for Dealing with Uneven Distribution

Richard L. Riley

4 Intrapulmonary Gas Mixing and Stratification

Peter Scheid and Johannes Piiper

5 Blood–Gas Equilibration in Lungs

Johannes Piiper and Peter Scheid

6 Kinetics of Pulmonary Gas Exchange
Robert A. Klocke

7 Ventilation–Perfusion Relationships
Peter D. Wagner and John B. West

8 Numerical Analysis of Gas Exchange
Albert J. Olszowka and Peter D. Wagner

9 Mathematical Analysis of Compartmental Lung Models
John W. Evans

List of Contributors

Numbers in parentheses indicate the pages on which the authors' contributions begin.

John W. Evans (307), Department of Mathematics, University of California, San Diego, La Jolla, California 92093

Robert A. Klocke (173), Department of Medicine, State University of New York at Buffalo, Buffalo, New York 14214

Albert J. Olszowka (263), Department of Physiology, State University of New York at Buffalo, Buffalo, New York 14214

Arthur B. Otis (33), Department of Physiology, University of Florida College of Medicine, Gainesville, Florida 32610

Johannes Piiper (87, 131), Abteilung Physiologie, Max-Planck-Institut für experimentelle Medizin, D-3400 Gottingen, Federal Republic of Germany

Hermann Rahn (33), Department of Physiology, State University of New York at Buffalo, Buffalo, New York 14214

Richard L. Riley (67), Departments of Environmental Health Sciences and Medicine, The Johns Hopkins Medical Institutions, Baltimore, Maryland 21205

Peter Scheid (87, 131), Abteilung Physiologie, Max-Planck-Institut für experimentelle Medizin, D-3400 Gottingen, Federal Republic of Germany

Peter D. Wagner (219, 263), Department of Medicine, School of Medicine, University of California, San Diego, La Jolla, California 92093

John B. West (1, 219), Department of Medicine, School of Medicine, University of California, San Diego, La Jolla, California 92093

Preface

The purpose of this two-volume treatise is to provide an up-to-date comprehensive account of pulmonary gas exchange, particularly in relation to the human lung. Interest in the lung has burgeoned over the last few years and dramatic advances have been made in the area of gas exchange. This is the cardinal function of the lung and is of interest and importance not only to physiologists but also to chest physicians, anesthesiologists, and cardiologists who are frequently confronted with problems of disordered gas exchange.

This first volume is devoted to the mechanisms of gas exchange in the lung, particularly the roles of ventilation, blood flow, and diffusion. The opening chapter briefly traces the emergence of our knowledge from ancient times; this is of interest because in the seventeenth and eighteenth centuries pulmonary gas exchange was the central preoccupation of some of the best scientists, and the history of pulmonary gas exchange is largely the history of chemistry and physics. The next two chapters are devoted to the momentous developments which took place near the end of the Second World War, advances which established the modern basis of gas exchange. We are fortunate that Dr. Richard Riley and Drs. Arthur Otis and Hermann Rahn were persuaded to contribute first-hand accounts of those pivotal times. Most of the remainder of the book is devoted to how gas gets to the alveoli, how it crosses the blood–gas barrier, and the way in which ventilation–perfusion relationships determine the efficiency of exchange.

The second volume deals with how gas exchange is altered in a variety of circumstances including exercise, high altitude, anesthesia, and lung disease. Two chapters are concerned with highly contentious areas— possible facilitated diffusion across the blood–gas barrier and the alleged reversed arterial–alveolar difference for carbon dioxide.

I am indebted to the contributors, who are all authoritative (and correspondingly busy), for keeping to the deadlines so effectively. It is a pleasure to thank the staff of Academic Press for their help.

John B. West

Contents of Volume II

1

Historical Development

John B. West

I. INTRODUCTION

In a book devoted to pulmonary gas exchange, it is worth tracing the historical development of the topic for at least two reasons. First, there is the intrinsic interest of the subject. For example, the evolution of ideas on respiration in the seventeenth and eighteenth centuries is one of the scientific sagas of civilized man. Indeed, the development of chemistry and physics during that time was largely the history of pulmonary gas exchange.

PULMONARY GAS EXCHANGE, VOL. I
Copyright © 1980 by Academic Press, Inc.
All rights of reproduction in any form reserved.
ISBN 0-12-744501-3

But perhaps a more compelling reason is that our modern understanding of any subject must reflect to some extent the way knowledge has developed, and it is important to be aware of this. In the future, historians will no doubt recognize where some of our current misconceptions had their origin, and a sense of history should help to keep us alert for change.

It is easy to forget how recently prejudices have been corrected. For example, only 80 years ago Bohr (1909) vehemently argued in one of his best-known papers that up to 60% of the oxygen consumption of an animal occurs in the tissue cells of the lung. If this were true it would mean that the Fick principle for measuring pulmonary blood flow from the arterial–venous oxygen difference and oxygen uptake would be invalid. Indeed, Bohr staunchly took this position. This seems a very bizarre attitude for one of the most distinguished physiologists of his time, until we realize that in the eighteenth century all oxygen consumption and heat production was thought to take place in lung tissue (an idea that is traceable to the early Greek philosophers) and that the site of oxygen usage in the body remained a contentious issue right through the nineteenth century (see Section IV,A).

Another notion that took an "unconscionable time adying" was active secretion of oxygen by the lungs against a partial pressure gradient. Only 50 or so years ago, Haldane and Priestley (1935) devoted a whole chapter in their book "Respiration" to the evidence for this long after the Kroghs and Barcroft had apparently clinched the issue in favor of passive diffusion. Was this a dying gasp of the vitalism that had had so enormous an influence on the whole history of respiration from the time of Aristotle, and that was thought to have received a mortal blow from Claude Bernard in the 1880s?

Of course, it is easy to be wise after the event and no doubt historians in the future will be able to point a finger at some of our modern prejudices. In any event a sense of history can be very humbling and smooths the way to accepting changes, even when these are in conflict with prevailing opinion.

In this chapter, the history of pulmonary gas exchange is briefly traced from ancient times. There is, however, no attempt at a comprehensive account; the ideas followed are those most relevant to the subject as we see it today. Most of the material is necessarily derivative, the chief sources being Clendening (1960), Foster (1901), Fulton (1930), Goodfield (1960), Perkins (1964), Singer (1957, 1959), and Stirling (1902).

II. KNOWLEDGE PRIOR TO THE SEVENTEENTH CENTURY

A. Greeks and Romans

A central notion of many of the Greek philosophers as early as the sixth century B.C. was that the essence of all things is "pneuma," which can be translated as air, breath, or spirit. This was seen to be essential for life. Empodocles (ca. 495–435 B.C.) taught that all matter was composed of four elements: earth, air, fire, and water. The purpose of respiration was to cool the heart and blood, and the blood was then responsible for distributing "innate heat" from the heart to the various parts of the body. The ideas of Empodocles are important because he greatly influenced Aristotle (384–322 B.C.), many of whose views held sway until the eighteenth century. In addition, Aristotle was a vitalist who believed that the presence of a peculiar spirit, which he called "psyche," was responsible for the different functioning of animate and inanimate things. This view was opposed by Democritus (470–400 B.C.), an atomist, who favored mechanistic, deterministic causes. Aristotle was a keen observer of many species of animals, but he was not an experimentalist. For example, he taught that the arteries normally contain air.

Galen (130–199 A.D.) was born in Asia Minor and became a physician to the emperor Marcus Aurelius. Through his writings he exerted an enormous influence on the way men thought for 1500 years, his teachings being embellished by Arabic and medieval commentators. Many of his views can be traced to Erasistratus (born ca. 304 B.C.), who is credited with originating the "pneumatic" theory of respiration. Galen believed that blood was formed in the liver from food absorbed in the gut (Fig. 1). In the liver, it was imbued with "natural spirit." The blood then flowed to the right ventricle, where some of it went through the pulmonary artery to nourish the lungs, while a portion passed through "invisible pores" in the interventricular septum into the left ventricle. Here it was mixed with "pneuma" from the inspired air, and the resulting "vital spirit" was distributed throughout the body by the arterial blood. Blood that reached the brain received "animal spirit" and was distributed from there through the nerves, which were thought to be hollow. Galen also believed that fuliginous (sooty) waste products were eliminated from the blood by the lungs, though the route was a strange one in that the blood was thought to travel back through the pulmonary vein.

Although much of what Galen taught now seems quaint, it can be argued that the elements of pulmonary gas exchange had been established. Blood was enriched with a vital element from the inspired air and distributed by means of the arteries throughout the body. Waste materials

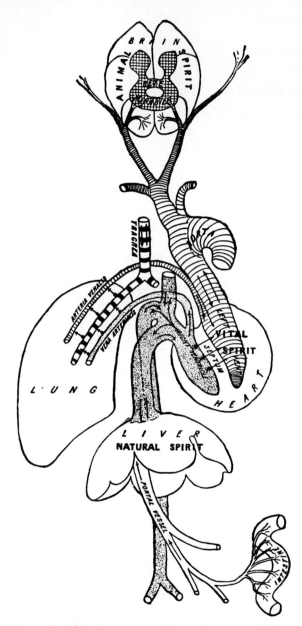

Fig. 1. Galen's cardiopulmonary system, which held sway for 1300 years. During inspiration, pneuma entered the lung through the trachea and reached the left ventricle via the pulmonary vein (arteria venalis). Blood was formed in the liver, and imbued there with natural spirit. A portion passed through minute channels in the interventricular septum to the left ventricle, where vital spirit was formed and distributed through arteries to the rest of the body. The blood that reached the brain was charged with animal spirit, which was distributed through the hollow nerves. (From Singer, 1957, reproduced by permission.)

in the blood were eliminated via the lungs. Unfortunately, the anatomical basis for these functions was in a very confused state, chiefly because the circulation of the blood was unsuspected.

B. The Dark Ages and Renaissance

For 1300 years, from the third to the sixteenth century, very little progress in physiology was made. The teachings of Galen and Aristotle were preserved chiefly in Arabic writings and were forgotten in much of Europe when the Roman civilization was destroyed. When the universities began to form in the twelfth century, medieval scholars started to discuss and embellish the knowledge inherited from the Arabs but little direct observation or experiment accompanied their theoretical studies.

A few events toward the end of this dismal period presaged the reawakening of science and the consequent rapid expansion of knowledge, which continues to the present day. Several of these advances were in the area of the pulmonary circulation, where the erroneous ideas of Galen and Aristotle so effectively stifled progress. For example, Ibn An-Nafis (ca. 1210–1288), a physician in Damascus, argued that blood did not go through the septum between right and left ventricles as Galen had taught, but through the lung. Because he could not see direct communications between the pulmonary artery and vein, he supposed that there must be invisible pores linking the two. Presumably this notion was not difficult to accept because the existence of invisible pores in the demonstrably solid interventricular septum was a central tenet in Galen's scheme (Fig. 1). Indeed, the possibility of pores between systemic arteries and veins had been suggested by Erasistratus in the fourth century B.C.

The manuscript of Ibn An-Nafis was not known to the medieval scholars and therefore Servetus (1511–1533) can be credited with independently discovering the pulmonary circulation (or more strictly the transit of blood through the lung), when he stated the blood passed from the right venticle to the left, not through the interventricular septum "as is commonly believed" but through the lungs from pulmonary artery to vein. He also wrote that the blood became reddish yellow in the process. However, his book "Christianismi Restitutio" was considered heretical by both Catholics and Calvinists, and Servetus and his books were burned at the stake in Geneva by the latter. Six years later Realdus Columbus (1516–1559) also clearly described the pulmonary transit, though it should be emphasized that the notion of the continuous circulation of blood through the lungs had not emerged at this time.

One of the most significant scientific events in the sixteenth century was the resurgence of anatomy, especially in the work of Vesalius

(1514–1564). There had been intimations before this; for example, the beautiful anatomical drawings of Leonardo da Vinci (1452–1519) broke some new ground, and he clearly understood the anatomy of the intra-pleural space (a subject that often confuses twentieth century medical students). But Vesalius' chief work "De Humani Corporis Fabrica" ("Mechanisms of the Human Body"), published in 1543 when he was 28, is considered to be the first clear break with the centuries-old tradition dominated by the teachings of Galen and Aristotle. This is not to say that Vesalius was not influenced by Galen (for example, he wondered uneasily how blood could get through the invisible interventricular pores) nor that Galen's teachings were abandoned (in some universities his writings were prescribed reading until the middle of the eighteenth century). But Vesalius' work typifies the fresh, inquiring spirit of the Renaissance, which was to provoke the explosion of learning in the seventeenth century.

III. SEVENTEENTH AND EIGHTEENTH CENTURIES

A. Harvey and the Microscopists

In many respects the seventeenth century was dominated by the work of William Harvey (1578–1657). His pivotal book "De Motu Cordis et Sanguinis" ("On the Motion of the Heart and Blood"), published in 1628, marks the beginning of the vigorous use of scientific method, which caused an abrupt acceleration of knowledge. Harvey was first at Cambridge but spent two formative years in Padua at the same time as Galileo. He then returned to London to become a lecturer in the new College of Physicians (soon to become the Royal College). He did not much concern himself directly with respiration but his discovery of the circulation of the blood immediately clarified the functions of the heart and lung to such an extent that the way was open for a century of dramatic progress.

The brilliant concept of Harvey was soon supplemented by momentous discoveries of the microscopic anatomy of the lung, notably by Malpighi (1628–1694) of Bologna. Although Harvey recognized that large quantities of blood moved from the arteries to the veins, he was perplexed by the route. But in 1661, Malpighi wrote two letters about microscopic observations he had made on the frog lung to his friend Borelli (1608–1679), who was professor of mathematics at Bologna and keenly interested in physiology. Malpighi begins disarmingly by referring to "a few little observations that might increase the things found out about the lungs" and blithely goes on to announce the discovery of the alveoli and the pulmonary capillaries! In the first letter he describes the alveoli as "an almost infinite number of orbicular bladders just as we see formed by wax plates in the walls of the honeycomb cells of beehives.'' And in the second letter he announces the discovery of the capillaries, remarking that the network of tiny vessels occupies not only the walls but also the floors of the alveoli and that as the blood flows through the tortuous vessels it is not "poured into spaces but always works through tubules.'' He adds wryly that for these experiments, "I have destroyed almost the whole race of frogs.'' Thus for the first time the anatomical basis for gas exchange was clearly established. Malpighi also saw red blood cells within the capillaries though he mistook them for fat globules. Their true nature was recognized by the Anton van Leeuwenhoek (1632–1723), another great microscopist, who communicated his discovery in 1674 to the recently founded Royal Society.

B. Oxford School

A notable group of scientists was working at Oxford in the mid-seventeenth century. At this time we begin to see the emergence of chemistry and physics as recognizable disciplines, but remarkably the central question on which much of their research centered was the nature of pulmonary gas exchange. Robert Boyle (1627–1691), often called the "father of modern chemistry,'' is perhaps the most familiar of this group; he moved to Oxford in 1654 where he made striking advances in physics, chemistry, and physiology. He carried out studies of the compressibility of gases ("Experiments . . . Touching the Spring and Weight of the Air") and discovered the inverse relationship between volume and pressure. Together with Robert Hooke (1635–1703), he investigated the length of time that animals could survive in closed vessels at different pressures and wrote "About 10 of the Clock in the morning, I included a Shrew-Mouse with common Air in a Receiver, fortified against the external air; about 11 the Mouse was brought to such straights, that he could hardly breathe" (Boyle, 1682). By reducing the pressure with an air pump, it was shown that the viable period was shortened but that in compressed air the animal lived longer. The two scientists argued that the purpose of respiration was to supply a life-giving substance present in the air to the body and that the respiratory movements were of secondary importance; indeed, a dog could be kept alive by blowing air through the lungs if holes were made in the pleural surface and the chest wall was open (Hooke, 1667).

The work of Boyle and Hooke was extended by two other eminent Oxford physiologists, Richard Lower (1631–1691) and John Mayow (1643–1679). Lower studied the change in color that occurred in blood exposed to air. He was able to show that the blood in the pulmonary vein became red before it reached the left heart, and that if the trachea was obstructed, the blood remained dark blue. He concluded that the change in color occurred as a result of some substance that the blood acquired from the air in the lungs.

This train of thought was pursued by Mayow, who argued that air contained a "nitro-aerial spirit," which was required for both respiration and combustion. He showed in a critical experiment that if a burning lamp is enclosed in a jar with an animal, death occurs more rapidly "for want of nitro-aerial particles." Both respiration and combustion were found to decrease the volume of air in a jar with a water seal (the carbon dioxide dissolving in the water). Moreover, Mayow reasoned that the nitro-aerial substance when it entered the blood via the lungs provided the means for the animal to produce muscular contraction. Finally he showed that when antimony is burned it gains weight, and he argued that this was because of incorporation of nitro-aerial particles.

Some historians believe that Mayow plagiarized many ideas from Boyle, Hooke, and Lower. Be that as it may, his writings represent a culmination of the intense activity of the seventeenth century. Mayow died in 1691, only 63 years after the publication of "De Motu Cordis." In that brief period, many of the essential features of pulmonary gas exchange had been established. Indeed it could well be argued that Mayow discovered oxygen, though this name was not introduced until about a century later when another comparable advance in understanding gas exchange was made by Lavoisier.

C. Phlogiston Theory

The ebb and flow that characterizes the progress of knowledge is well illustrated by the events that occurred following the introduction of phlogiston theory by Stahl (1660–1734). This ingenious but totally erroneous theory had an insidious effect on the thinking of even the greatest scientific minds of the mid-eighteenth century with the result that knowledge took a backward step and the work of Boyle, Hooke, Lower, and Mayow was largely forgotten.

Stahl argued that all combustible materials are composed of ash (calx) and phlogiston, and that the phlogiston escaped on burning. In a closed container, a fire died out because the air became saturated with phlogiston. A metal oxide could be reconstituted as metal by heating it with charcoal because the latter contributed phlogiston. The apparently insuperable objection that metals increased in weight during ashing was countered by the ingenious assertion that phlogiston had negative weight!

It is difficult for the modern physiologist to understand how the dramatic advances of the Oxford School could be reversed by such a contrived theory, but it should be remembered that the communication of scientific ideas was much more haphazard than it is today. For example, some of the proponents of the phlogiston theory were hardly aware of the work of Mayow done many years before. Also, the theory was in essence a mirror image of reality (the supposed loss of phlogiston from burning material being actually the combination of oxygen with it) and, erroneous as it was, it was possible to mold the theory to fit many experimental observations. Certainly in the mid-eighteenth century it had a stranglehold on progress.

D. Carbon Dioxide and Oxygen

Scientific historians often cite 1750 as a nadir in the development of chemistry and physiology because of the sinister influence of the phlogiston theory. Lively minds, however, were certainly at work; one of these was Stephen Hales (1677–1761), whose contributions to respiratory physiology are much underrated. Hales was the vicar of the parish of Teddington, then a small village 15 miles from London. He was a man of exceptionally broad interests. In addition to ministering to the needs of his parish, he made important contributions to plant physiology, sanitary engineering, hemodynamics, and respiration. He measured the size of the alveoli in the lung of a calf (reporting a diameter of one-hundredth part of an inch), remarked on the enormous surface area of the blood–gas barrier, observed the pulsatility blood in the pulmonary veins, developed the pneumatic trough for collecting gases over water, clarified the difference between gases in their "elastick," that is, free state, compared with their "fixed" condition in chemical combination, and was aware that expired air contained a gas that soon was shown to be carbon dioxide. Perhaps his most important contribution was to emphasize the quantitative ("statical") approach to physiology in which we "must in all reason . . . number, weight and measure."

During the next few years, investigations on the respiratory gases developed at an accelerating rate to culminate in the work of Lavoisier. Joseph Black (1728–1799) was a chemist who rediscovered carbon dioxide (it had been described 100 years earlier by van Helmont) and laid the foundation for the overthrow of the phlogiston theory with his work on the chemistry of alkalis. He found that "fixed air" (carbon dioxide) was produced by respiration, burning charcoal, and fermenting beer. In a colorful experiment he collected air from the ceiling of a church in Glasgow where a congregation of 1500 pious Scots remained at their devotions for 10 hours and showed that this contained considerable amounts of "fixed air." His experiments on lime and its chemical derivatives rendered the phlogiston theory unnecessary though Black himself did not in fact interpret them in this way.

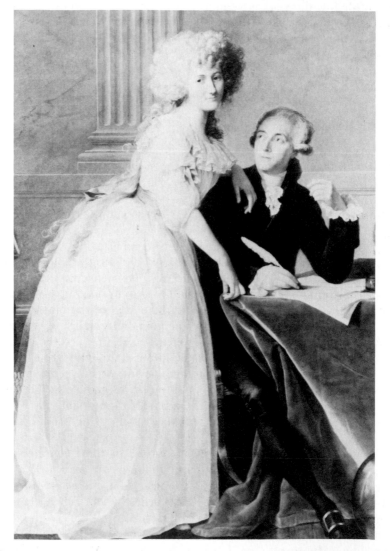

Fig. 2. Antoine Lavoisier (1743–1794) in his laboratory with his wife, who also acted as his laboratory assistant. Lavoisier first clearly described the nature of the respiratory gases, oxygen, carbon dioxide, and nitrogen. (From the portrait by David.)

The discovery of oxygen independently by Priestley and Scheele should have sounded the death knell of the phlogiston theory, although curiously it did not. Joseph Priestley (1733–1804) was a Unitarian minister at Leeds and Birmingham whose political views made him so unpopular that he eventually moved from England to Pennsylvania. In a classical experiment carried out in August 1774, he heated red mercuric oxide and was astonished to find that the gas that was released caused a candle to burn "with a remarkably vigorous flame." He went on to show that a mouse could survive longer in this gas than ordinary air, and actually surmised that it might be useful for people with disease ("this pure air . . . might be peculiarly salutary to the lungs in certain morbid cases"). He also was surprised to find that whereas animals consumed the new air he had discovered, plants such as a sprig of mint produced it. However, he interpreted all his findings in the light of the prevailing theory and called the new gas "dephlogistinated air." Priestley visited Lavoisier in Paris and no doubt stimulated the latter's research. Scheele (1742–1786) in Sweden also prepared oxygen which he called "fire–air" and also communicated his discovery to Lavoisier. The time was opportune for the true nature of the respiratory gases to be revealed.

E. Lavoisier

Antoine Lavoisier (1743–1794) showed early promise as a chemist and was elected at the age of only 25 years to the Académie des Sciences (Fig. 2). It was to this august society that from 1772 until his death by the guillotine in 1794 he communicated a series of memoirs that formed the basis of our modern knowledge of pulmonary gas exchange.

After Priestley's visit to Paris in 1774, Lavoisier began to experiment with red mercuric oxide and by 1775 could state "the substance which combines with metals during calcination, thereby increasing their weight is nothing else than the pure portion of the air which surrounds us and which we breathe." Moreover, he added, "the principle called up to now 'fixed air,' is the combination of the portion of eminently respirable air with the carbon." In 1777, he communicated his memoir on "Expériences sur la respiration des animaux, et sur les changemens qui arrivent à l'air en passant par leur poumon," an event that can be regarded as marking the definitive discovery of the respiratory gases. In it Lavoisier stated

Eminently respirable air that enters the lung, leaves it in the form of chalky aeriform acids [CO_2] . . . in almost equal volume. . . . Respiration acts only on the portion of pure air that is eminently respirable . . . , the excess, that is its mephitic portion [nitrogen], is a purely passive medium which enters and leaves the lung . . . without change or alteration. The respirable portion of air has the property to combine with blood and its combination results in its red color.

He later named the eminently respirable air "oxygine," meaning acid-producer.

In subsequent memoirs, Lavoisier emphasized the essential similarity between respiration and combustion stating, for example, "Respiration is a slow combustion of carbon analogous to that operating in a lamp or a lighted candle, and . . . from this point of view animals which breathe are really combustible substances burning and consuming themselves." With the mathematician Laplace, he carried out calorimetry to compare the heat production of respiration and combustion. One of his few erroneous conclusions was that combustion actually took place in the lungs, being assisted by a special fluid secreted into the bronchi, and that the resulting heat was carried away by the blood. "This combustion" wrote Lavoisier and Laplace "is produced within the lungs, without evolving perceptible light, because the substance of the fire thus liberated is immediately absorbed by the moisture of these organs; the heat developed in this combustion is communicated to the blood which traverses the lungs and is dispersed in the whole animal system."

With Lavoisier, the phlogiston theory, which had proved to be so tenacious for nearly 100 years, was finally routed. Now that the nature of the respiratory gases was clear, attention began to be focused on more specific aspects of metabolism, including the elusive problem of the site of heat production. It is curious that this should have proved to be such a knotty problem. Another vexing question was how the respiratory gases were carried by the blood. But in many ways it now appears that Lavoisier's work was a watershed. Many of the notions discussed prior to his time seem very quaint today, whereas once we reach the nineteenth century, the arguments have a much more familiar ring.

IV. NINETEENTH CENTURY

A. Site of Respiration

Although Lavoisier clearly understood the nature of the respiratory gases, oxygen, carbon dioxide, and nitrogen, there was little notion that metabolism took place in peripheral tissues and that oxygen and carbon dioxide were transported to and from the lungs by the blood. Indeed, as noted above, Lavoisier and Laplace believed that all combustion (i.e., metabolism) occurred in the lungs and that the resulting heat was carried away from them by the blood. This problem of the site of production of "animal heat" preoccupied physiologists for a surprisingly long time.

Perhaps we see here a legacy of Aristotle's "innate heat" teachings, which held sway for 2000 years. A central feature of that scheme was that the main vital processes occurred in the heart and lungs. At any event, in a typical textbook of physiology published just over 100 years ago (Dalton, 1867) a whole chapter is devoted to "animal heat." There is also a section describing a peculiar "pulmonic acid," which is synthesized in the lungs and assists the elimination of carbon dioxide. Even in this century Bohr (1909) contended that up to 60% of all the oxygen consumption of the body can occur in lung tissue.

The Italian zoologist Spallanzani (1729–1799) was one of the first to turn attention away from the lungs to the peripheral tissues by demonstrating that various organs from freshly killed animals were able to take up oxygen and eliminate carbon dioxide. Spallanzani's wide interests led him to study a great variety of animals including insects, worms, snails, frogs, fish, birds, mice, and man. Animals without lungs were shown to take up oxygen and give off carbon dioxide by means of their skin.

But two conceptual problems delayed the acceptance of the peripheral tissues as the site of respiration. One was the argument that the respiratory gases could not penetrate the membranes lining the lung and that therefore the conversion of oxygen to carbon dioxide must take place on the surface of the airways. Actually there had been clear demonstrations by both Borelli in the seventeenth and Priestley in the eighteenth century that gases could diffuse through living membranes but this evidence was apparently forgotten. The other impediment was the mistaken belief that there was no carbon dioxide in venous blood. If true, this was strong evidence that all the conversion of oxygen to carbon dioxide must take place in the lung.

A key advance here was the work of Gustav Magnus (1802–1870), who in 1837 bubbled hydrogen through venous blood collected from human volunteers and demonstrated that large amounts of carbon dioxide could be extracted in this way. He went on to construct a blood–gas analyzer that allowed him to measure the amounts of oxygen, carbon dioxide, and nitrogen in arterial and venous blood. The finding that arterial blood contained more oxygen and less carbon dioxide than venous blood strongly supported the notion that the conversion took place peripherally and he wrote "it is probably that the inhaled oxygen is absorbed in the lungs by the blood which transports it then throughout the body, where, given up in the capillary vessels, it determines the formation of carbonic acid" (Magnus, 1837).

Another approach to the problem of the site of oxygen usage was the measurement of heat production in tissues. By inserting a thermocouple needle into the muscles of the arm after strenuous exercise it was possible to show a rise in temperature. The further demonstration by von Helmholtz (1821–1894) that even a single twitch of isolated muscle caused the liberation of measurable heat clearly suggested that the "animal heat" of exercise was formed peripherally. Claude Bernard (1813–1878) extended these observations by reporting that blood was warmed by the gut and the liver, thus showing that digestion was associated with a rise in temperature. Moreover, by careful measurements he found that the temperature of pulmonary venous blood was slightly less than that of pulmonary artery blood, thus finally disposing of the controversy that had existed since the time of Empedocles 2300 years earlier! It is only fair to add that more recent investigators have been unable to confirm Bernard's results on the temperature difference between pulmonary arterial and venous blood.

There were still some physiologists who believed until the end of the nineteenth century that substantial metabolism occurred within the blood vessels as opposed to within the peripheral tissues themselves. This belief was partly attributable to the demonstration that shed blood continued to take up oxygen and eliminate carbon dioxide. However, the great German physiologist Eduard Pflüger (1829–1910) was able to prove that the rate of metabolism of blood itself was very low, and one of his students showed that frogs which had had their blood replaced by saline continued to consume oxygen and produce carbon dioxide at the same rate. Thus the primary role of the blood as a transport system was established, though it was still many years before the way in which oxygen and carbon dioxide are carried by the blood was fully understood.

B. Energy Production

It was one thing to accept that oxygen was taken up and carbon dioxide eliminated by peripheral tissues, but another to accept that these events were parts of ordinary chemical processes obeying simple laws. Ever since the time of Aristotle, many philosophers and scientists had assumed that living things possessed a vital principle which was essential for life and which set animate beings apart from inanimate objects. An early controversy between the proponents of the vitalistic and deterministic views occurred in Greece in the fifth century B.C., and the argument was still being waged in the nineteenth century A.D! The issue was finally settled by careful simultaneous measurements of oxygen consumption and heat production, thus proving that living things obey the law of conservation of energy.

Von Mayer (1814–1878), a German country doctor, became interested in the relationship between metabolism and heat production while he was a ship's doctor on a voyage to the tropics. He noticed that the venous blood which he drew was a brighter red than he was accustomed to seeing in Europe, and he argued that this was because of the lower body metabolism required in a hot climate. Subsequently he developed the theory that the heat of animals is the result of chemical oxidative processes, and that the energy derived from metabolism appears either as mechanical work or heat, though chiefly the latter. However, he was never able to prove this.

The remarkable mathematician, physicist, and physiologist, von Helmholtz enunciated the first law of thermodynamics in 1847. He proposed that all forms of energy are interchangeable, and that in the process energy is neither lost nor gained. Moreover, he argued that this principle could be tested in living animals. However, it was not until physiologists such as Rubner (1854–1932) were able to perform direct calorimetry on intact animals and to demonstrate the relationship between oxygen consumption and heat production that vitalism was finally disproved.

Toward the end of the nineteenth century, the physiology of pulmonary gas exchange as we know it today was firmly established, and some of the papers published in the 1890s, for example, contain ideas that are still fresh and untested. This period is notable for some colorful controversies, for example, the magnitude and nature of the respiratory dead space, and the secretion versus diffusion theories of oxygen transfer in the lung. It was also a period when advances in the field of blood gas transport were very rapid, and exciting new information was becoming available about the effects of low and high pressures on pulmonary gas exchange.

V. ALVEOLAR GAS AND DEAD SPACE

A. Size of Dead Space

Alveolar gas has long been used to obtain information about pulmonary gas exchange because it is much easier to obtain than arterial blood, and it is also much easier to analyze. One of the first to use alveolar gas for physiological measurements was the chemist Humphrey Davy, who inhaled a hydrogen mixture to measure his lung volumes in 1800. He analyzed his expired gas for hydrogen, oxygen, carbon dioxide, and nitrogen and reported that his vital capacity was 213 in.³ (3490 ml) whereas his residual volume was 41 in.³ (672 ml). He added, "this capacity is probably below the medium; my chest is narrow, measuring in circumference but 29 inches, and my neck rather long and slender" (Davy, 1800).

Alveolar gas was the subject of a great deal of controversy from about 1890 until World War II. The aim of the investigators was to solve the apparently simple problem of the size of the respiratory dead space but the root of the disagreement was confusion about the composition of alveolar gas. The controversy brought into conflict two of the leading schools of respiratory physiology, one led by J. S. Haldane in Oxford and the other by August Krogh of Copenhagen.

These investigators believed that the lung behaved essentially as a large volume of alveoli in which gas exchange took place, connected to the atmosphere by a system of airways in which no gas exchange occurred. This latter volume was termed the respiratory dead space. The concept had been introduced by Zuntz in 1882, who had determined its anatomical volume on a cadaver and found a value of 140 ml. A further series of measurements were made by Loewy in 1894. In 1891 Bohr introduced his mixing equation from which the dead space (V_D) can be calculated if the expired tidal volume (V_T) and fractional concentrations of any component in inspired, expired, and alveolar gases (F_{I_X}, F_{E_X}, F_{A_X}) are known. It was derived as follows:

The total amount of any gas expired is equal to the amount in the dead space plus the amount expired from the alveoli.

Therefore,

$$V_T F_{E_X} = V_D F_{I_X} + (V_T - V_D) F_{A_X}$$

from which

$$\frac{V_D}{V_T} = \frac{F_{A_X} - F_{E_X}}{F_{A_X} - F_{I_X}}$$

Krogh and Lindhard (1914, 1917) used hydrogen as the indicator gas following its introduction in this context by Siebeck (1911). To reduce the effects of errors in gas analysis on the calculated dead space volume, inspiratory concentrations of 20–30% hydrogen were used; expiratory samples were collected after relatively small volumes (about 500 ml) had been exhaled. Haldane and co-workers (1919, 1920) concentrated on carbon dioxide; their method of sampling was to collect gas by a rapid full expiration at the end of either a normal expiration or inspiration. The subject exhaled into a rubber tube that had a bore of about 1 in. and length of about 3 ft. At the end of the expiration the proximal end of the tube was closed with the tongue, and a sample of the last expired gas was taken under mercury. This so-called Haldane–Priestley sample was used extensively to collect alveolar gas under a variety of situations, for example, at high altitude, and the method is still occasionally employed.

There was substantial agreement between Krogh and Haldane on the magnitude of the dead space volume during quiet breathing; the average value was about 150 ml, in agreement with the earlier results of Zuntz (1882) and also those of Rohrer (1915), who had made painstaking measurements on a cadaver lung. However, the results reported on exercise disagreed widely. Douglas and Haldane (1912) claimed increases in the dead space volume of 500 ml, but Krogh and Lindhard (1917) found much smaller rises and argued that the large values were erroneous. They thought that an important source of error was the increase in carbon dioxide concentration of alveolar gas that occurred during the course of the expirations. They added that though this rise might well be insignificant at rest, it could become large on exercise when the rate of carbon dioxide production was so much higher. The hydrogen method they argued was not influenced by this error. They further claimed that if the dead space volume on exercise was 600 ml, as Haldane claimed, hydrogen from an inspiration of 500 ml would not enter the alveoli at all, whereas they noted from 300 to 400 ml hydrogen in alveolar gas after such an inspiration. On mechanical grounds, too, they considered it unlikely that the bronchial tree could dilate to the degree implied.

Haldane replied that the limitations Krogh placed on the tidal volume on exercise distorted the results and he objected to the use of a nonphysiological gas such as hydrogen. He pointed out that Krogh had shown that some parts of the lung received less hydrogen than others on inspiration (that is, that ventilation was uneven) and that on expiration, the concentration tended to fall steadily. There was no reason to suppose that gas expired at 600–800 ml was a better sample of alveolar gas than that expired later. The apparent paradox of appreciable alveolar ventilation at low tidal volumes in the presence of a large dead space volume had been resolved, he said, by Henderson and co-workers (1915), who demonstrated that air in the respiratory tract did not move with a square front but in a conelike fashion.

The controversy, which continued for many years, will not be followed in detail. Krogh's contention was that the dead space volume was a static property of the lungs that varied little with large tidal volumes, hyperventilation, or exercise, whereas Haldane saw it as a much more functional entity capable of physiological adaptations. The great increase on exercise, for example, reflected the dilatation of the airways, which therefore offered less resistance to the high flow.

The controversy emphasized the difference in the measurement of dead space between the use of an exchanging gas such as carbon dioxide, and a gas such as hydrogen, which is merely diluted in the alveolar gas. Today we draw a distinction between the *physiologic dead space,* which is the volume of the lung that does not eliminate carbon dioxide (or some other gas that exchanges with the blood), and the *anatomic dead space,* which is the volume of the conducting airways down to the level where the rapid dilution of an inspired insoluble gas occurs with gas already in the lung. This latter reflects the geometry of the airway system, which expands rapidly with distance from the mouth, and thus it is determined by the morphology of the lung. However, it is interesting that when Fowler (1948) described what is now the accepted method for measuring the anatomic dead space by the single-breath nitrogen washout, he used the term "physiological" for the dead space he found. The measurement of physiologic dead space was greatly facilitated when Enghoff (1938) suggested using the arterial P_{CO_2} rather than the alveolar value in the Bohr equation. This modification was extensively developed by Riley and co-workers (see this volume, Chapter 3 by Riley) and is in constant use today.

B. Inhomogeneity of Alveolar Gas

The Haldane–Krogh controversy also highlighted the confusion that can occur if we assume that there is an entity "alveolar gas" that can be sampled, is homogeneous, and is representative of all alveoli. It is now accepted that there are substantial topographical differences in P_{O_2} and P_{CO_2} within the normal lung and that there are also temporal differences in the course of the respiratory cycle, especially on exercise. In the diseased lung the normal topographical pattern is often abolished but is replaced by more more nonuniformity at the alveolar level as a result of ventilation–perfusion inequality. The result is a large spectrum of values for alveolar P_{O_2} and P_{CO_2}. Much of the research on pulmonary gas exchange since World War II has been directed at a better understanding and expression of the inhomogeneity of alveolar gas and capillary blood. Thus in a sense the Haldane–Krogh controversy, which at first sight appeared to be confined to the somewhat sterile subject of the size of the dead space, promoted much of the most important work on gas exchange over the last 30 years.

One of the first suggestions that inspired gas is not evenly distributed to all parts of the lung was made over 70 years ago by Keith (1909). He made a careful anatomical study and distinguished three zones of tissue: (a) radical zone with bronchi and blood vessels; (b) intermediary zone with ramifying bronchi and blood vessels and the lung tissue between them; and (c) an outer zone 25–30 mm in thickness consisting mainly of alveoli. He thought that the outer zones were able to expand more freely and therefore ventilated more than the inner zones. Tendeloo reached similar conclusions in 1902 and also suggested that the asymmetrical thoracic cavity limited expansion of the upper lobes. Rohrer (1915), who did some most painstaking dissections, was able to make calculations of the degree of the inequality of ventilation.

It was soon appreciated that arguing from anatomical structure to function was hazardous, and most of our knowledge about uneven ventilation has come from alveolar gas analysis. Some of the first experiments were those of Krogh and Lindhard (1913, 1914, 1917). They made analyses of the expirate following a single inspiration of a hydrogen mixture and concluded that "the distribution of a gas in the alveolar air after an inspiration of it is not uniform. The last portion of an expiration will contain less of the gas then the earlier." Haldane *et al.* (1919), however, did not accept this: "We can get pure alveolar air by making a deep expiration. This alveolar air is contained in the air sacs (but not in the atria) of the lungs and is of constant composition throughout these at any given moment." But Sonne and his pupil Roelsen (1938, 1939) confirmed the Scandinavian work by a series of experiments in which they collected successive samples during expiration into evacuated tonometers by means of a rotating tap with several outlets. After an inspiration of pure hydrogen, the concentration of this gas in the expirate fell in direct proportion to the volume expired. In normal subjects, the variation was up to 20%; in patients with asthma or emphysema it rose to as high as 100%.

One of the main points of controversy was to what extent inequality of ventilation was due to variation in gas composition along the airway (stratified inhomogeneity) and how much was caused by variations between different anatomical parts of the lung (regional inequality). This question is not yet completely resolved and is discussed in more detail by Scheid and Piiper (this volume, Chapter 4).

Information about ventilatory inequality was greatly extended by the introduction of rapidly responding gas analyzers such as the nitrogen meter and the helium katharometer. The single-breath nitrogen method was introduced by Fowler (1949) and the use of the helium katharometer and multibreath methods is discussed by Briscoe (Volume II, Chapter 8). Topographical information on the inequality of ventilation and ventilation–perfusion ratios followed the introduction of radioactive gas studies by Knipping and colleagues (1955).

VI. SECRETION VERSUS DIFFUSION

Another English–Danish controversy enlivened the physiological scene at the turn of the century. This time the issue was whether oxygen and carbon dioxide are actively secreted by the alveolar epithelium against a concentration gradient, or whether these gases pass across the blood–gas barrier by simple diffusion. Christian Bohr (1855–1911) was one of the chief proponents of the secretion hypothesis. In his 1891 paper "Über die Lungenathmung" ("On Pulmonary Respiration") he compared the P_{O_2} and P_{CO_2} of alveolar gas exhaled from the lungs of dogs with the P_{O_2} and P_{CO_2} of gas in a tonometer equilibrated with arterial blood taken at the same time. In some instances, the alveolar P_{O_2} was reported to be as much as 30 mm Hg below, and the P_{CO_2} as much as 20 mm Hg above the arterial blood values. The anomalous behavior of carbon dioxide was particularly marked if the animals were given gas mixtures containing carbon dioxide to breathe. Bohr concluded,

> In general, my experiments have shown definitely that the lung tissue plays an active part in gas exchange; therefore the function of the lung can be regarded as analogous to that of the glands. It is true that this theory is incompatible with the presently prevalent views in physiology, at least those concerning oxygen. On the other hand, this concept does not seem to me actually to contradict any of the experimental facts published to date.

In a later paper, Bohr (1909) referred to the secretion ability of the lung as its "specific function." Ironically in the same paper he presented the mathematical basis for the calculation of the time course of P_{O_2} in the pulmonary capillary, and this "Bohr integration" became the cornerstone for analyses of oxygen transfer in the competing diffusion hypothesis.

Haldane visited Bohr in Copenhagen and also became convinced of the secretion theory, at least as far as oxygen was concerned. In 1897, Haldane and Lorraine Smith wrote "In the animals investigated the normal oxygen tension in the arterial blood is always higher than the alveolar air, and in some animals higher than the inspired air. The absorption of oxygen by the lungs thus cannot be explained by diffusion alone" (Haldane and Smith, 1897). Haldane remained a staunch supporter of oxygen secretion for many years, and even as late as 1935 the second edition of his book, "Respiration," written with J. G. Priestley contained a whole chapter devoted to the subject. In this he argues that active gas secretion occurs elsewhere in nature, for example, in the unicellular organism *Arcella,* and in the swim bladders of certain fish, though it is now believed that the swim bladder accumulates gas by a countercurrent exchange mechanism rather than active secretion. As evidence against oxygen secretion accumulated, Haldane retreated into a more and more defensive position maintaining, for example, that it principally occurred at altitude, and that even there it was seen only after a sufficient period of acclimatization.

The hypothesis of oxygen secretion was tested in several ways, particularly on expeditions to high altitudes and in low-pressure chambers, where it was argued that active transport of oxygen would be most beneficial and most easily observed. A series of measurements by Douglas *et al.* (1913) on Pikes Peak, Colorado (altitude 4300 m; 14,100 ft), apparently supported the secretion hypothesis. The investigators calculated the arterial P_{O_2} by an indirect method that involved breathing enough carbon monoxide to saturate as much as 20% of the hemoglobin with this gas and concluded that the arterial P_{O_2} was an average of 35 mm Hg higher than the alveolar value during exercise.

In response, Joseph Barcroft (1872–1947) conducted a dramatic experiment on himself using a gas-tight chamber, in which he exposed himself for 6 days to conditions of hypoxia and exercise similar to those of Haldane's expedition to Pikes Peak (Barcroft *et al.*, 1920). His left radial artery was exposed and blood was taken at intervals for the measurement of oxygen saturation. The results were consistent with the diffusion hypothesis though Haldane would not accept them because of the short time that Barcroft allowed for acclimatization. However, in 1921 Barcroft organized a high-altitude expedition to Cerro de Pasco in Peru, where additional data supporting the diffusion hypothesis were obtained.

The controversy stimulated Marie Krogh (wife of August) to develop a method for measuring the pulmonary diffusing capacity using small concentrations of carbon monoxide (Krogh, 1915). A single breath of this gas was inspired and the amount of carbon monoxide that was taken up by the pulmonary capillary blood was measured. Since the partial pressure of carbon monoxide in the blood remained extremely low because of the avidity of the blood for this gas, the amount removed from the alveoli was assumed to be solely determined by the diffusion properties of the blood–gas barrier. The general conclusion was that the enormous diffusion properties conferred on the blood–gas barrier by its large area and small thickness were sufficient to allow passive diffusion of oxygen under all conditions. An interesting question raised by Comroe (1975) is why the test of the diffusing capacity for carbon monoxide, which is now a standard one in pulmonary function laboratories, lay virtually dormant for 35 years until it was resurrected by Forster and co-workers in the 1950s. The answer may be the great technical difficulty of measuring carbon monoxide before the introduction of the infrared analyzer.

August Krogh was one of the most articulate opponents of the secretion theory and one of his most trenchant papers was published in 1910, a year before Bohr died. Since Krogh had been a student of Bohr and has assisted him in his experiments on gas secretion from 1899 to 1908, and bearing in mind that Bohr was very jealous of his secretion theory, the introductory section of Krogh's paper required an unusually delicate touch. He wrote Krogh (1910),

> I shall be obliged in the following pages to combat the views of my teacher Prof. Bohr on certain essential points and also to criticize a few of his experimental results. I wish here not only to acknowledge the debt of gratitude which I, personally, owe to him, but also to emphasize the fact, patent to everybody, who is familiar with the problems here

discussed, that the real progress, made during the last twenty years in the knowledge of the processes in the lungs, is mainly due to his labours and to that refinement of methods, which he has introduced. The theory of the lung as a gland has justified its existence and done excellent service in bringing forward facts, which will survive any theoretical construction, which has been put or shall hereafter be put upon them.

In retrospect, the notion that the lung was like a gland in that it could actively secrete substances such as gases it not particularly surprising when we look at the development of ideas about pulmonary function. As we have seen, it was believed from early Greek times that the actual energy transformation that resulted from inspiring some active element in air took place in the lungs themselves. Even Lavoisier who so strongly broke with traditional thinking on the nature of the respiratory gases believed that "combustion" or oxidation took place in the lungs as a result of a special substance within them, and that the resulting heat was carried away by the blood. Incidentally, a corollary of Bohr's view of active secretion of oxygen and carbon dioxide was that the lung tissue used large amounts of oxygen—up to 60% of the total requirements of the body. Thus there were plenty of historical precedents for proposing that the lung did more than allow passive diffusion of gases to occur. Indeed today we know that in addition to its chief role of gas exchange, the lung is involved in the active metabolism of a range of substances such as angiotensin 1, serotonin, bradykinin, and some prostaglandins. Moreover, the possibility that the transfer of carbon dioxide across the blood–gas barrier involves more than passive diffusion has received increasing attention in the last few years, as discussed by Hlastala and Robertson (Volume II, Chapter 7).

VII. BLOOD GASES

A. Carriage of Oxygen

As we have seen, the earliest physiologists believed that the function of the blood was to carry heat away from the lungs, a notion that eventually survived beyond Lavoisier. The first intimations that oxygen was transported by the blood were given by the Oxford school in the seventeenth century. Lower was aware that venous blood became red when exposed to air and Mayow was actually able to extract some of his nitro-aerial spirit from blood. But few further advances were made for the next 150 years until 1837, when Magnus, using a new mercury pump, exposed blood to a partial vacuum and showed that it contained both oxygen and carbon dioxide. The carbon dioxide was measured by absorbing it in potassium hydroxide, while the remaining gas was detonated with hydrogen to determine the volume of oxygen. Gasometric analysis of blood then developed apace with important advances by Ludwig and Pflüger. The latter developed the aerotonometer, a glass bulb in which a small bubble of air was equilibrated with blood and subsequently analyzed. This was further developed by Krogh (1908) and Roughton and Scholander (1943) and the principle formed the basis of the Riley bubble method, which played such an important part in the development of pulmonary gas exchange in the period following World War II (see this volume, Chapter 3).

The gradual discovery of the role of hemoglobin in oxygen transport by the blood is a saga in itself. The microscopist Leeuwenhoek recognized in 1674 that the red blood corpuscles were responsible for the blood's color, and the presence of iron in blood was demonstrated in 1747 by showing its magnetic behavior when ashed. Justus Liebig in 1842 was aware that the iron was in the erythrocytes and he believed that the iron formed a compound with oxygen, which he called "protoxide." He also suggested that carbon dioxide is carried by the red cells and that this carriage is interfered with by the presence of oxygen, thus anticipating the Haldane effect.

The eminent biochemist Hoppe-Seyler (1825–1895) was responsible for elucidating much of the chemistry of hemoglobin. He prepared the substance in a crystalline form and determined the absorption spectra of the oxygenated and reduced forms. He showed that it formed a loose association with oxygen and that carbon monoxide could displace the oxygen, an observation also made by Claude Bernard.

The first dissociation curves for oxygen and carbon dioxide were constructed by Paul Bert (1833–1886), a remarkably versatile physiologist who was a pupil of Bernard. Holmgren had earlier shown that the amounts of oxygen and carbon dioxide increased as the partial pressures were raised, but Bert was the first to explore the behavior of blood over a wide range of gas pressures (Fig. 3). He carried out experiments both on samples of blood *in vitro* and on animals exposed to various pressures in a chamber, removing the arterial blood by cannulas. One of Bert's chief interests was the physiological effects of high altitude and he was the first to show that it was the partial pressure of oxygen that was responsible for the deleterious consequences of high altitude. This he proved by subjecting animals to low barometric pressures of air on the one hand and low concentrations of oxygen on the other. "Oxygen tension is everything, barometric pressure in itself does nothing or almost nothing," he concluded, though the issue remained controversial for many years.

The peculiar S shape of the oxygen dissociation curve was first recog-

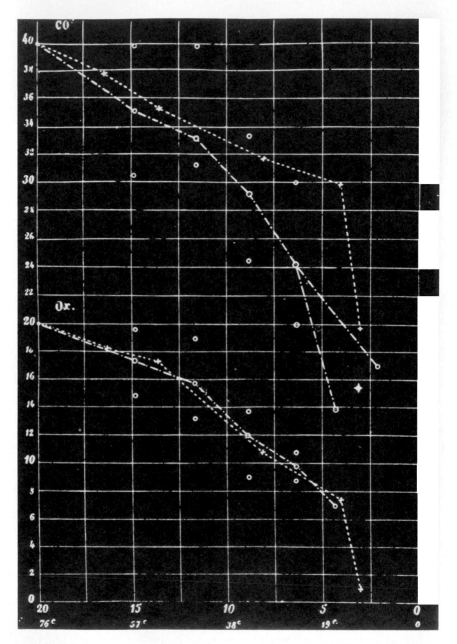

Fig. 3. First dissociation curves for oxygen and carbon dioxide. These were published in 1878 by Paul Bert (1833–1886). The concentrations on the ordinate have been normalized to bring the control value in each case to 40 m/100 ml for CO_2 and 20 ml/100 for O_2. The circles with alternating dots and dashes show data obtained from arterial blood of dogs during decompression; the crosses and dotted lines were from dogs rebreathing air through a CO_2 absorber. The abscissa shows barometric pressure in centimeters of mercury in the decompression experiments and percentage of oxygen concentration in the rebreathing experiments (Bert, 1878).

nized by Bohr. In 1886 he found that purified hemoglobin gave a curve that resembled a hyperbola though there were no values below 30% saturation. Hüfner (1890) took up the question and, assuming that only one molecule of oxygen combined with each molecule of hemoglobin, predicted a rectangular hyperbola. These calculations were apparently confirmed by a few points that he determined experimentally. However, Bohr subsequently mapped the curve carefully over the whole range of partial pressures and revealed its S-shaped character.

Another major advance occurred in 1904 when Bohr, Hasselbalch, and Krogh discovered that the addition of carbon dioxide to blood reduced its affinity for oxygen, although Stokes (1863) had actually anticipated this 40 years before. The possibility that the reverse process occurs, that is, the addition of oxygen drives out carbon dioxide, was considered but the investigators could not prove this. The "Bohr effect" as it became known was shown to be caused by the change in pH of the blood. It was not until 1933 that Margaria and Green (1933) showed that carbon dioxide has a small additional effect of its own on oxygen affinity.

The influence of temperature on the oxygen dissociation curve was suggested by early measurements of Holmgren and Bert, but Barcroft and King (1909) studied the problem in detail and showed that relatively small rises of temperature resulted in substantial increases in P_{50}, that is, the P_{O_2} for 50% saturation. Subsequently Barcroft made an extensive study of hemoglobin and described his work in three classical volumes entitled "The Respiratory Function of the Blood" (Barcroft, 1914, 1925, 1928). His theoretical studies were facilitated by the use of the Hill equation suggested by A. V. Hill (1910). This was before the molecular weight and number of iron atoms in the hemoglobin molecule were known, but the form of the equation still remains useful. Another important step was the formulation of the intermediate compound hypothesis by Adair (1925), which took account of the sequential combination of four atoms of oxygen with a molecule of hemoglobin. The last major physiological factor for determining the position of the oxygen dissociation curve was not discovered until 1967, when Chanutin and Curnish (1967) and Benesch and Benesch (1967) demonstrated that an increased intracellular concentration of 2,3-diphosphoglycerate shifts the curve to the right.

B. Carriage of Carbon Dioxide

Reference has already been made to the key experiments of Gustav Magnus in 1837, in which he exposed venous blood to a partial vacuum by using a new mercury pump and showed that it contained large amounts of carbon dioxide. Prior to that time there had been several sporadic demonstrations of carbon dioxide in blood but many physiologists believed that all oxidation and therefore carbon dioxide production took place in the lungs. Magnus thought that all of the carbon dioxide was in the free rather than the combined form because it was released so easily. However, Zuntz found that much of the carbon dioxide was carried within the red cells and also that the presence of red cells increased the amount of carbon dioxide carried by the serum itself. This was explained when the movement of bicarbonate and chloride ions across the red cell membrane that accompanies the uptake of carbon dioxide by the blood was gradually elucidated. The name of Hamburger is associated with the discovery of the chloride ion shift into the cells in exchange for the outward movement of bicarbonate ions but whether he should be given credit for this is disputed.

The fact that increasing the oxygen saturation of hemoglobin reduces the carbon dioxide content of blood (for a given P_{CO_2}) was reported by Christiansen, Douglas and Haldane (1914), although as stated earlier, Holmgren had anticipated this as early as 1863. The phenomenon is generally known as the "Haldane effect" despite some efforts to rename it the "CDH effect." L. J. Henderson (1878–1942), an outstanding physiologist and biochemist who developed an elaborate scheme of blood as a physicochemical system, has mused on why it took 10 years after the discovery of the Bohr effect to find its reverse, which is predictable on theoretical biochemical grounds. In fact, in their original paper, Bohr and co-workers (1904) looked for the phenomenon but observed "In any case where such an effect is at all present, it must be very slight."

Carbonic anhydrase, the enzyme that accelerates the hydration and dehydration of carbon dioxide within the red cells, was discovered by Meldrum and Roughton (1933). The study of the kinetics of oxygen and carbon dioxide in blood was much facilitated by the introduction of the rapid-reaction apparatus by Hartridge and Roughton (1923). Much work continued to be done in this area and only in the last few years has it been generally recognized that because carbonic anhydrase is limited to the interior of the red cells, plasma pH changes remarkably slowly when carbon dioxide is added to or removed from blood (see this volume, Chapter 6).

C. Measurement of Blood Gases

Although extensive measurements of oxygen and carbon dioxide in expired gas in man were made in the last part of the nineteenth century, advances in the understanding of pulmonary gas exchange were held up because of the difficulty of obtaining arterial blood. Venous blood was no problem; Magnus in 1837 described how he collected venous blood from "common people who for a modest sum permitted themselves to be bled" though it was later recognized that peripheral venous blood was of limited value in analyzing pulmonary gas exchange because its composition depended so much on local metabolism. The collection of mixed venous blood in man had to wait on the introduction of the cardiac catheter by Cournand and co-workers (1945) following the pioneering work of Forssmann (1929).

The first arterial punctures in man were made by Hürter (1912). He reported measurements of arterial oxygen and carbon dioxide content in four normal subjects and found that the arterial oxygen saturation was between 93 and 100%. He also made a series of measurements in patients with various types of heart and lung disease and showed that the procedure was harmless. However, the significance of his contribution was overlooked until 1919, when Stadie introduced the technique at the Rockefeller Institute and carried out an extensive investigation of the relationship between arterial oxygen saturation and cyanosis in patients with pneumonia (Stadie, 1919). A 19- or 20-gauge needle was used to enter the radial or brachial artery percutaneously, in most instances without local anesthesia. The only complication was an occasional hematoma at the site of the puncture but this could be avoided by applying pressure after the needle was withdrawn. Stadie taught the technique to Harrup (1919), who studied patients with anemia and heart disease at Johns Hopkins Hospital in 1919. A number of measurements in patients with lung disease were reported by Meakins and Davies (1925) in their book "Respiratory Function in Disease." Meakins was a pioneer in the application of physiological methods to the problems of clinical medicine and in 1923 had set up one of the first respiratory function laboratories in the Royal Victoria Hospital, Montreal.

A particularly enterprising arterial puncture was made by J. H. Talbot during the 1935 International High Altitude Expedition. The sample was taken from Ancel Keys, who was lying in the snow at an altitude of 6100 m (Keys, 1936). Nevertheless the technique of arterial puncture was not widely used until the late 1950s because of its reputation of being hazardous and therefore unjustified. When the method was gaining acceptance in the United States in 1956, I can vividly remember being warned in England by the late Colin McKerrow that there were many one-armed men walking around New York City as a result of the injudicious use of arterial puncture!

Initially most laboratories had to be content with reporting the arterial oxygen saturation, which was usually obtained from the oxygen content as measured by the Van Slyke method (Van Slyke and Neill, 1924). It is still occasionally possible to recognize the investigators who were active in those days by their penchant for arterial oxygen saturation (Bates *et al.*, 1971). However, the information that was really needed was the arterial partial pressures of oxygen and carbon dioxide. While the P_{O_2} can be estimated from the oxygen saturation and the pH of the blood, this is an inaccurate procedure above a P_{O_2} of about 60 mm Hg because the oxygen dissociation is so flat in this region.

Unfortunately direct measurements of arterial P_{O_2} and P_{CO_2} were very difficult to make prior to the introduction of blood gas electrodes. The earliest measurements were made by using the aerotonometer, in which a small bubble of air was equilibrated with blood and then analyzed. This was introduced by Pflüger and was used as early as 1872 by Strassburg. Variants were developed by Bohr (1891), Krogh (1908), Comroe and Dripps (1944), and Aksnes and Rahn (1957). Roughton and Scholander (1943) introduced a syringe method for gas analysis in which a bubble of gas was equilibrated with a small sample of blood in a tuberculin syringe and the volume of gas was measured in a fine capillary tube. This prompted Riley *et al.* (1945) to develop their bubble equilibration technique (see this volume, Chapter 3), which made the measurement of arterial P_{O_2} practicable for clinical investigation.

The introduction of the Riley bubble method for blood P_{O_2} and P_{CO_2} had an enormous impact on the physiology of gas exchange and prompted the development of the three-compartment model for analyzing the behavior of the diseased lung (see this volume, Chapter 3). However the method required a good deal of adroitness and it was often said that only investigators who had done time at Hopkins could expect accurate results! Thus although the technique stimulated a tremendous amount of interest in gas exchange, it was actually used in only a few relatively few laboratories.

The measurement of arterial P_{O_2} was revolutionized by the introduction of the polarographic oxygen electrode. The principle is that a small potential difference (0.6 V) is maintained between two electrodes, and the current that then flows is proportional to the P_{O_2}. Early forms of the device used a dropping mercury electrode and this was successfully employed by Berggren (1942) for measuring alveolar–arterial P_{O_2} differences in a series of normal subjects. However, the device was difficult to work with and never became popular. The breakthrough was the introduction of the platinum electrode by Clark and co-workers (1953). In their original description, a small platinum electrode was covered with cellophane and immersed in a sample of blood. Early models showed errors caused by oxygen depletion near the electrode unless the blood was stirred rapidly, but in later developments this problem was avoided by using a very small electrode tip.

Soon after the introduction of the oxygen electrode, Severinghaus and Bradley (1958) described an electrode for measuring P_{CO_2}. In this technique, carbon dioxide diffused from the blood through a Teflon membrane into a small volume of electolyte solution in which the changes of pH were measured by a glass electrode. It was not long before both oxygen and carbon dioxide electrodes were mounted in a single water jacket in a commercially available package. This method could be used effectively by well-trained technician and the way was opened up for measurements of arterial P_{O_2} and P_{CO_2} on a routine clinical basis. These measurements are so valuable and are so frequently made today that the modern hospital resident can hardly imagine that they were not available 15 years ago.

REFERENCES

Adair, G. S. (1925). The hemoglobin system. The oxygen dissociation curve of hemoglobin. *J. Biol. Chem.* **63**, 529–545.

Aksnes, E., and Rahn, H. (1957). Measurement of total gas pressure in blood. *J. Appl. Physiol.* **10**, 173–178.

Barcroft, J. (1914). "The Respiratory Function of the Blood." Cambridge Univ. Press, London.

Barcroft, J. (1925). "The Respiratory Function of the Blood. Part 1: Lessons from High Altitudes." Cambridge Univ. Press, London.

Barcroft, J. (1928). "The Respiratory Function of the Blood. Part 2: Haemoglobin." Cambridge Univ. Press, London.

Barcroft, J., and King, W. O. R. (1909). The effect of temperature on the dissociation curve of blood. *J. Physiol. (London)* **39**, 374–418.

Barcroft, J., Cook, A., Hartridge, H., and Parsons, T. R. (1920). The flow of oxygen through the pulmonary epithelium. *J. Physiol. (London)* **53**, 450–472.

Bates, D. V., Macklem, P. T., and Christie, R. V. (1971). "Respiratory Function in Disease," pp. 136, 140, 148. Saunders, Philadelphia, Pennsylvania.

Benesch, R., and Benesch, R. E. (1967). The effect of organic phosphates from the human erythrocyte on the allosteric properties of hemoglobin. *Biochem. Biophys. Res. Commun.* **26**, 163, 167.

Berggren, S. (1942). The oxygen deficit of arterial blood caused by non-ventilating parts of the lung. *Acta Physiol. Scand.* **4**, Suppl. No. 11.

Bert, P. (1878). "La pression barométrique." Masson, Paris. (Engl. transl. by M. A. Hitchcock and F. A. Hitchcock. College Book Co., Columbus, Ohio, 1943. Reprinted by the Undersea Med. Soc., 1978.)

Bohr, C. (1891). Über die Lungenatmung. *Skand. Arch. Physiol.* **2**, 236–268. [Engl. transl. in "Translations in Respiratory Physiology" (J. B. West, ed.), pp. 655–680. Dowden, Hutchinson & Ross, Stroudsburg, Pennsylvania, 1975.]

Bohr, C. (1909). Über die spezifische Tätigkeit der Lungen bei der respiratorischen Gasaufnahme und ihr Verhalten zu der durch die Alveolarwand stattfindenden Gasdiffusion. *Skand. Arch. Physiol.* **22**, 221–280. [Engl. transl. in "Translations in Respiratory Physiology" (J. B. West, ed.), pp. 691–735. Dowden, Hutchinson & Ross, Stroudsburg, Pennsylvania, 1975.]

Bohr, C., Hasselbalch, K. A., and Krogh, A. (1904). Ueber einen in biologischer Beziehung wichtigen Einfluss, den die Kohlensäurespannung des Blutes auf dessen Sauerstoffbindung übt. *Skand. Arch. Physiol.* **16**, 402–412. [Engl. transl. in "Translations in Respiratory Physiology" (J. B. West, ed.), pp. 681–690. Dowden, Hutchinson & Ross, Stroudsburg, Pennsylvania, 1975.]

Boyle, R. (1682). "A Continuation of New Experiments Physico-Mechanicall, Touching the Spring and Weight of the Air, and Their Effects," 2nd Printing. Miles Flesher, London.

Chanutin, A., and Curnish, R. R. (1967). Effect of organic and inorganic phosphates on the oxygen equilibrium of human erythrocytes. *Arch. Biochem. Biophys.* **121**, 101–102.

Christiansen, J., Douglas, C. G., and Haldane, J. S. (1914). The absorption and dissociation of carbon dioxide by human blood. *J. Physiol. (London)* **48**, 244–271.

Clark, L. C., Wolf, R., Granger, D., and Taylor, Z. (1953). Continuous recording of blood oxygen tension by polarography. *J. Appl. Physiol.* **6**, 189–193.

Clendening, L. (1960). "Source Book of Medical History." Dover, New York.

Comroe, J. H. (1975). Retrospectroscope. Pulmonary diffusing capacity for carbon monoxide ($D_{L_{CO}}$). *Am. Rev. Respir. Dis.* **111**, 225–228.

Comroe, J. H., and Dripps, R. D. (1944). The oxygen tension of arterial blood and alveolar air in normal human subjects. *Am. J. Physiol.* **142**, 700–720.

Cournand, A., Riley, R. L., Breed, E. S., Baldwin, S. de F., and Richards, D. W. (1945). Measurement of cardiac output in man using the technique of catheterization of the right auricle or ventricle. *J. Clin. Invest.* **24**, 106–116.

Dalton, J. C. (1867). "A Treatise on Human Physiology," 4th ed. Henry C. Lea, Philadelphia.

Davy, H. (1800). "Researches, Chemical and Philosophical, Chiefly Concerning Nitrous Oxide." J. Johnson, London.

Douglas, C. G., and Haldane, J. S. (1912). Capacity of the air passages under varying physiological conditions. *J. Physiol. (London)* **45**, 235–238.

Douglas, C. G., Haldane, J. S., Henderson, Y., and Schneider, E. C. (1913). Physiological observations made on Pike's Peak, Colorado, with special reference to adaptation to low barometric pressure. *Philos. Trans. R. Soc. London, Ser. B* **203**, 185–318.

Enghoff, H. (1938). Volumen inefficax. Bemerkungen zur Frage des schädlichen Raumes. *Upsala Laekarefoeren. Foerh.* **44**, 191–218.

Forssmann, W. (1929). Die Sondierung des rechtens Herzens. *Klin. Wochenschr.* **8**, 2085–2087.

Foster, M. (1901). "Lectures on the History of Physiology." Cambridge Univ. Press, London.

Fowler, W. S. (1948). Lung function studies. II. The respiratory dead space. *Am. J. Physiol.* **154**, 405–416.

Fowler, W. S. (1949). Lung function studies. III. Uneven pulmonary ventilation in normal subjects and in patients with pulmonary disease. *J. Appl. Physiol.* **2**, 283–299.

Fulton, J. F. (1930). "Selected Readings in the History of Physiology." Thomas, Springfield, Illinois.

Goodfield, G. J. (1960). "The Growth of Scientific Physiology." Hutchinson, London.

Haldane, J. S. (1920). "Methods of Air Analysis," 3rd ed. Griffin, London.

Haldane, J. S., and Priestley, J. G. (1935). "Respiration," 2nd ed. Oxford Univ. Press (Clarendon), London and New York.

Haldane, J. S., and Smith, J. L. (1897). The absorption of oxygen by the lungs. *J. Physiol. (London)* **22**, 231–158.

Haldane, J. S., Meakins, J. C., and Priestley, J. G. (1919). The effects of shallow breathing. *J. Physiol. (London)* **52**, 433–453.

Harrop, G. A. (1919). The oxygen and carbon dioxide content of arterial and venous blood in normal individuals and in patients with anemia and heart disease. *J. Exp. Med.* **30,** 241–157.

Hartridge, H., and Roughton, F. J. W. (1923). A method of measuring the velocity of very rapid chemical reactions. *Proc. R. Soc. London, Ser. A* **104,** 376–394.

Henderson, Y., Chillingworth, F. P., and Whitney, J. L. (1915). The respiratory dead space. *Am. J. Physiol.* **38,** 1–19.

Hill, A. V. (1910). The possible effects of the aggregation of the molecules of haemoglobin on its dissociation curves. *J. Physiol. (London)* **40,** iv–vii.

Hooke, R. (1667). An account of an experiment made by M. Hooke of preserving animals alive by blowing through their lungs with bellows. *Philos. Trans. R. Soc. London* **28,** 539.

Hürter (1912). Untersuchungen am arteriellen menschlichen Blute. *Dtsch. Arch. Klin. Med.* **108,** 1–34.

Hüfner, G. V. (1890). Ueber das Gesetz der Dissociation des Oxyhaemoglobins und über einige sich knüpfende wichtige Fragen aus der Biologie. *Arch. Anat. Physiol., Physiol. Abt.* **1,** 1–27.

Keith, A. (1909). *In* The Mechanism of Respiration in Man. "Further Advances in Physiology" (L. Hill, ed.). Arnold, London.

Keys, A. (1936). Physiology of life at high altitudes. *Sci. Mon.* **43,** 289–312.

Knipping, H. W., Bolt, W., Venrath, H., Valentin, H., Cudes, H., and Endler, P. (1955). Eine neue Methode zur Prufung der Herz- und Lungenfunction. *Dtsch. Med. Wochenschr.* **80,** 1146–1147.

Krogh, A. (1908). Some new methods for the tonometric determination of gas tensions in fluids. *Skand. Arch. Physiol.* **20,** 259–278.

Krogh, A. (1910). On the mechanism of gas exchange in the lungs. *Skand. Arch. Physiol.* **23,** 248–278.

Krogh, M. (1915). The diffusion of gases through the lungs of man. *J. Physiol. (London)* **49,** 271–300.

Krogh, A., and Lindhard, J. (1913). The volume of the "dead space" in breathing. *J. Physiol. (London)* **47,** 30–44.

Krogh, A., and Lindhard, J. (1914). On the average composition of the alveolar air and its variations during the respiratory cycle. *J. Physiol. (London)* **47,** 431–445.

Krogh, A., and Lindhard, J. (1917). The volume of the dead space in breathing and the mixing of gases in the lungs of man. *J. Physiol. (London)* **51,** 59–90.

Magnus, H. G. (1837). Ueber die im Blute enthaltenen Gase, Sauerstoff, Stickstoff und Kohlensäure. *Ann. Phys. Chem.* **40,** 583–606.

Margaria, R., and Green, A. A. (1933). The first dissociation constant, pK_1, of carbonic acid in hemoglobin solutions and its relation to the existence of a combination of hemoglobin with carbon monoxide. *J. Biol. Chem.* **102,** 611–634.

Meakins, J. C., and Davies, H. W. (1925). "Respiratory Function in Disease." Oliver & Boyd, Edinburgh.

Meldrum, N. U., and Roughton, F. J. W. (1933). Carbonic anhydrase. Its preparation and properties. *J. Physiol. (London)* **80,** 113–142.

Perkins, J. F. (1964). Historical development of respiratory physiology. *In* "Handbook of Physiology. Sect. 3: Respiration" (H. Rahn and W. O. Fenn, eds.), Vol. 1, pp. 1–62. Am. Physiol. Soc., Washington, D.C.

Riley, R. L., Proemmel, D. D., and Franke, R. E. (1945). A direct method for determination of oxygen and carbon dioxide tensions in blood. *J. Biol. Chem.* **161,** 621–633.

Roelsen, E. (1938). Fractional analysis of alveolar air after inspiration of hydrogen as a method for the determination of the distribution of inspired air in the lungs. *Acta Med. Scand.* **95,** 452–482.

Roelsen, E. (1939). The composition of the alveolar air investigated by fractional sampling. *Acta Med. Scand.* **98,** 141–171.

Rohrer, F. (1915). Der Strömungswiderstand in den menschlichen Atemwegen und der Einfluss der unregelmässigen Verzweigung des Bronchialsystems auf den Atmungsverlauf in verschiedenen Lungenbezirken. *Pfluegers Arch. Ges. Physiol.* **162,** 225–229. [Engl. transl. in "Translations in Respiratory Physiology" (J. B. West, ed.), pp. 3–66. Dowden, Hutchinson & Ross, Stroudsburg, Pennsylvania, 1975.]

Roughton, F. J. W., and Scholander, P. F. (1943). Micro gasometric estimation of the blood gases. I. Oxygen. *J. Biol. Chem.* **148,** 541–550.

Severinghaus, J. W., and Bradley, A. F. (1958). Electrodes for blood P_{O_2} and P_{CO_2} determination. *J. Appl. Physiol.* **13,** 515–520.

Siebeck, R. (1911). Ueber den Gasaustausch zwischen Aussenluft und Alveolen. Zwitte Mitteilung. Ueber die Bedeutung und Bestimmung des "schädlichen Raumes" bei der Atmung. *Skand. Arch. Physiol.* **25,** 81–95.

Singer, C. (1957). "A Short History of Anatomy and Physiology from the Greeks to Harvey." Dover, New York.

Singer, C. (1959). "A Short History of Scientific Ideas to 1900." Oxford Univ. Press, London.

Stadie, W. C. (1919). The oxygen of the arterial and venous blood in pneumonia and its relation to cyanosis. *J. Exp. Med.* **30,** 215–240.

Stirling, W. (1902). "Some Apostles of Physiology." Waterlow, London.

Stokes, G. G. (1863–1864). On the reduction and oxidation of the colouring matter of the blood. *Proc. R. Soc. London* **13,** 355–364.

Strassburg, G. (1872). Die Topographie der Gasspannungen im thierischen Organismus. *Arch. Gesamte Physiol. Menschen Tiere* **6,** 65–96.

Van Slyke, D. D., and Neill, J. M. (1924). The determination of gases in blood and other solutions by vacuum extraction and manometric measurement. I. *J. Biol. Chem.* **61,** 523–573.

Zuntz, N. (1882). Physiologie der Blutgase und des respiratorischen Gaswechsels. *In* "Handbuch der Physiologie" (L. Hermann, ed.), Vol. 4, part 2, pp. 1–162. Vogel, Leipzig.

2

Development of Concepts in Rochester, New York, in the 1940s

Arthur B. Otis and Hermann Rahn

I. INTRODUCTION

If in the fall of 1941, anyone had suggested to us that a year hence we would be working as colleagues in a study of human respiration, specifically of the physiology of pressure breathing, we would, with some bewilderment, have dismissed the proposition as a most unlikely possibility. To begin with, we had never heard of each other, and, furthermore, little in our previous training, experience, or inclination would appear to have prepared us for such work. We did know that human beings like many other organisms consumed oxygen and gave off carbon dioxide but our special knowledge of respiration in this species was limited indeed. As to "pressure breathing" we would have had to admit complete ignorance. Even had we been completely familiar with the medical physiology text-

PULMONARY GAS EXCHANGE, VOL. I

33

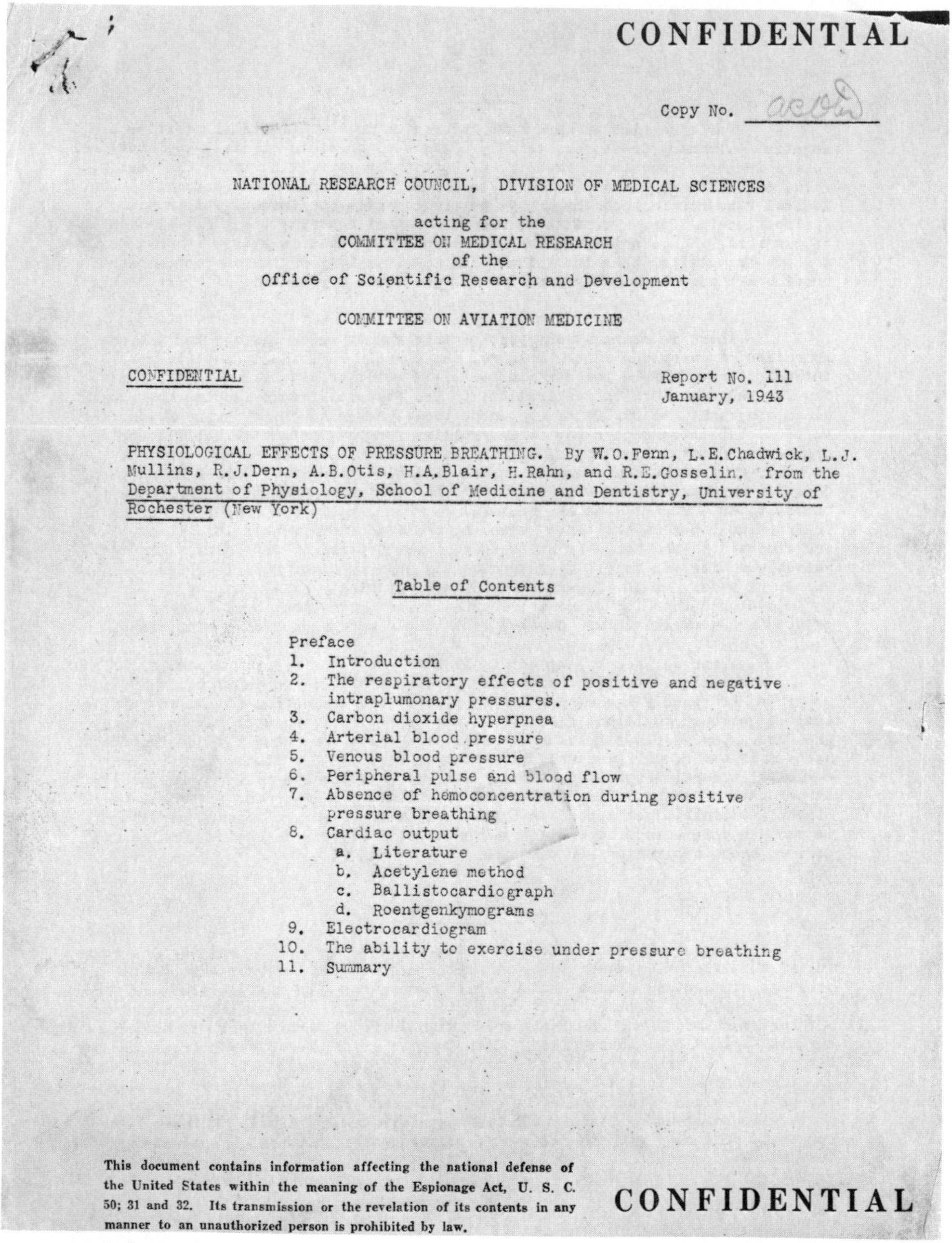

CONFIDENTIAL

Copy No. _____

NATIONAL RESEARCH COUNCIL, DIVISION OF MEDICAL SCIENCES

acting for the
COMMITTEE ON MEDICAL RESEARCH
of the
Office of Scientific Research and Development

COMMITTEE ON AVIATION MEDICINE

CONFIDENTIAL   Report No. 111
                                                               January, 1943

PHYSIOLOGICAL EFFECTS OF PRESSURE BREATHING. By W.O.Fenn, L.E.Chadwick, L.J.
Mullins, R.J.Dern, A.B.Otis, H.A.Blair, H.Rahn, and R.E.Gosselin. from the
Department of Physiology, School of Medicine and Dentistry, University of
Rochester (New York)

Table of Contents

Preface
1. Introduction
2. The respiratory effects of positive and negative
    intrapulmonary pressures.
3. Carbon dioxide hyperpnea
4. Arterial blood pressure
5. Venous blood pressure
6. Peripheral pulse and blood flow
7. Absence of hemoconcentration during positive
    pressure breathing
8. Cardiac output
    a. Literature
    b. Acetylene method
    c. Ballistocardiograph
    d. Roentgenkymograms
9. Electrocardiogram
10. The ability to exercise under pressure breathing
11. Summary

CONFIDENTIAL

Fig. 1.   Cover page of our first report (No. 111) on the physiology of pressure breathing.

books of that era we would not have found listed a number of terms, which are commonplace today, e.g., positive pressure breathing, pressure–volume diagram, O_2–CO_2 diagram, work of breathing, pulmonary compliance, airway resistance, alveolar ventilation, ventilation–perfusion ratio. Nevertheless, our names appeared with a number of others as coauthors on a report entitled "Physiological Effects of Pressure Breathing" dated January, 1943, with W. O. Fenn as first author (Fig. 1). Acknowledgment of our contribution was given in the preface, from which we now quote:

> For some time we have been interested in the effects of positive and negative pulmonary pressures, chiefly because of possible clinical applications. We are indebted however to Prof. H. C. Bazett for suggesting to us the possible value to aviation. We are grateful to Dr. A. N. Richards and the Committee on Medical Research for encouraging us to proceed with our investigations with this application in mind. Herewith we submit a report covering the first six months of our work. We do not claim to have learned much that is really new but we hope to have brought together the information now available on the subject so as to provide a theoretical background for the practical application of pressure breathing.
>
> There is scarcely any part of this report which has not had the cooperation of every one of the authors, but certain individuals have been more intimately responsible for certain parts. Special credit is due to Dr. Chadwick and Dr. Rahn for work on respiration, to Dr. Chadwick for developing the finger plethysmograph; to Dr. Otis for venous blood pressure, CO_2 hyperpnoea, and the vertical ballistocardiograph, to Dr. Mullins for the horizontal ballistocardiograph, the Roentgenkymographs, and the acetylene method for cardiac output, and to Mr. Dern for the measurements on arterial blood pressure. Dr. Rahn and Mr. Gosselin were associated with us during the first three months and Dr. Otis for the last three months. We are grateful to Mr. J. Kelly for measuring for us the refractive index of the blood plasma before and after pressure breathing. We are indebted to Dr. Nolan P. Kaltreider of the Department of Medicine for much valuable advice and to Mr. Meermagen of the Department of Radiology for the X-rays. Dr. G. H. Ramsay of the Department of Radiology kindly examined many of our experimental subjects for pulmonary abnormalities before they were allowed to participate in the experiments. Several individuals were rejected as poor risks.
>
> A special acknowledgment is also due to Major A. P. Gagge and Lt. Molomut of the Aeromedical Research Laboratory at Wright Field. In their hands pressure breathing is rapidly becoming a highly practicable and useful method of gaining altitude with an addition of 1000 feet for every 5 cm of water extrapulmonary pressure. During a visit to Wright Field they have very kindly demonstrated their methods to two of us (Fenn and Blair) and we have had the pleasure of setting up our ballistocardiograph in their high altitude chamber and making a few preliminary experiments on the effects of pressure breathing on the cardiac output at the highest attainable altitudes. A brief account of these preliminary experiments is contained in a separate report. From these practical demonstrations we have derived much inspiration for our work.

This preface was, of course, entirely written by Wallace Fenn and we present it here because of the clarity with which it sets forth the background of the work that was to involve us for the next decade and because, together with the table of contents, it suggests the variety of directions from which the pressure-breathing problem was being approached in the Rochester laboratory. Also it indicates the modest and gracious nature of Wallace Fenn and his direct but imaginative approach to a problem.

Report 111 deals entirely with the mechanical effects of positive pressure on breathing and circulation. All of the experiments were performed at ground level because our altitude chamber was not yet ready for use. Problems related to gas exchange remained to be dealt with later. Some of the topics in this report, such as stroke volume estimates from roentgen-kymograms (Fig. 2), were not investigated in further detail and were never published elsewhere. Others such as the studies of respiratory effects of positive and negative intrapulmonary pressures and of venous blood pressure were the basis for further exploration, refinement, and elaboration of concepts related to the pressure–volume diagram of the chest and lungs and to work of breathing.

Early in 1943, our altitude chamber became functional and during the next 2 years our efforts became concentrated on studying the effects of pressure breathing at simulated altitude with our attention focused mainly on gas exchange rather than mechanics. It was during this 2-year period that the alveolar gas equations and their graphic representation on the CO_2–O_2 diagram became developed and refined. They were first presented in OSRD Report No. 304, May 22, 1944. Problems of mechanics had not been forgotten, however, because a later report dated May 10, 1945, dealt entirely with the work of breathing, with intermittent as compared to continuous pressure breathing, and with a method for estimating the distensibility of the lung from a simultaneous measurement of peripheral venous and relaxation pressures.

Up to this point no publication of our work had been made in the open literature but shortly after the end of World War II in the summer of 1945, the material was declassified, and we were free to publish in the open literature. In the spring of 1946, we made the first public oral presentations of our work at the Federation Meetings in Atlantic City and shortly thereafter our first published papers appeared (Rahn et al., 1946a; Otis et al., 1946a; Fenn et al., 1946).

During these early days, the project had been supported largely by funds from contracts with the Office of Scientific Research and Development (OSRD), the initial contract for a sum of $500.00. With the return to peacetime, the OSRD was discontinued, but thanks to a contract negotiated for us by Colonel Pharo Gagge with the Air Force Material Command at Wright Field, continued support of our work was ensured. For the remainder of the decade covered in this chapter and for some years

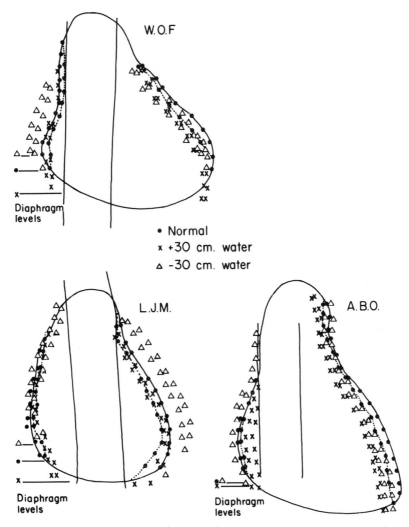

Fig. 2. Roentgenkymograph tracings used for estimation of cardiac output during pressure breathing in three subjects: Wallace O. Fenn, Lorin J. Mullins, and Arthur B. Otis. The different symbols indicate the outline of the heart under pulmonary pressures of 0, +30, and −30 cm H_2O. Note that the symbols appear in pairs; the innermost member of a pair indicates systole, the outermost diastole. Thus, the dotted line represents the cardiac outline during systole and the solid line during diastole under conditions of no applied pressure. Diaphragmatic levels are also indicated. Note that in WOF and LJM, the levels changed with the different conditions. In ABO the level is constant because he was instructed to bring his chest volume under each condition to a constant value as registered by a pneumograph on a mercury manometer.

thereafter, a growing number of people contributed their efforts to the project for various periods of time. During the war years we and, of course, Wallace Fenn were the only ones who were continuously with the project to the war's end in 1945, although Leigh Chadwick was a member of the team for much of the period. Our association continued for several years longer and was enriched by the presence of a number of postdoctoral fellows and visiting investigators who came from abroad as well as from various places in our own country.

II. EQUIPMENT

Most of the equipment available in the laboratory would be regarded as primitive by current standards. Among the more useful items were a few assorted spirometers, two or three Haldane machines, an equal number of Van Slykes, and several U-tube manometers. There were also several sensitive galvanometers suitable for use with thermocouples, an excellent camera for optical recording, two or three electrocardiographs with string galvanometers, and a two-channel Brush ink writing recorder in which the pens were driven piezoelectrically by large crystals.

Our first acquisition of a more sophisticated instrument was a Milliken oximeter on loan from the Air Force. Accompanying it was a security classification but no instruction manual. It took considerable time and finally a visit to Glenn Milliken himself at the Johnson Foundation in Philadelphia before any of us were able to make proper use of it. Another valuable piece of advanced instrumentation, also obtained through the Air Force and also highly classified, was a Pauling oxygen tensimeter, which had been invented by Linus Pauling. We understand that the instrument was originally intended for analyzing exhaust gases from airplace engines rather than those from humans. Our fleet of exotic instruments was rounded out by a thermal conductivity meter, originally designed for the analysis of CO_2 in flue gas, which we purchased from Cambridge Instrument Company.

Later in the decade, we obtained a couple of Statham pressure transducers and a Hathaway oscillograph for the recording of dynamic pressures. For such recording in the earlier days, we relied on glass spoon manometers or membrane manometers of our own fabrication. Usually we chose the latter because with our limited glass-blowing abilities we found them easier to construct. The basic feature of this device is an elastic membrane fitted snugly over the end of a rigid tube. When a pressure is applied to the open end of the tube the membrane bulges. By attaching a small mirror to the membrane near its periphery, one can record a reflected light beam on a roll of moving photographic paper. For membranes we used whatever bits of sheet rubber we could obtain. Rubber gloves, dental dam, and gasket material all became useful. For the mirror, we broke chips from a concave galvanometer mirror usually with a focal length of 1 m and preferable front-surfaced to minimize extraneous reflections.

We also built our own version of the Fleisch pneumotachograph. In our first model, a cluster of soda straws encased in a brass tube served as the flow-resistive element. The pressure drop was recorded by a differential manometer constructed from a sensitive membrane manometer, a two-hole rubber stopper, and a section of brass tubing to one end of which a glass window was sealed in an airtight fashion with De Khotinsky cement (see Fig. 3). In later versions of the pneumotachograph, we used as resistive elements glass wool enclosed in a lady's hair net (suggested to us by John Lilly and John Pappenheimer), disks of sintered brass, and finally Monel metal mesh screening.

We also constructed our own breathing valves. One method of doing this was to start with a piece of brass tubing about $\frac{3}{4}$ in. diameter and to solder a flat piece of brass over one end. The center of this plate was then drilled out to leave a narrow annular ring, which served as the valve seat. The valve itself consisted of a disk of rubber of appropriate thickness fastened to the seat at one point with a small drop of rubber cement. At the cost of an hour or two of time and a few burned fingers, one would, with a

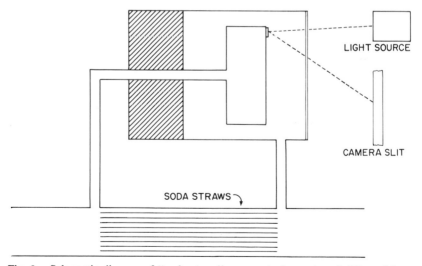

Fig. 3. Schematic diagram of "soda straw" pneumotachograph and differential membrane manometer.

little luck, produce a valve that opened and closed as it was supposed to do and that allowed no back flow. Later, we were able to obtain much better valves by extracting them from Air Force masks.

All in all neither the equipment nor the investigators were very impressive, and it seems doubtful that by present standards the project could have qualified for an NIH grant. The one big asset was Wallace Fenn himself. He was not put off by the lack of ready-made equipment. He was well endowed with Yankee ingenuity and he loved to improvise. He could, with whatever components happened to be handy, construct an apparatus that might not be beautiful but would do the job. We have many memories of him in the laboratory surrounded by what at first sight appeared to be an unrelated jumble of strange wires and rubber bands, tubing, pulleys, lenses, light sources, mirrors, and other assorted bits and pieces. More careful examination might suggest that there was possibly some order in the arrangement and further observation would reveal that

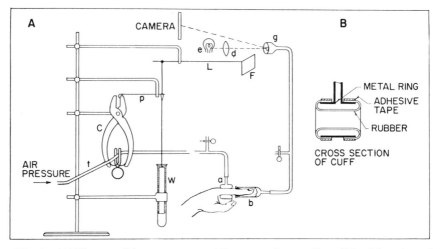

Fig. 4. (A) Diagram of the apparatus used for automatic recording of blood flow through the finger by the plethysmography method. (B) Cross-sectional diagram of the pneumatic cuff: "This is essentially a method of obstructing the recording light beam a given interval of time after the pressure is admitted to the cuff so that the height of the excursion in the optical record is a direct measure of the rate of blood flow. When the clamp, D, is squeezed this releases the tube, t, leading from the pressure reservoir to the finger cuff. At the same time it pulls a pin, p, which releases a weight, w. The weight sinks slowly in a test tube full of oil or water. After falling a fixed distance it exerts tension on a heart lever, L, by means of a thread. On the end of the lever is a flag, F, which rises and cuts off the recording beam of light. As soon as the light is obstructed, the operator releases the cuff pressure, opens the plethysmograph to the air, raises the weight and resets the apparatus for another test. These tests can be repeated every 15 seconds or oftener if desired". (From Fenn and Chadwick, 1947, reproduced by permission.)

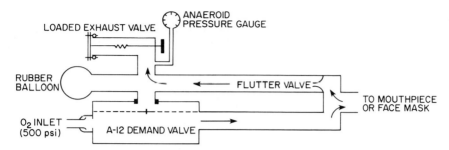

Fig. 5.   Device for delivering positive pressure breathing (see method no. 6 in text quotation from Report 111). Pressure demand regulators were not yet available to us. This was our improvised version. Exhalation occurred through a flutter valve down a tube, which terminated with an adjustable spring-loaded valve, which determined the magnitude of the expiratory pressure. This pressure was applied to the diaphragm of the demand regulator through an air-tight connection, and was maintained during inspiration by the action of the flutter valve. The balloon served as an elastic reservoir which compensated for leakage that might occur through the exhaust valve. The demand valve delivered whenever the pressure at the mouth was less than that in the expiratory tube beyond the flutter valve.

something of physiological interest was actually being measured and perhaps graphically recorded. A relatively refined example is a device for the automatic recording of blood flow through the finger. It was used by Fenn and Chadwick (1947) to study the effect of pressure breathing on the circulation (see Fig. 4). Other examples are described in the following description quoted from our report 111 (see also Fig. 5):

Methods

Although we were not concerned primarily with the development of methods for applying positive pressure we were nevertheless forced to devise a variety of methods in order to study their effects. These methods were not however designed particularly with a view to using them outside the laboratory. They were selected more for our own convenience than for that of the aviator. Six different methods will be described although combinations of these methods were often used.

Method No. 1.   *Drinker respirator* with constant negative pressure around the body. The intermittent gears are disconnected and the extent of the negative pressure was regulated by adjusting the short circuit between the input and output of the pump. With positive pressure around the body this serves also to produce negative intrapulmonary pressure. The subject must be in the supine position and must wear a rubber collar around his neck which must be fairly tight to avoid excessive leakage. The method is useful for experiments where the head and mouth need to be accessible.

Method No. 2.   *Body box* with electrical pressure control. A cubical box of sheet steel was constructed about 4 feet on a side with an air tight door at one end. A hole in the top permits the subject's head to protrude through a rubber collar as in the Drinker respirator. The subject is in a sitting position. The pressure around the body is made either positive or negative by connecting it either to the laboratory air blast or the suction. Pressure in the box was adjusted by an electrically controlled air valve activated by an electrical contact on a mercury manometer column. The method is convenient for many purposes, especially for respiratory studies, but the subject is somewhat immobilized, and in case of collapse "rescue" is somewhat delayed. [This comment is not merely academic. Fenn himself indeed collapsed during an experiment. Considerable anxiety ensued during the awkward process of extricating and reviving him.]

Method No. 3. *Helmet.* This apparatus was constructed from a large ether can, 10 inches in diameter and 13 inches high. The bottom was cut out and replaced by a collar of sponge rubber. A large window was cut out of the front and was sealed air tight with a sheet of lucite 15″ by 9½″ and ¼ inch thick. An inlet and outlet tube were inserted in the top, the former projecting down along the inside of the can to open near the level of the rubber collar to insure good mixing. Straps were attached to the helmet so that it could be strapped down under the arms to prevent it from rising up when the pressure was applied. When used without pressure it was found convenient to support it by a rope and overhead pulley although this was not altogether necessary. A much smaller and lighter helmet could be made with success. Pressure was maintained inside the helmet by retarding the outflow, the inflow being connected to the air blast. For this purpose we used a loaded valve as illustrated in Fig. 0. A similar helmet but of larger capacity was also used. With the larger helmet the pressure remained fairly constant but with the smaller one there were considerable variations of pressure due to the breathing so that a strong rubber balloon was added to the circuit to stabilize the pressure. When connected to the suction the helmet was also used for negative pulmonary pressures in certain experiments. The helmet is very convenient and on the whole very comfortable, if the collar is properly adjusted. It has the disadvantage that the air blast is rather noisy and the subject cannot hear the instructions of the operator.

Method No. 4. *Mouthpiece.* Pressure is maintained by connecting the mouth piece to the air supply and permitting it to escape through a loaded valve (see method 3) or a variable leak. It can also be permitted to escape under water in a large tank. A rubber balloon stabilizes the pressure. The mouth piece can also be used in a closed circuit maintained at an elevated pressure and circulated by a pump. An absorber for carbon dioxide is necessary and a constant influx of air with a variable leak. With a sufficiently large reservoir not too far from the mouth piece the pressure can be kept very constant. The method is convenient for short and quick observations but it is very tiring to the cheeks and lips and enhances very much the sensation of respiratory difficulty. It is impossible to use this method for prolonged periods.

Method No. 5. *Pneumatic vest.* This may be used in conjunction with any of the methods already described. We used a standard U.S. Navy aviation pneumatic life-vest with the CO_2 cylinders removed. The vest was strapped fairly snugly to the chest without actually limiting the movement and the air input was connected to the helmet or mouth piece so that the outside of the chest was exposed to the same pressure as the lungs inside. Furthermore when the subject inhaled the pressure fell in the mouth piece or helmet so that air was drawn out of the pneumatic vest thus making room for the expansion of the chest. This reciprocating device if carefully designed can be very helpful in relieving any sense of respiratory difficulty which may be present with the higher pressures.

Method No. 6. *Demand valve,* Pioneer Instrument Co., A-12. This instrument was used to deliver oxygen to a mouth piece or face mask according to the diagrams in figs. 0–00. The expired air passes through a Y-tube and a flutter valve to a loaded expiratory valve. The pressure built up in this expiratory valve is applied to the outside of the demand valve itself by making the cover of the instrument air tight. Thus the demand valve delivers oxygen whenever the pressure falls below the pressure set by the expiratory valve. The flutter valve prevents a fall of pressure in the expiratory valve during inspiration. This method has worked well in tests but we have not had time to use it in any of our experiments as yet.

III. THE HIGH-ALTITUDE CHAMBER

Our high-altitude chamber was perhaps the crowning masterpiece of Fenn's ingenuity. The initial contract with the OSRD provided the sum of $500.00 for special research equipment. From this budget eked out by a small contribution from departmental funds Fenn bought a steel tank designed for the processing or transport of beer. He then persuaded the University Grounds Department to loan us the pump from its only tree sprayer, reversed its valves, and connected pump to tank, and the result was a chamber that could go to simulated altitudes at the rate of 5000 ft/min (see Fig. 6). As he later said "It surely was the worst high altitude chamber in the country but a rare atmosphere is the same wherever you find it" (Fenn, 1962).

One had to enter the chamber by lowering himself through a small circular hatch located at the top. Inside there was barely room for two subjects seated side by side on folding chairs, facing a small shelf, which held equipment of one sort of another depending on the mission of the particular "flight." When preliminary preparations were completed the hatch was closed, the pump was turned on, and the chamber was evacuated until the desired altitude was reached. This was controlled by an outside observer who kept one eye on a mercury manometer, which indicated the pressure inside the chamber, and the other eye on the subject by peering through one of the small portholes in the side of the chamber. Communication was partly by a two way microphone–loud speaker system and partly by sign language. We did not always have enough functional microphones to allow both subjects to have one.

With this chamber, we explored limits of performance and of consciousness. When the outside observer no longer obtained from a subject a reasonable response to his interrogation over the loudspeaker, he would open a valve to admit air into the chamber until the subject demonstrated satisfactory activity. For the reassurance of subjects who might wish to have personal control of their destinies, there was also a "dump" valve that could be operated from inside the chamber. No emergency requiring the use of this valve ever arose, but we did use it occasionally just for fun to see how fast we could recompress and still keep out ears clear.

Most of our flights were carried out between 18,000 and 25,000 ft, breathing air, and between 40 and 46,000 ft, breathing oxygen. On two occasions, two of us reached an altitude of 50,000 ft by vigorous hyperventi-

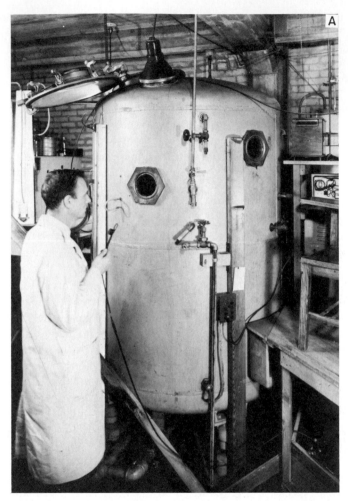

Fig. 6. Two views of the high-altitude chamber. (A) Note the hatch in the top, which was the only access. The two ports on the side of the chamber were used for visual monitoring of the subjects. The box galvanometer on the right was for reading percentage saturation from the ear oximeter. (Hermann Rahn is holding the microphone.) (B) One of the mercury manometers, which served as altimeters, is located just to his left, the other is left of center. The lamp on the far right could be focused on the mirror of a membrane manometer within the chamber and the reflected beam recorded outside on the photokymograph (not shown). The smoked drum kymograph was used for recording a variety of events via signal magnets. (Arthur Otis is the observer.)

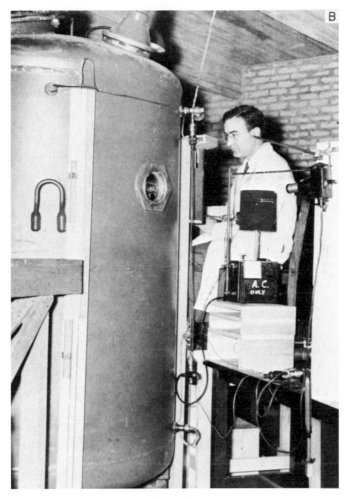

Fig. 6B.

lation combined with positive pressure breathing, and we were able to maintain a convincing semblance of consciousness for 5 to 10 min. The total barometric pressure at this altitude is 87 Torr. Mean lung pressurization was about 15 torr, which meant that the total intrapulmonary gas pressure was 102 torr. Allowing 46 torr for water vapor leaves 55 torr, which had to be divided between O_2 and CO_2 in the alveoli. Thus, by sufficient hyperventilation to reduce the alveolar CO_2 to 15 torr, we would theoretically have had an alveolar O_2 of 40 torr, which was just at the edge of consciousness. To ventilate sufficiently to maintain a P_{CO_2} of 15 torr for any length of time required a tremendous concentration of effort and, as soon as one tired and P_{CO_2} rose, alveolar P_{O_2} fell and one reached a state of semiconscious sublimity that rended him irresponsive to the outside world. We also remember having some symptoms of bends at this altitude and being able to feel bubbles of gas under the skin of our fingers.

In the early days of our altitude chamber operations, Wallace Fenn was always the first to volunteer when a new procedure was to be tried out, but when the dean of our school, Dr. George Whipple, one day came by at an inopportune time to see Wallace passing out from a mask leak at high altitude, he immediately gave strict orders to us that Fenn should henceforth not be allowed to enter the chamber. Fortunately for us, human experimentation committees did not exist at that time for they surely would have stopped all of our research at simulated high altitudes.

IV. SAMPLING AND ANALYSIS OF ALVEOLAR GAS

By comparison with today's technology, the sampling and analysis of alveolar gas was in those days a rather formidable task. A single experiment such as an altitude chamber run might produce half a dozen samples, each taken from a single forced expiration according to the Haldane procedure (Fig. 7). This meant that someone (frequently one of us rather than a technician) would spend the rest of the day doing duplicate or triplicate analyses on a Haldane gas analyzer. Each sample was collected over mercury and stored in a Haldane sampling tube under slight positive pressure to prevent any inboard leaks. The Haldane method has a high degree of accuracy but was tedious and time-consuming, and it was the end of the day before we had the answers. On-line data processing was carried out by us with our slide rules. An inevitable side effect of the Haldane procedure was that sooner or later mercury became generously distributed over the floor and benches of the laboratory and in the space under the floor boards of our altitude chamber. Various rumors circulated about the possibilities of mercury poisoning but apparently none of us suffered any ill effects.

The urgency of military needs for multiple gas samples required in high-altitude chambers of the U.S. Air Force for exploring the limits of decompression and for testing mask leaks led to a search for quicker if less accurate methods of gas analysis. One method devised by Scholander was used by us for CO_2 analyses at altitude. A 10-ml gas sample was injected from a syringe into a vessel container KOH. The unabsorbed volume was measured in a graduated tube sealed to the vessel. Another method widely adopted was that devised by Professor F. Fry, a zoologist

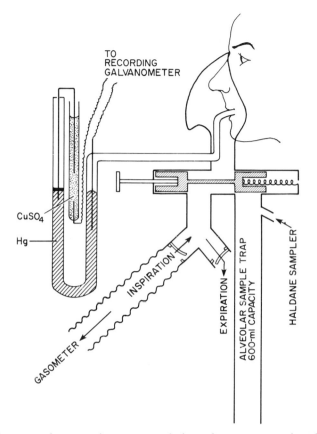

TO
RECORDING
GALVANOMETER

CuSO$_4$

Hg

GASOMETER

INSPIRATION

EXPIRATION

ALVEOLAR SAMPLE TRAP
600-ml CAPACITY

HALDANE SAMPLER

Fig. 7. Apparatus for measuring pressures during voluntary pressure breathing and for sampling alveolar gas. The subject inspired through the inspiratory valve, voluntarily exerted pressure while closing his lips around the pipe stem, and then exhaled through the expiratory valve. The pressure exerted was recorded from the mercury manometer. A float in the open arm of the manometer supported a wire that dipped into a dilute copper sulfate solution. When the wire moved in response to pressure changes, the electrical resistance of the circuit changed proportionately and was registered on a recording galvanometer outside the altitude chamber. When an alveolar sample was desired, the subject pressed the plunger, exhaled down the sample trap, and released the plunger. The sample was then drawn into an evacuated Haldane tube, which could be located either inside or outside the chamber. (From Fenn *et al.*, 1949a, reproduced by permission.)

at Toronto (Fry *et al.*, 1949). In this procedure, the gas sample was collected in a syringe and then injected into a modified 1-ml pipet filled initially with an acid rinsing solution. By adding sequentially strong base and oxygen absorber one could in turn obtain relatively quickly values for carbon dioxide and oxygen. Although the accuracy of the Fry analyzer was not as good as that of the Haldane, the analysis took less time and could easily be performed even in the limited space of our high altitude chamber. We will never forget the surprise of our discovery while seated at 40,000 ft altitude breathing pure oxygen that in the analysis of a normal alveolar sample nearly half the gas volume disappeared when the CO_2 absorber was added. The CO_2 concentration was indeed 40%: $P_B = 147$, $P_B - 47 = 100$, $P_{A_{CO_2}} = 40$, $F_{A_{CO_2}} = 0.40$.

Our ability to gather alveolar gas data was tremendously enhanced by our development of a device that sampled automatically 10 ml of the last part of each expiration and delivered it for continuous analysis into the Pauling oxygen tensimeter and the Cambridge CO_2 meter. Although the sampling device in its final version was exceedingly simple (Fig. 8), it took us several weeks of trial and error effort to produce a satisfactory prototype. An essential moving element in its operation was a condom, which we delicately refer to in our original description (Rahn *et al.*, 1946c) as a

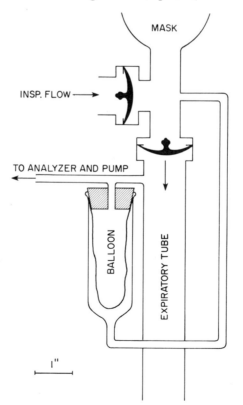

Fig. 8. The end-tidal gas sampler. (From Rahn and Otis, 1949a, reproduced by permission.)

"thin walled rubber balloon." The time taken in developing this sampler was well spent, however, because we were now able for the first time to explore steady state alveolar gas composition, not only during quiet resting breathing but also during a wide variety of perturbations such as exercise, voluntary hyperventilation, inhalation of CO_2 mixtures, anesthesia, and ascent to altitude.

V. THE OXYGEN–CARBON DIOXIDE DIAGRAM

By the time our system for the continuous analysis of alveolar gas was operational, Wallace Fenn had already developed the essential features of the oxygen–carbon dioxide diagram (Figs. 9 and 10). These were indeed exciting days for us, because the large amount of data that we could generate were not merely numbers but brush strokes forming part of a congruent painting or perhaps musical notes arranged in harmony, which could be interpreted with reference to RQ, alveolar ventilation, blood gas contents and hydrogen ion concentration, and percentage saturation of hemoglobin. It allowed us for the first time to perceive clearly the nature of the simultaneous changes in blood and alveolar gas. It permitted us to

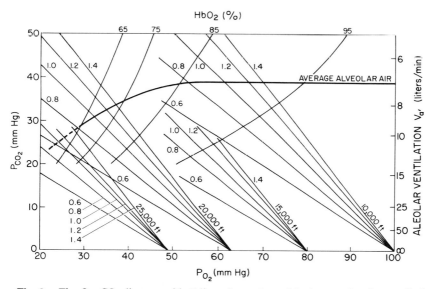

Fig. 9. The O_2–CO_2 diagram with R lines for various altitudes, an alveolar ventilation scale, and percentage saturation isopleths. The alveolar air line was based on our altitude chamber data. The alveolar ventilation scale is based on an assumed value for CO_2 production of 315 ml/min STPD. (From Fenn *et al.*, 1946, reproduced by pemission.)

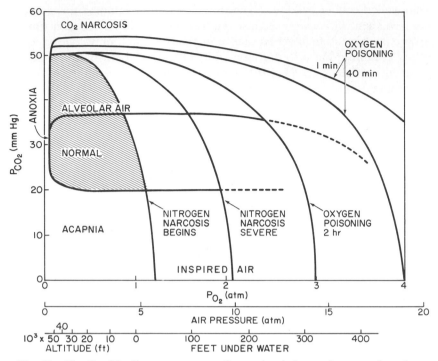

Fig. 10. The O_2-CO_2 diagram as a map of normal and abnormal ranges of respiratory gases. (From Fenn *et al.*, 1946, reproduced by permission.)

follow the changes during acute (Rahn and Otis, 1947) (Fig. 11) and chronic exposure to altitude (Rahn and Otis, 1949a,b) (Fig. 12), during breath holding at sea level and at altitude (Otis *et al.*, 1948), and during anesthesia (Ament *et al.*, 1949). It also allowed a clear portrayal of the effects of hypocapnia and hypoxia, singly and combined on human psychomotor performance (Fig. 13) (Otis *et al.*, 1946a; Rahn *et al.*, 1946b). Application of the diagram to the physiology of abnormal respiratory gas concentrations was elegantly presented by Fenn (1948) before a meeting of the American Philosophical Society in a lecture for which he was awarded the John F. Lewis prize.

Although the oxygen–carbon dioxide diagram may be regarded merely as a nomogram useful for computational purposes, it is much more than that. We prefer to think of it as a sort of map of the domain of gas exchange on which latitude and longitude are represented by P_{CO_2} and P_{O_2}, respectively, and on which any number of parameters can be represented by isopleths. On this map, one can start at a normal steady state value ($P_{O_2} = 100$, $P_{CO_2} = 40$) and move from there by a variety of pathways.

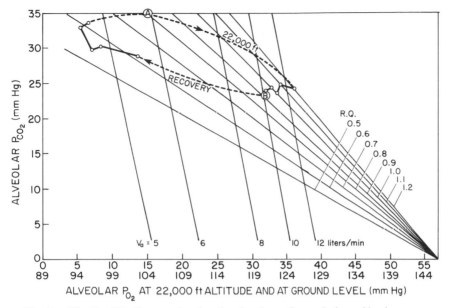

Fig. 11. The O_2–CO_2 diagram showing the alveolar pathway during a 30-min exposure to 22,000 ft and subsequent recovery. The points located around the loop are based on measurements obtained at 5-min intervals during exposure to altitude and during subsequent recovery at ground level. The dashed line beginning at A indicates the 5-min ascent and that beginning at B the 5-min descent. The alveolar ventilation lines were calculated using an assumed value for oxygen consumption of 300 ml/min STPD. (From Rahn and Otis, 1947, reproduced by permission.)

One can, for example, increase or decrease barometric pressure while breathing air, or substitute abnormal gas compositions, or both. This map guided us on our first mountain expedition to Wyoming in 1946, where we explored chronic exposure to altitude (Rahn and Otis, 1949b). It led to the elaboration and quantitation of the ventilation–perfusion ratio concept (Rahn, 1949) (Fig. 14) and later to that of the $a - A$ N$_2$ difference. It allowed us to assess quantitatively the differences between breathing air at altitude and breathing a so-called equivalent oxygen–nitrogen mixture at sea level (Rahn and Otis, 1949c); to analyze the effects of adding CO_2 to inspired gas on tolerance to high altitude (Otis *et al.*, 1949); and to ascertain the limits of altitude during the use of special breathing devices (Fenn *et al.*, 1949b) and voluntary pressure breathing (Fenn *et al.*, 1949a). Especially it allowed one to predict limits of tolerable gas composition at any ambient pressure and this was perhaps the practical result of most importance to the Air Force.

It is, of course, not possible for us to state what went on in Wallace

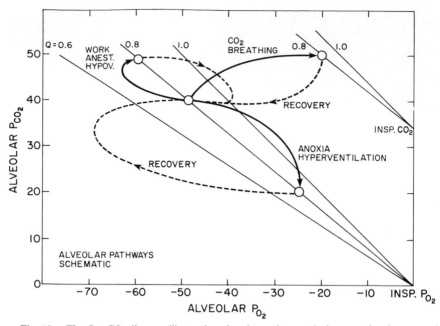

Fig. 12. The O_2–CO_2 diagram illustrating alveolar pathways during exercise, hyper- and hypoventilation, CO_2 breathing, hypoxia, and anesthesia. (From Rahn and Otis, 1949a, reproduced by permission.)

Fenn's mind during the conception of the O_2–CO_2 diagram. We do know that he was seeking to clarify a problem about which there was considerable confusion at the time, namely, the problem of equivalent altitude. Practically, this problem arose in connection with attempts to compare effects of breathing low oxygen mixtures at sea level with those of exposure to high altitude. Various related questions can be formulated. What inspired mixture of oxygen and nitrogen at sea level is equivalent to air breathing at a given altitude? What altitude, breathing pure oxygen, is equivalent to sea level breathing air? At a given altitude, how much oxygen must be added to the inspired gas so that sea level equivalence is obtained? The answer to each of these questions is simple enough, if one accepts identical values of $P_{I_{O_2}}$ under the various conditions as the criterion of equivalency. Physiologically, however, the important equivalence is not that between inspired gas pressures but rather in the composition of alveolar gas. The answer now is not as simple, but the problem can be readily visualized and understood by application of the O_2–CO_2 diagram with its R lines and ventilation lines. The following quotation is from our

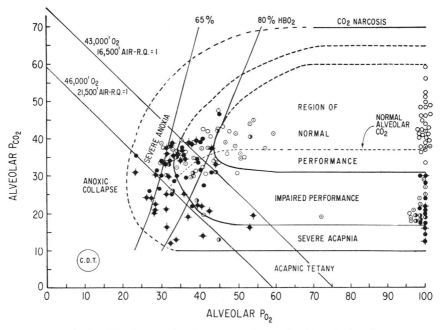

Fig. 13. The O_2–CO_2 diagram showing ranges of normal and impaired performance on a visual contrast discrimination test. Measurements were made under normal conditions, and with various alterations of alveolar gas composition. The results of each experimental series were compared by Fisher's t test with those obtained in the control situation during normal breathing at ground level. Each type of symbol represents a probability (p value) that the experimental score was not different from the control. The darker the symbol the lower the p value and the greater the likelihood that performance was impaired. Solid circle with cross, $P < 0.01$. Solid circle, $0.01 < P < 0.05$. Half solid circle, $0.05 < P < 0.1$. Open circle with dot $0.1 < P < 0.5$. Open circle $P > 0.5$. (From Otis *et al.*, 1946a, reproduced by permission.)

report 304 to the Committee on Aviation Medicine of the OSRD entitled "A Study of Hyperventilation as a Means of Gaining Altitude":

> In the light of this discussion, it is evident that calculations of equivalent altitude breathing air are meaningless for practical purposes if they are based upon the assumption of a steady state and an RQ and metabolic rate which are independent of altitude. When hyperventilation begins, the RQ remains considerably above normal for 15 to 20 minutes and somewhat above normal for even longer periods. Tests lasting only 15 to 20 minutes therefore are deceptive. In our own experience, 45,000 feet on pure oxygen is far worse than 18,500 breathing air, although the calculated alveolar O_2 should be the same if $RQ = 1.0$. The reason for the difference seems to be that CO_2 which is blown off dilutes the nitrogen when air is breathed while this is impossible on pure O_2. In other words, the high RQ increases the sum of the CO_2 and O_2 in air breathing. But on pure O_2 this sum must remain constant as long as the altitude remains constant. The altitude for

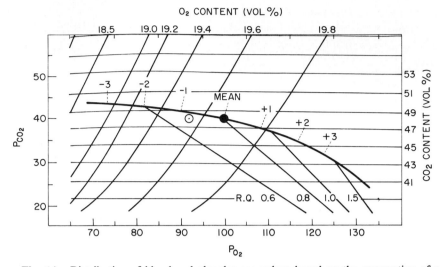

Fig. 14. Distribution of blood and alveolar gas values based on the assumption of a log-normal distribution of the ventilation–perfusion ratio around the mean value shown by the solid circle. Each dotted line indicates the locus corresponding to the stated number of standard deviations from the mean, when the value of one standard deviation is arbitrarily fixed as log 1.3. The resulting value for arterial blood is indicated by the open circle. (From Rahn, 1949, reproduced by permission.)

oxygen breathing which is simulated by breathing air at a given altitude is decreased when the apparent RQ is increased and overventilation is capable of causing large increases in the RQ.

It seems to us impossible to predict in advance what proportion of nitrogen and oxygen will be required to simulate a given altitude breathing oxygen. This will depend upon the sum of P_{CO_2} and P_{O_2} in the alveoli which is dependent upon the true metabolic RQ, the reserve CO_2 in the body, and the rate at which it can blow off. The greatest simplification of the problem of equivalent altitude is achieved in our opinion by *defining equivalent altitudes as those in which the sums of P_{CO_2} and P_{O_2} in the alveolar air are equal.* If equivalent altitudes are defined as those in which the alveolar P_{O_2} values are equal, that presupposes some particular rate of ventilation and makes it possible theoretically for a subject breathing pure oxygen at high altitude to change his equivalent altitude by merely changing his ventilation rate.

This was Wallace Fenn's clear and definitive answer to the problem of equivalent altitudes.

VI. THE VENTILATION–PERFUSION RELATIONSHIP

Our long preoccupation with alveolar gas recording led us to ask the obvious question, What is the mean alveolar gas concentration? We became quite aware of the fact that even during quiet breathing at rest, the composition showed small temporal fluctuations. Did these occur because of changes in ventilation, or could they be due to changes in lung perfusion or both? Our observation that these fluctuations also involved a cyclic change of the exchange ratio eventually led us to consider the exchange ratio in terms of blood as well as of alveolar gas and to the realization that a particular exchange ratio depended upon the delivery of certain quantities of blood and gas. The exchange ratio lines for gas had already been developed by Fenn on his original version of the O_2–CO_2 diagram. What now was needed was a set of exchange ratio lines for blood originating at the mixed venous point. The intersection of the same R lines for blood and gas became obviously the only point on the O_2–CO_2 diagram where such an exchange could take place and which was determined by the precise ratio of the perfusion to ventilation.

In 1948, Dick Riley from Cournand's laboratory came to visit us at Rochester to discuss his own solution to the same problem, using the four-quadrant diagram (see this volume, Chapter 3, by Riley). We agreed to exchange final manuscripts before submitting them for publication and furthermore agreed as a convention to refer to the V_A–Q ratio rather than the Q–V_A ratio.

With millions of alveoli each receiving its own perfusion and ventilation it is obvious that even in a normal lung, all alveoli are not likely to have precisely the same V_A–Q ratio. Thus, one might suspect that there exists some sort of distribution of V_A–Q ratios where alveoli with high ratios were balanced out by those low ones. Furthermore, it was quite reasonable to assume that this ratio could actually vary from 0 to infinity. It was therefore proposed (Rahn, 1949) that in a lung the V_A–Q ratio of the separate units are log normally rather than linearly distributed (see Fig. 14). This suggestion has frequently evoked much eye-brow lifting, to which R. A. Bagnold (1941) would have answered, "The linear scale, since it was first cut on the wall of an Egyptian temple, has come to be accepted by man almost as if it were the unique scale with which nature builds and works. Whereas it is nothing of the sort." In personal conversation with us, J. H. Gaddum emphasized that in nature, all functions and dimensions are log normally distributed and only if their range is small will a linear distribution scale suffice to describe it. To quote from Gaddum's (1945) article, "In some cases, the normal (linear distribution) curve gives very close approximation to the observed facts. These cases are the exception rather than the rule but it is usually possible to transform the distribution by means of some function of the actual observation which is normally distributed." With ventilation–perfusion ratios, of course, if we can assume that some alveoli at any moment are not being perfused and others are not being ventilated, the range would be zero to infinity and the log normal distribution would appear to be the scale of choice. Further discussion of this problem may be found in the book by Aitchison and Brown (1957).

VII. THE PRESSURE–VOLUME DIAGRAM

The pressure–volume diagram is to the mechanics of breathing as the O_2–CO_2 diagram is to gas exchange. Although the basic diagram had been previously presented by Rohrer, Fenn conceived it independently and elaborated it. It became for us the navigational chart for approaching a variety of problems of respiratory mechanics. On it, we could define physiological boundaries, limiting values for muscle forces and for the corresponding volumes of gas and blood (Fig. 15). Within these limits lay the normal operating range of pulmonary mechanics and the displacements that might result from the response of the system to perturbing forces such as postural changes, continuous or intermittent pressure breathing either positive or negative, or various types of artificial ventilation. On the diagram the mechanical properties of the lung and of the chest wall, acting separately and in combination, can be represented. The

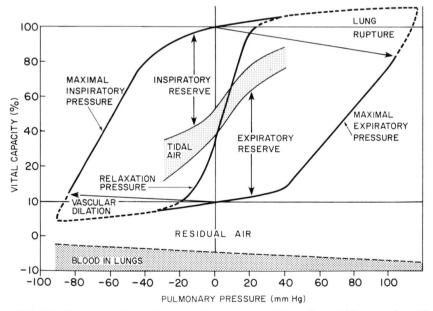

Fig. 15. Pressure–volume diagram of human chest. (From Fenn, 1951, reproduced by permission.)

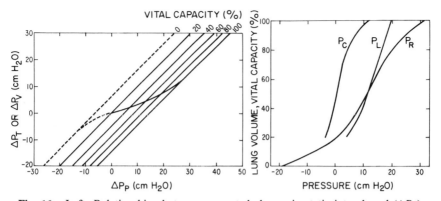

Fig. 16. Left: Relationships between expected change in static intrapleural (ΔP_T) or peripheral venous pressure (ΔP_V) with change in intrapulmonary pressure (ΔP_P). Lung volumes are shown as isopleths. At constant lung volume the magnitude of ΔP_T or ΔP_V is equal to ΔP_P, i.e., the relationship follows an isopleth. The curved line indicates the relationship when intrapulmonary pressures are relaxation pressures. Right: Pressure–volume diagram showing a measured relaxation pressure curve (P_R), with lung tension (P_L) and chest wall tension (P_C) curves calculated from venous pressure measurements assuming that $\Delta P_V = \Delta P_T$ and that when $P_P = 0$, $P_2 = 4$ cm H_2O. (From Otis *et al.*, 1946b, reproduced by permission.)

mechanical work involved in breathing can be quantitatively indicated and analyzed in terms of areas on the diagram. The consequences of gas compressibility to the mechanics of breathing can also be portrayed. Our venous pressure measurements were originally made merely to get evidence regarding the effect of pressure breathing on venous return. It was only after plotting the results on the pressure volume diagram that we conceived the notion of estimating pulmonary compliance from our data (Fig. 16).

The diagram has application in the description and analysis of such respiratory maneuvers as diving, singing, and the playing of wind instruments. (One of us helped a graduate student from the Eastman School of Music measure the pressures developed during French horn playing.) It is also useful in connection with the wide variety of ventilatory devices and procedures currently employed by anesthesiologists and respiratory therapists.

VIII. OTHER CONTRIBUTIONS TO RESPIRATORY PHYSIOLOGY

Although the pressure–volume and oxygen–carbon dioxide diagrams and their applications represent to us the great masterpiece of Fenn's sci-

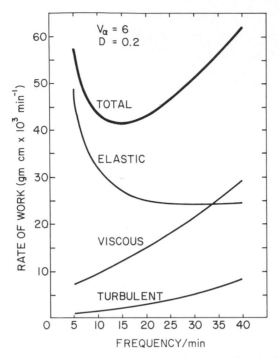

Fig. 17.   Relationships between rate of work done in overcoming elastic, viscous, turbulent, and total forces as a function of breathing frequency (indicated in breaths/min on the abscissa) when alveolar ventilation = 6 liters/min and dead space = 200 ml. The curves are calculated from a theoretical equation using empirically estimated constants. (From Otis *et al.*, 1950, reproduced by permission.)

entific artistry, he initiated, inspired, encouraged, or contributed to many other works during this period. To give a few examples: development of the concept of an optimal breathing frequency (Fig. 17), measurement of alveolar pressure (Fig. 18 is probably the first recording in this county using the interrupter method), dynamic pressure–volume curve (Fig. 19 is probably the first recorded on a cathode ray oscilloscope), development of an infrared CO_2 meter by Dr. Richard Fowler (Fig. 20a is probably the first published continuous recording of CO_2 changes during single breaths under various conditions). The prototype of Fowler's instrument, which predated the one developed by Liston, was during its development spread out on a table in bread-board fashion (a feature that enhanced our understanding or how it worked) and utilized as its recording instrument the string galvanometer and camera from one of our electrocardiographs.

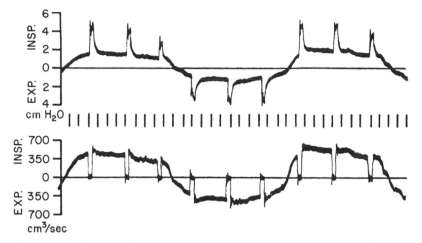

Fig. 18. Simultaneous changes of mouth pressure (upper curve) and flow (lower curve) with abrupt brief interruptions during resting breathing. Vertical lines between the two recordings indicate 0.2 sec intervals. When the tube through which the subject breathed was suddenly occluded, flow dropped to zero, and the mouth pressure rose or fell depending on the phase of the breathing cycle. The immediate change in mouth pressure was taken as approximating the alveolar-mouth pressure difference existing at the moment of interruption. From such pressure changes and the corresponding flows airway resistance was estimated. (Otis and Proctor, 1948, reproduced by permission.)

IX. RETROSPECT

In retrospect, and at the time, the decade from which we have attempted to sketch some glimpses was an exciting and productive period for us. What were the factors that made it so? It may seem incongruous that a group of individuals with such diverse and unrelated interests (Lee Chadwick was studying *Drosophila* flight, Herman Rahn was developing a bioassay method in frogs for testing intermedin hormone of the pituitary, and Arthur Otis was studying the activation and inhibition of the enzyme tyrosinase in grasshopper eggs) could put aside these activities to participate and collaborate effectively in a project on pressure breathing. None of us had any previous training in human physiology (we were not certain which lung volume was, in the terminology of the day, *complemental air* and which was *supplemental air*). But our education had developed in us an appreciation of scholarship and investigation, our horizons had not been restricted by narrowly prescribed learning objectives, nor

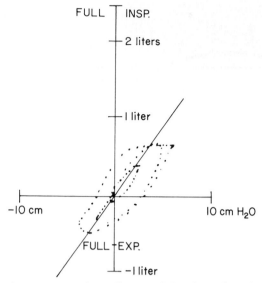

Fig. 19. Dynamic pressure–volume diagram of the chest of a relaxed human subject being ventilated by a Drinker respirator.

had we been required to qualify for anything by obtaining certain scores on standardized multiple choice examinations.

The national climate of those years during World War II was quite different from that of our more recent involvement of the 1960s. Nearly everyone seemed to have an attitude of quiet determination. The war was a disaster to be dealt with and everyone had to do what he could.

In a strange way, the intellectual atmosphere was perhaps actually enhanced. Many of today's common distractions were present to a limited degree or not at all. Television did not exist, automobiles were unobtainable, and gasoline was strictly rationed. Rents were controlled. Some foods were rationed but there were no serious shortages. Most luxury items were not being manufactured and on our salaries, which initially were only a fraction of the stipend received today by part-time graduate assistants, we could not have afforded to buy them anyway, but the laboratory was always open and there were interesting things to do. Moreover we had wives who, liberated to follow their own professional or academic interests, encouraged us in ours.

The doors of the laboratories and offices (except for that of the secretary) were never locked and were usually open. We could and did talk freely with such people as Edward Adolph, Harry Blair, and Bob Ramsay and received valuable lessons from each of them. Bureaucratic procedures were minimal or nonexistent. Purchasing procedures were simple.

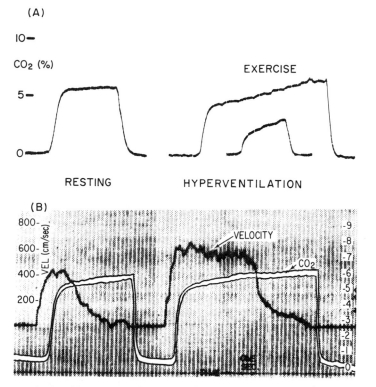

Fig. 20. (A) Continuous recordings of CO_2 in expired gas during rest, exercise and hyperventilation. (B) Continuous recording of CO_2 and flow during expiration. Normal exhalation followed by a complete exhalation. The white curve is the CO_2 concentration as recorded from Fowler's infrared analyzer by a string galvanometer. The dark curve is flow rate of exhalation as recorded from a pneumotachograph by a sensitive membrane manometer. Left-hand ordinate: expiratory flow (ml/sec). Right-hand ordinate: exhaled CO_2 concentration (%). This figure is from Fowler (1946), but for improved clarity the CO_2 record has been retouched by inking the margins of the tracing and new labels have been added.

There were no percentage effort forms, no leave forms, no human investigation forms, and no forms for evaluating our colleagues.

Wallace Fenn has been quoted (Lape, 1955) as saying before the war that research in his Physiology Department "has been organized as little as possible and depends entirely on the interests of the individual members of the staff." This policy of minimal organization was continued even during the war years. On one of our first days in the laboratory, he suggested that the elastic recoil of the thorax could be measured by inspiring a given volume of gas and then relaxing against a mercury manometer. One of us had the temerity to say that this would probably not yield any useful results. Fenn did not argue but quietly turned and walked out of the room. By the end of the afternoon, however, we had our first crude diagram of respiratory pressure–volume relationships. Wallace Fenn led by example and suggestion, never by command.

Although we contributed to the periodic progress reports and submitted them on time, there was no pressure on us to publish papers. In fact, because our project had a security classification, we were not permitted to appear in the open literature until the war had ended. By this time, we had a considerable backlog of material on which to base our publications. The enforced delay, by allowing time for thought and reflections, may indeed have improved the quality of our writings.

For whatever reasons we worked well together as a team (see Fig. 21) yet at the same time were able to maintain our individualities. We were able to collaborate closely without being intrusive. Our ideas were freely pooled and mutually criticized.

Although we personally had no problems regarding our separate identities, we were the object of a certain amount of confusion for others.

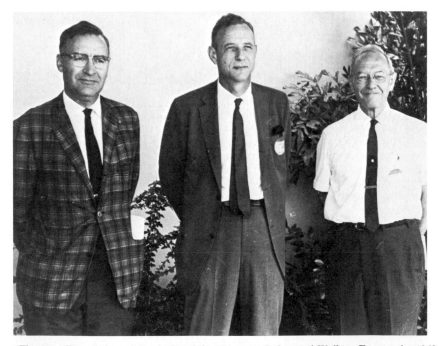

Fig. 21. From left to right: Arthur Otis, Hermann Rahn, and Wallace Fenn at the 1963 Fall Meeting of the American Physiological Society in Coral Gables, Florida.

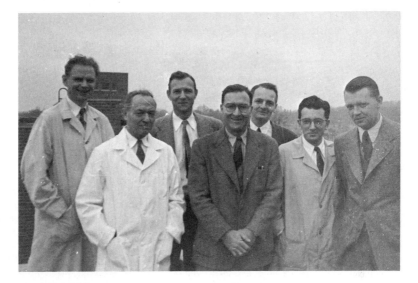

Fig. 22. Picture taken on the roof of the University of Rochester School of Medicine in the fall of 1951. From left to right: H. Bjurstedt (Sweden), Wallace Fenn, Hermann Rahn, Arthur Otis, Paul Sadoul (France), Pierre Dejours (France), and H. Heemstra (Holland).

When, in 1946, we attended the first postwar Federation Meetings, we were frequently recognized as being "Rahn and Otis" but no one seemed to be sure which of us was which. This situation continued to some extent for several years but eventually, everyone got us sorted out.

Between 1941 and 1956 more than 100 publications in pulmonary physiology were published from Fenn's laboratory (Fenn *et al.*, 1951; Rahn and Fenn, 1955; Rahn, 1956). Among the many postdoctoral fellows and visiting faculty from the United States and abroad (see Fig. 22) who collaborated with him, as well as staff members at the School of Medicine, were the following, listed in approximate chronological order: A. B. Otis, H. Rahn, L. E. Chadwick, R. J. Dern, A. H. Hegnauer, V. de Lalla, Jr., L. J. Mullins, M. B. Sheldon, G. A. Culver, D. F. Proctor, W. C. Bembower, C. C. Cain, A. B. DuBois, B. Ross, M. A. Epstein, S. W. Hunter, M. Hodge, R. Galambos, R. C. Fowler, M. Suskind, R. A. Bruce, M. E. Mc-Dowell, P. N. Yu, F. W. Lovejoy, Jr., R. Ament, F. J. Herber, A. Soffer, A. G. Britt, J. F. Muxworthy, Jr., H. T. Bahnson, J. M. Hagen, R. S. Stroud, D. Hammond, W. J. Osher, M. Guillet, R. T. Clark, Jr., J. N. Stannard, H. Bjurstedt, H. Heemstra, C. M. Hesser, P. Dejours, H. D. Van Liew, R. Gramiak, W. A. Dale, C. E. Tobin, M. Lategola, P. Sadoul, L. E. Farhi, J. Shapiro, S. M. Tenney, J. C. Mithoefer, J. L. Chapin, R.

E. Nye, Jr., J. E. Drorbaugh, R. E. Canfield, F. G. Carpenter, C. M. Mathews, M. S. Bitter, E. G. Aksnes, W. H. Massion.

APPENDIX

In response to a query from the editor as to how we happened to join Fenn at Rochester we offer the following recollections.

Hermann Rahn: My appointment to Fenn's Department occurred rather suddenly in the late summer of 1941 as I passed through Rochester on my way from Woods Hole to the University of Wyoming where I was an instructor, teaching zoology and physiology. At that time I realized that my preparation in physiology was minimal and I needed a good basic grounding. I talked this over with my friend, Robert W. Ramsey, at that time an Assistant Professor in Fenn's Department, and he suggested that I see Fenn about a possible assistantship. Whereupon we walked into the machine shop, where Fenn was frequently found, and I was introduced. Fenn stopped the lathe, lowered his bifocal glasses, looked me over, and finally said that there might be an opening but it would pay only $60 per month. I accepted on the spot, Fenn went back to his lathe, and three weeks later, in September, I started to work in his Department on a problem of my choice, namely, intermedin hormone assays. It was only two months later, on Pearl Harbor Day, that he talked to me quietly and mentioned that I might be interested in switching my research to problems related to the war effort. That afternoon my first job was to see whether one could record with a mercury manometer the intrapulmonary pressure at different lung volumes when completely relaxed. This was my initiation into pulmonary physiology.

The rather sudden switch was due to the fact that Fenn had been confidentially briefed by Washington many months previously concerning an impending national emergency and the possible role that he might play in exploring the pressurization of the lung as a means for gaining altitude in fighter planes. Thus Fenn, in his quiet way, was ready and prepared upon declaration of war to implement a plan of action: What is the pressure–volume relationship of the chest, what physiological changes would ensue upon pressurization, what were the physiological limits?

Arthur Otis: In the Spring of 1941 I was completing my doctoral work in the Biology Department at Brown University. My dissertation research was a study of effects of drugs and ions on the oyster heart, and I had come to realize how limited was my understanding of muscle contraction.

I knew Fenn's reputation, had read some of his papers, and had heard him participate in two symposia. Consequently I wrote him inquiring about the possibilities of working in his laboratory. Although his reply was encouraging it was delayed and I had in the meantime become committed to a postdoctoral year at Iowa with Dr. Joseph Bodine to work in his program "Enzymes in Ontogenesis," which was based on grasshopper eggs.

I responded to Fenn that I would be interested in going to Rochester at some future time, and there the matter rested until near the close of my year at Iowa. At that time, in the second week of August 1942, I received a telegram, followed by a letter offering me an appointment as an instructor. In the letter Fenn wrote "Dr. Adolph of this department has just received a contract for work on thirst in the desert and is taking two members of the department with him. This has given rise to the vacancy which now exists." One of the members referred to was Hermann Rahn. Thus it looks as though my opportunity to go to Rochester at that particular time resulted from Hermann's participation in the desert expedition. At any rate, I accepted the offer and arrived in Rochester about one month later.

REFERENCES

Aitchison, J., and Brown, J. A. C. (1957). "The Log Normal Distribution." Cambridge Univ. Press, London and New York.

Ament, R., Suskind, M., and Rahn, H. (1949). An evaluation of respiratory depression by alveolar gas changes during pentothal sodium anesthesia. *Proc. Soc. Exp. Biol. Med.* **70**, 401–406.

Bagnold, R. A. (1941). "The Physics of Blown Sand and Desert Dunes." Methuen, London.

DuBois, A. B., and Ross, B. B. (1951). "A New Method for the Pressure–Volume Diagram of the Chest and Lungs by Means of a Cathode Ray Oscilloscope," Tech. Rep. No. 6528, pp. 202–203. U. S. Air Force, Dayton, Ohio.

DuBois, A. B., Fowler, R. C., Soffer, A., and Fenn, W. O. (1951). "Alveolar CO_2 Measured by Expiration into the Rapid Infra-red Gas Analyzer," Tech. Rep. No. 6528, pp. 410–418. U.S. Air Force, Dayton, Ohio.

Fenn, W. O. (1948). Physiology of exposures to abnormal concentrations of the respiratory gases. *Proc. Am. Philos. Soc.* **92**, 144.

Fenn, W. O. (1951). Mechanics of respiration. *Am. J. Med.* **10**, 77–90.

Fenn, W. O. (1962). Born fifty years too soon. *Annu. Rev. Physiol.* **24**, 1–10.

Fenn, W. O., and Chadwick, L. E. (1947). Effect of pressure breathing on blood flow through the finger. *Am. J. Physiol.* **151**, 270.

Fenn, W. O., Rahn, H., and Otis, A. B. (1946). A theoretical study of the composition of the alveolar air at altitude. *Am. J. Physiol.* **146**, 637–653.

Fenn, W. O., Otis, A. B., Rahn, H., Chadwick, L. E., and Hegnauer, A. H. (1947). Displacement of blood from the lungs by pressure breathing. *Am. J. Physiol.* **151**, 258–269.

Fenn, W. O., Rahn, H., Otis, A. B., and Chadwick, L. E. (1949a). Voluntary pressure breathing at high altitudes. *J. Appl. Physiol.* **1**, 752–772.

Fenn, W. O., Rahn, H., Otis, A. B., and Chadwick, L. E. (1949b). Physiological observations on hyperventilation at altitude with intermittent pressure breathing by the pneumolator. *J. Appl. Physiol.* **1**, 773–789.

Fenn, W. O., Otis, A. B., and Rahn, H. (1951). "Studies in Respiratory Physiology," Tech. Rep. No. 6528. U.S. Air Force, Dayton, Ohio.

Fowler, R. C. (1946). A rapid infra-red analyzer. *Rev. Sci. Instrum.* **20**, 173–176.

Fry, F. E., Burton, A. C., and Edholm, O. G. (1949). A simple gas analyzer. *Can. J. Res. Sect. E* **27**, 188–194.

Gaddum, J. H. (1945). Log normal distributions. *Nature (London)* **156**, 463–465.

Lape, E. E., ed. (1955). "Medical Research: A Midcentury Survey. Vol. I: American Medical Research in Principle and Practice." Little, Brown, Boston, Massachusetts.

Otis, A. B., and Proctor, D. F. (1948). Measurement of alveolar pressure in human subjects. *Am. J. Physiol.* **152**, 106–112.

Otis, A. B., Rahn, H., Epstein, M. A., and Fenn, W. O. (1946a). Performance as related to composition of alveolar air. *Am. J. Physiol.* **146**, 207–221.

Otis, A. B., Rahn, H., and Fenn, W. O. (1946b). Venous pressure changes associated with positive intra-pulmonary pressures; their relationship to the distensibility of the lung. *Am. J. Physiol.* **146**, 307–317.

Otis, A. B., Rahn, H., Brontman, M., Mullins, L. J., and Fenn, W. O. (1946c). Ballistocardiographic study of changes in cardiac output due to respiration. *J. Clin. Invest.* **25,** 413–421.

Otis, A. B., Rahn, H., and Fenn, W. O. (1948). Alveolar gas changes during breath holding. *Am. J. Physiol.* **152,** 674–686.

Otis, A. B., Rahn, H., and Chadwick, L. E. (1949). Effects of adding carbon dioxide to inspired oxygen on tolerance to high altitudes. *Proc. Soc. Exp. Biol. Med.* **70,** 487–490.

Otis, A. B., Fenn, W. O., and Rahn, H. (1950). Mechanics of breathing in man. *J. Appl. Physiol.* **2,** 592–607.

Rahn, H. (1949). A concept of mean alveolar air and the ventilation-bloodflow relationships during pulmonary gas exchange. *Am. J. Physiol.* **158,** 21–30.

Rahn, H. (1956). "Studies in Respiratory Physiology," 3rd Ser., WADC Tech. Rep. 56–466, ASTIA Doc. No. AD 110487. U.S. Air Force, Dayton, Ohio.

Rahn, H., and Fenn, W. O. (1955). "Studies in Respiratory Physiology," 2nd Ser., WADC Tech. Rep. 55–357. U.S. Air Force, Dayton, Ohio.

Rahn, H., and Otis, A. B. (1947). Alveolar air during simulated flights to high altitudes. *Am. J. Physiol.* **150,** 202–221.

Rahn, H., and Otis, A. B. (1949a). Continuous analysis of alveolar gas composition during work, hyperpnea, hypercapnia and anoxia. *J. Appl. Physiol.* **1,** 717–724.

Rahn, H., and Otis, A. B. (1949b). Man's respiratory response during and after acclimatization to high altitude. *Am. J. Physiol.* **157,** 445–462.

Rahn, H., and Otis, A. B. (1949c). Survival. Differences breathing air and oxygen at equivalent altitudes. *Proc. Soc. Exp. Biol. Med.* **70,** 185–186.

Rahn, H., Otis, A. B., Chadwick, L. E., and Fenn, W. O. (1946a). The pressure–volume diagram of the thorax and lung. *Am. J. Physiol.* **146,** 161–178.

Rahn, H., Otis, A. B., Hodge, M., Epstein, M. A., Hunter, S. W., and Fenn, W. O. (1946b). The effects of hypocapnia on performance. *J. Aviat. Med.* **17,** 164–172.

Rahn, H., Mohney, J., Otis, A. B., and Fenn, W. O. (1946c). A Method for the Continuous Analysis of Alveolar Air. *J. Aviat. Med.* **17,** 173–179.

Rahn, H., Fenn, W. O., and Otis, A. B. (1949). Daily variations of vital capacity, residual air, and expiratory reserve including a study of the residual air method. *J. Appl. Physiol.* **1,** 725–736.

3

Development of the Three-Compartment Model for Dealing with Uneven Distribution

Richard L. Riley

PULMONARY GAS EXCHANGE, VOL. I

67

I. CAST OF CHARACTERS DURING WORLD WAR II

A. Joseph L. Lilienthal, Jr.

In 1944, at the U.S. Naval School of Aviation Medicine in Pensacola, Florida, an urgent need arose to reduce the number of fatal crashes occurring during flight training. Carbon monoxide toxicity was a possible explanation, and so Joseph L. Lilienthal, Jr., Lt., USNR, was ordered to study CO levels in the air of the cockpit and in the blood of aviation cadets. Thus began studies to reduce airplane accidents, which involved use of a recently developed syringe analyzer for blood CO determination (Scholander and Roughton, 1943) and led to the exploitation of the syringe analyzer to deal with the question of uneven distribution of blood and gas in the lungs.

B. Roughton and Scholander

The story goes that in the early days of World War II F. J. W. Roughton and P. F. Scholander met in a bar in Harvard Square to talk about a field method for determination of blood gases. With the aid of a pocket slide rule and a few beers, they designed an analyzer consisting of a 1-ml tuberculin syringe attached to a calibrated capillary with a small cup on the end. Scholander, noted for his ingenuity in devising analytic techniques and supported by the country's best glass blower, James D. Graham, was soon able to test the Roughton–Scholander design. It worked as expected, and techniques for determining the contents of O_2 and CO in blood were published in 1943 (Roughton and Scholander, 1943; Scholander and Roughton, 1943).

C. Riley and Earlier Bubblers

Richard L. Riley, Lt. (jg), USNR, worked across the hall from Lilienthal at the Naval School of Aviation Medicine. He was fresh from the pulmonary function laboratory at Bellevue Hospital under the direction of Dickinson W. Richards and Andre Cournand. Riley was familiar with classical tonometry, where a small amount of blood is equilibrated with a large amount of gas. Observing Lilienthal measuring bubbles in the Roughton–Scholander syringe analyzer, he wondered about reversing the process. Why not equilibrate a small bubble of gas with 1 ml of blood in the syringe analyzer? If the bubble were small enough in relation to the volume of blood, the partial pressures of gases in the bubble should, after equilibration, approximate those of the blood before equilibration. The bubble could then be analyzed for CO_2 and O_2 by measuring its length in the capillary before and after absorption of the respective gases, and the resultant fractional concentrations could be converted to partial pressures (Riley *et al.,* 1945).

There was nothing new about either the theory or practice of bubble equilibration. August Krogh published on the aerotonometer in 1908 (Krogh, 1908), and Comroe and Dripps presented a method in 1944 in which a tonometer was used for bubble equilibration and a microanalyzer for bubble analysis (Comroe and Dripps, 1944). According to Rossier *et al.* (1960a), "the aerotonometer of Pflueger . . . was used by Strassburg as early as 1872." The method using the Roughton–Scholander syringe analyzer proved simpler than previous methods because the same instrument served as both tonometer and analyzer.

The bubble method provided new possibilities for studying alveolar–arterial relationships and focused the efforts of Lilienthal and Riley on these matters. The prospect of gaining knowledge of importance to aviation medicine convinced the Office of Naval Research to support these fundamental studies during war time.

D. Fenn, Rahn, and Otis

At the University of Rochester, in Rochester, New York, the famous team of Wallace Fenn, Hermann Rahn, and Arthur Otis was systematically deriving the mathematical equations describing pulmonary gas exchange (Fenn *et al.,* 1946), developing and applying an apparatus for continuous sampling and analysis of end-tidal alveolar samples (Rahn and Otis, 1949), and, of particular importance to the story that follows, calling the attention of other physiologists to the O_2–CO_2 diagram for displaying complex aspects of gas exchange (Fenn *et al.,* 1946). Both the Rochester group and the Pensacola group relied heavily on the earlier work of Dill, who in 1937 had published nomograms describing blood–gas relationships in the blood of man at sea level and at altitude (Dill *et al.,* 1937a,b).

E. Rossier

In Zurich, developments were taking place independently that in some respects paralleled those in Pensacola. Rossier and his colleagues were concerned with the respiratory dead space and the problems of direct sampling of alveolar gas. They calculated arterial P_{CO_2} using the Henderson–Hasselbalch relationship and used this value for alveolar P_{CO_2}, apparently as early as 1942 (Rossier *et al.,* 1960b). First publication of this work came in 1946 (Rossier and Blickenstorfer, 1946). The idea is believed to have appeared in print for the first time in 1938 (Enghoff, 1938).

II. ALVEOLAR GAS AND END-CAPILLARY BLOOD

A. Direct Alveolar Samples

To study the alveolar–arterial P_{O_2} difference, a reliable and definable measure of alveolar P_{CO_2} and P_{O_2} was needed. The classical Haldane– Priestley sample, obtained by having the subject exhale maximally and by sampling the last air out, was highly dependent on the speed of exhalation and on the state of lung inflation from which the exhalation was begun (Haldane and Priestley, 1935; Riley et al., 1946). The technique of Sonne and Nielsen, in which small samples from the ends of several normal expirations were combined, minimized these difficulties (Nielsen and Sonne, 1932). Rahn and Otis devised an ingenious automatic device for sampling the ends of expirations, and used this method for continuous measurements of alveolar P_{CO_2} and P_{O_2} under a variety of physiological conditions in normal people (Rahn and Otis, 1949). A problem, however, remained: alveolar P_{CO_2} and P_{O_2} were known to vary in different parts of the lungs and at different times in the respiratory cycle, and it was difficult to know the effects of these "space" and "time" factors on directly obtained alveolar samples, particularly in the presence of lung disease.

B. Effective Alveolar P_{CO_2}

The arterial P_{CO_2} provided an indirect approach that was not plagued by these problems (Riley et al., 1946). Because of the steepness of the physiological CO_2 dissociation curve of blood, the spread of CO_2 values in gas and blood from different parts of the lungs is remarkably small. Furthermore, because of the high diffusivity of CO_2, gas and blood leaving any given alveolus have virtually identical P_{CO_2} values. Thus, blood in the systemic arteries provides a good measure of mean alveolar P_{CO_2}. To be sure, the arterial P_{CO_2} is blind to the P_{CO_2} of nonperfused alveoli. This difficulty can be overcome, however, by defining the arterial P_{CO_2} as the "effective" alveolar P_{CO_2}, a mean value excluding nonperfused alveoli but including all alveoli taking part in gas exchange. The effective alveolar P_{CO_2} so defined has three important advantages: it is precisely definable; it is not subject to the time and space errors inherent in direct alveolar samples; and no respiratory maneuvers are required. It turned out subsequently that the effective alveolar P_{CO_2} could be even more precisely defined and that it had physiological significance beyond what was originally appreciated.

C. Effective Alveolar P_{O_2}

The effective alveolar P_{O_2} cannot be equated with arterial P_{O_2}. The spread of P_{O_2} values between alveoli with high and low ventilation–perfusion (V/Q) ratios is much greater than in the case of P_{CO_2} because the O_2 dissociation curve of blood is much less steep than the CO_2 curve. Thus, in contrast to P_{CO_2}, the mixed blood in the systematic arteries has a P_{O_2} that is significantly lower than the alveolar gas. The difference is the alveolar–arterial P_{O_2} gradient.

The calculation of the effective alveolar P_{O_2} requires knowledge of the effective alveolar P_{CO_2} (arterial P_{CO_2}) and the composition of inspired and expired air, from which the CO_2/O_2 exchange ratio (R) can be obtained. Given this information, the alveolar gas equation can be used to determine a value for effective alveolar P_{O_2} that has the same meaning for oxygen as the arterial P_{CO_2} has for carbon dioxide. It provides a mean alveolar value for the lung as a whole, excluding nonperfused alveoli but including all alveoli taking part in gas exchange. The following is a convenient form of the alveolat gas equation:*

$$\text{Effective alveolar } P_{O_2} = P^e_{E_{O_2}} = P_{I_{O_2}} + F_{I_{O_2}} P_{a_{CO_2}} \frac{(1-R)}{R} - \frac{P_{a_{CO_2}}}{R} \qquad (1)$$

These relationships, though now famililar, were confusing in 1945. After the derivation by Fenn et al. (1946), Riley and Cournand (1949) changed to the above form of the alveolar gas equation. In earlier work in Pensacola a slightly inaccurate form of the equation had been used (Riley et al., 1946).

Minor uncertainties remained. Was the CO_2/O_2 exchange ratio R as determined from analysis of expired gas strictly applicable to alveolar gas? This was more or less settled in the affirmative when R as calculated using

---

* We have elected to use the standard symbols for respiratory physiology in slightly modified form for greater precision of meaning (Riley and Permutt, 1965, 1973). The subscript E will be used not only for mixed expired gas but also for all other contributions to the expired mixture. The source, whether dead space or alveolar, will be identified by the superscript. Similarly, all contributions to the arterial blood will be identified by the subscript a with appropriate superscripts. Effective alveolar P_{O_2}, when symbolized by $P^e_{E_{O_2}}$, is the P_{O_2} of gas expired from the effective compartment. This system was introduced by Riley and Permutt in 1965 and differs from the symbols used in the original papers. Since the original papers differ from one another, there seems no persuasive reason to perpetuate their symbols even though some readers may be distressed by lack of familiarity with the usage in this chapter.

end-tidal alveolar samples in normal people was found to be indistinguishable, on the average, from R as calculated from the mixed expired gas (Bateman, 1945; West *et al.*, 1957a,b). Thus evidence from direct alveolar sampling helped to validate the indirect method, which was itself devised to avoid errors in the direct methods.* Was it correct to use arterial P_{CO_2} for effective alveolar P_{CO_2} when there was a large right-to-left shunt bypassing the alveoli? Clearly it was not (Severinghaus and Stupfel, 1957). Fortunately a correction could be made for this error (Riley *et al.*, 1951).

D. The Effective Alveolar–Arterial P_{O_2} Gradient (AaP_{O_2} Gradient)

Having developed techniques for determining alveolar and arterial partial pressures of respiratory gases, Lilienthal *et al.* (1946) undertook a major study of the AaP_{O_2} gradient during rest and exercise at sea level and during low O_2 breathing. The subjects were naval officers from the research division, ages ranging from 28 to 36 years, all presumed to be normal and in good health. At rest, the AaP_{O_2} difference both during air breathing and low O_2 breathing averaged approximately 9 mm Hg, and with exercise (average O_2 consumption approximately 1.6 liters/min) it averaged 17 mm Hg both during air breathing and low O_2 breathing. One subject who increased his O_2 consumption to approximately 3 liters/min on air had an AaP_{O_2} gradient of 36 mm Hg; with an O_2 consumption of 2.5 liters/min on low O_2, the AaP_{O_2} gradient was 27 mm Hg. Thus, a significant AaP_{O_2} difference was shown to be present at all times.

This was the last joint effort of Lilienthal and Riley in Pensacola and in many ways the high point of their collaboration. Most of the subsequent elaboration concerning the AaP_{O_2} gradient was foreshadowed in this paper. The venous admixture component and the diffusion component were discussed in detail, the Bohr integration was invoked to calculate the mean diffusion gradient for oxygen, and the diffusing capacity (then called the diffusion constant) was derived. The findings were discussed in the context of the carbon monoxide diffusing capacity measurements of Marie Krogh, the calculations of Roughton regarding diffusion at high altitude, and the integrative concepts of Murray and Morgan. Of particular relevance to the three-compartment model was the assertion (Lilienthal *et*

---

* Fenn *et al.* (1951) turned the argument around and used correspondence with the effective values as validation for their direct alveolar sampling technique: "Experiment has shown that our method of sampling alveolar air gives values which are very close to this effective mean alveolar air point and very close, also, to the measured arterial CO_2 tension. This provides, therefore, a valuable validation of the method."

al., 1946) "that the total venous admixture component, although arising from sources with various oxygen saturations, may, nevertheless, be expressed as though it were all the result of the addition of mixed venous blood."

Lilienthal was discharged from the Navy before the 1946 manuscript was completed. He assumed major responsibilities at The Johns Hopkins School of Medicine, where he worked closely with the new professor of medicine, A. McGehee Harvey. He arranged to have Riley invited to join the Hopkins faculty in 1950, but the Pensacola era of day-to-day collaboration had passed. Lilienthal was made professor and chairman of the Department of Environmental Medicine. He traveled widely for the Navy trying to stimulate research on burns, suddenly raised to high priority by the atom bomb. In 1955 he died with but a few days' warning, following a happy evening at the Baltimore Museum Ball. Thus, Joseph L. Lilienthal, Jr., a truly brilliant star and unquestioned leader, dropped suddenly from sight.

Riley stayed on in the Navy through most of 1946 to take part in Operation Everest with Charles S. Houston of mountaineering fame. Operation Everest was a study of acclimatization to simulated high altitude in a low-pressure chamber, where AaP_{O_2} gradients were studied over a period of a month at progressively higher altitudes, reaching briefly to 29,000 ft (Houston and Riley, 1947). Riley then returned for 3 years with Dickinson W. Richards and Andre Cournand at Bellevue Hospital and 1 year with New York University before making the final academic move to Baltimore.

Richards and Cournand, who later shared the Nobel Prize with Forssmann for the development of cardiac catheterization, were primarily concerned with their expanding cardiovascular research in the late 1940s. Riley was given a free hand and the support of the laboratory to apply three-compartment principles to the study of patients from the Chest Service with all types of pulmonary dysfunction. This was done in collaboration with Kenneth Donald, Attilio Renzetti, John McClement, Robert Austrian, and others. Cournand was involved in every step of the proceedings with incisive criticism and discussions verging on pitched battles. It was with Cournand that the next advances in theory were pulled together in 1949 and 1951.

E. The O_2–CO_2 Diagram and the V/Q Curve

The effective alveolar gas concept seemed a little obscure until relationships were clarified by graphic presentation. The O_2–CO_2 diagram, often called the Fenn diagram, was the chief instrument for general enlighten-

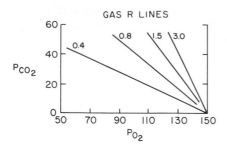

Fig. 1. Gas κ lines: P_{CO_2} and P_{O_2} as coordinates.

ment (Fenn *et al.*, 1946; Rahn and Fenn, 1955). When P_{O_2} and P_{CO_2} are the coordinates, a given O_2–CO_2 exchange ratio R describes a straight line originating at the inspired air point. Different R values plotted on the same graph describe a family of straight lines radiating from the inspired air point (Fig. 1). When O_2 content and CO_2 content of the blood are the coordinates, different R values describe a family of straight lines radiating from the mixed venous blood point (Fig. 2). To transpose the blood R lines to the $P_{O_2} - P_{CO_2}$ diagram, the relationships between blood gas content and partial pressure are needed for both O_2 and CO_2. The O_2 and CO_2 dissociation curves of blood, corrected for Bohr and Haldane effects, provide these relationships and are used to make the transposition. With P_{O_2} and P_{CO_2} as coordinates, the blood R lines become a family of curves radiating from the mixed venous P_{O_2}–P_{CO_2} point. Each blood R curve intersects a corresponding gas R line, defining the only point on the diagram that is compatible with the given R value for both alveolar gas and end-capillary blood. When all the points of intersection of corresponding blood and gas R lines are connected, a curve extending from the mixed venous blood point to the inspired air point is described (Fig. 3). This curve defines the locus of all possible alveolar gas and end-capillary blood values. It is called the distribution curve (or the ventilation–perfusion line) because the effects on alveolar gas and blood of all possible variations of V/Q ratio (and of R) are displayed along its course.

In 1949 Rahn (1949) and Riley and Cournand (1949) both published deri-

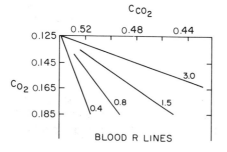

Fig. 2. Blood R lines: C_{CO_2} and C_{O_2} as coordinates.

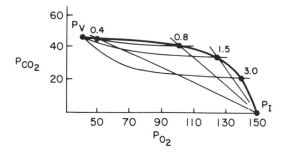

Fig. 3. The V/Q curve, passing through the intersections of gas and blood R lines: P_{CO_2} and P_{O_2} as coordinates.

vations of the V/Q line. Rahn's derivation was simpler and made better use of previous work. Instead of constructing O_2 and CO_2 dissociation curves, he made use of the Dill blood nomogram, which contains in a single-line chart the necessary information concerning R and the O_2 and CO_2 dissociation curves.

In 1948 Riley had one of those breaks in the academic struggle for survival that others achieve only through sabbatical leave or old age retirement. He was sent to bed for an extended period to cure a tuberculous lesion that was barely visible on a chest X ray. Having no symptoms and a physician for a wife, he was allowed to rest at home, where he could spend his days and nights pondering the mysteries of the V/Q line. He argued with Rahn by mail, developed graphs to show the reciprocal changes in the diffusion gradient and the venous admixture gradient at different levels of oxygenation, and played with the notion of a four-quadrant diagram. Members of Cournand's laboratory kept him abreast of daily developments and showed him data from the earliest applications of the three-compartment analysis to patients. He had time to let his imagination wander and data to anchor flights of fancy to reality. Never was enforced confinement given more profitable psychotherapy.

F. The Four-Quadrant Diagram

In 1951 Riley and Cournand (1951) extended the Fenn diagram into a four-quadrant diagram in which the interrelationships between gas and blood could be visualized more easily. As in the Fenn diagram, P_{O_2} and P_{CO_2} were used as coordinates in the upper left-hand quadrant (quadrant 1), but in the lower right-hand quadrant (quadrant 3) blood CO_2 and O_2 contents were the coordinates (Fig. 4). In quadrant 1 the origin in the center of the diagram was the inspired air point, and in quadrant 3 it was

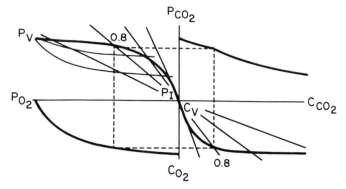

Fig. 4. The four quadrant diagram, with V/Q curves in quadrants 1 and 3, CO_2 dissociation curve in quadrant 2, and O_2 dissociation curve in quadrant 4. Broken lines connect simultaneous values in each quadrant.

the mixed venous blood point. Thus the gas and blood R lines in quadrants 1 and 3 were families of straight lines radiating in opposite directions from a common origin. Quadrants 2 and 4 had suitable coordinates for CO_2 and O_2 dissociation curves, with the range of each curve extending from mixed venous blood to inspired air. The dissociation curves could be used for graphic conversion of any blood gas content values in quadrant 3 into units of P_{O_2} and P_{CO_2} in quadrant 1, and vice versa. Blood R lines were readily transposed from quadrant 3 to quadrant 1, and the distribution curve drawn through the points of intersection of gas and blood R lines of equal value. The distribution curve itself could then be transposed to quadrant 3, where, as will be seen, it proved useful in visualizing certain aspects of the three-compartment model.

In 1960, Ross and Farhi (1960) called attention to the fact that the gas inhaled into the alveoli is not pure inspired air but a mixture of inspired air and the alveolar gas that occupied the dead space at the end of the preceding expiration. The gas R lines in quadrant 1 should thus radiate from a corrected inspired point. This change was included in the 1965 presentation by Riley and Permutt (1965) in the "Handbook of Physiology." It does not lead to a change in the effective alveolar point since the gas R line for the lung as a whole is unchanged. Other points on the V/Q curve are altered slightly.

The point on the distribution curve where R is the same as for the lung as a whole is of particular interest because, if all alveoli were identical with respect to R (and V/Q) and if in all equilibrium were reached between gas and blood, they would all have to have the P_{O_2} and P_{CO_2} values represented by this point. This would be the "ideal" composition for alveolar gas and end-capillary blood.

G. Ideal versus Effective Values

On the O_2–CO_2 diagram the effective values, derived from arterial P_{CO_2} and the expired gas R value, and the ideal values, identified by the point of intersection of blood and gas R lines, can both be visualized (Fig. 5). The blood R line is so nearly horizontal in the range between the arterial blood point and the ideal point that the effective and ideal P_{CO_2} values are virtually the same in normal people. The graphic representation of the effective alveolar P_{O_2}, as calculated using the alveolar gas equation [Eq. (1)], is the P_{O_2} on the gas R line when P_{CO_2} equals arterial P_{CO_2}. Thus the effective P_{O_2} is also virtually the same as the ideal P_{O_2}. If the blood R line were truly horizontal in the range under consideration, the effective and ideal points would be identical. However, since the blood R line becomes less horizontal as the mixed venous point is approached and since the arterial blood of patients with extreme dysfunction is displaced toward the mixed venous point, the arterial P_{CO_2} may be 2 or 3 mm Hg higher than the ideal P_{CO_2} in such cases. The associated large alveolar–arterial P_{O_2} difference calls attention to this possibility and an appropriate correction can be applied (Riley et al., 1951). The operationally determined effective values can thus be used to determine the theoretically defined ideal values, and the laborious process of constructing intersecting blood and gas R lines for the lung as a whole can be avoided.

An exception to this happy conclusion exists when a diffusion gradient remains between the alveolar gas and the blood leaving the alveolar capillary, as occurs when a low concentration of oxygen is breathed (Riley and Cournand, 1951). Under this circumstance the effective P_{O_2} of the alveolar gas (P_E^e) differs from the effective P_{O_2} of the end-capillary blood (P_a^e) by the amount of the alveolar–end-capillary diffusion gradient. The ideal point falls below and to the right of the effective points (Fig. 6).

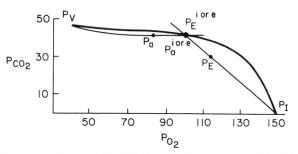

Fig. 5. V/Q curve, and gas and blood R lines for the lung as a whole. The P_{CO_2} and P_{O_2} values for the ideal or effective point, for expired gas, and for arterial blood are shown.

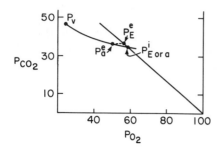

Fig. 6. Gas and blood R lines for the lung as a whole during low O_2 breathing, showing the end-capillary diffusion gradient for O_2 between P_E^e and P_a^e. The ideal point differs from the effective points.

H. The Ideal Compartment

The ideal compartment forms the cornerstone of the three-compartment model since ideal P_{O_2} and P_{CO_2} values would exist in all functioning alveoli if gas exchange took place under ideal conditions. In quantifying deviations from the ideal, it has proved useful to consider the amount by which the P_{O_2} and P_{CO_2} values in expired gas and arterial blood differ from the values in the ideal compartment. The function of real lungs in health or disease can thus be assessed by comparison with hypothetical ideal lungs.

III. THE THREE-COMPARTMENT MODEL

A. The Concept

If there is uneven distribution of gas and blood to the alveoli, causing scatter of alveolar values along the distribution curve, the mixed gas and the mixed blood from the alveoli cannot have the ideal values. The mixed effluents, called the alveolar component of the expired gas (P_E^{ac}) and the alveolar component of the arterial blood (P_a^{ac}, C_a^{ac}), must have values that lie within the concavity of the distribution curve and also on the appropriate R lines for the lung as a whole. Thus, P_E^{ac} lies on the gas R line and is displaced away from the ideal point in the direction of the inspired air point (Fig. 7). P_a^{ac} and C_a^{ac} lie on the blood R line and are displaced away from the ideal point in the direction of the mixed venous point (Fig. 7). These displacements, representing in real life the net effects of a myriad of different contributions, can be simulated by adding inspired air (dead space air) (P_I) to ideal alveolar gas (P_E^i) and by adding mixed venous blood (C_v) to ideal end-capillary blood (C_a^i). Thus, the lung can be thought of as containing some alveoli that are nonventilated (the venous admixture or shunt compartment), some that are nonperfused (the dead space

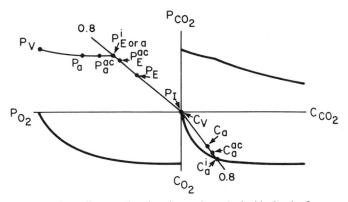

Fig. 7. Four-quadrant diagram showing, in quadrant 1, the ideal point for gas and blood, the alveolar component of the expired gas, and the mixed expired gas; and in quadrants 1 and 3, the ideal point, the alveolar component of the arterial blood, and the mixed arterial blood.

compartment), and the rest that are evenly ventilated and perfused (the ideal compartment). This three-compartment model is attractive because the concentration of O_2 and CO_2 in each compartment is definable and the unevenness of distribution can be quantified.

Although the term "three-compartment model" was not used at the time, the basic elements of the concept were described diagrammatically and in words in 1949 (Riley and Cournand, 1949):

> The cyclic nature of the ventilatory process tends to obscure certain fundamental relationships between alveolar air and the blood in the alveolar capillaries. Let us therefore consider a schematic representation of ventilation, perfusion and gas exchange in which these processes are conceived of as continuous [Fig. 8]. Inspired air and mixed venous blood pass into the alveoli where they approach equilibrium with respect to partial pressures of oxygen and carbon dioxide by diffusion of gases across the pulmonary membrane. The blood leaving the alveolar capillaries is modified slightly by the admixture of a small amount of venous blood which can be thought of as a shunt. The alveolar air leaving the alveolar spaces is modified by the admixture of dead space air, which has the composition of inspired air and may also be thought of as a shunt.

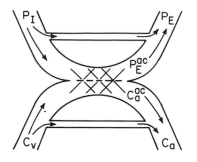

Fig. 8. Model of lung gas exchange with ventilation and perfusion both represented as continuous flow systems. Dead space ventilation and venous admixture are both represented as shunts.

Not stated in this quotation is the essential fact that variations in V/Q ratios produce net effects that are dead-space-like and venous-admixture-like and therefore representable as additions to anatomic dead space and anatomic venous admixture. The shunts in Fig. 8 are intended to include both anatomic and alveolar components.

B. Dead Space

Quantification of the dead space effect was based on the amount of dead space gas that would have to be added to ideal alveolar gas to produce a mixture with the composition of expired gas. The Bohr equation expresses this relationship in mathematical terms that have a graphic counterpart on the O_2–CO_2 diagram:

$$\frac{V_E^{D \text{ anat+alv}}}{V_E} = \frac{P_E^i - P_E}{P_E^i - P_I} = \frac{P_{a_{CO_2}} - P_{E_{CO_2}}}{P_{a_{CO_2}} - O} \tag{2}$$

The ratio of dead space volume ($V_E^{D \text{ anat+alv}}$) to total expired volume (tidal volume, V_E) equals the ideal-expired difference ($P_E^i - P_E$) divided by the ideal-inspired difference ($P_E^i - P_I$). These differences correspond to distances along the gas R line and are equally valid using CO_2 or O_2 data (Fig. 7). A correction for apparatus dead space is required.

C. Venous Admixture

A similar form of the mixing equation was used to quantify the venous blood shunt, i.e., the ratio of venous admixture ($Q_a^{S \text{ anat+alv}}$) to total arterial blood flow ($\dot{Q}_a$):

$$\frac{\dot{Q}_a^{S \text{ anat+alv}}}{\dot{Q}_a} = \frac{C_a^i - C_a}{C_a^i - C_v} = \frac{S_{a_{O_2}}^i - S_{a_{O_2}}}{S_{a_{O_2}}^i - S_{c_{O_2}}} \tag{3}$$

The differences in Eq. (3) correspond to distances along the blood R line in quadrant 3 (Fig. 7) and are equally valid using CO_2 or O_2 data. Since the quantity of blood gas in a mixture (C_a) depends on the quantities in the aliquots being mixed (C_a^i and C_v), the equation is valid only when the units are proportional to the quantity of gas per unit volume of blood. Thus the units can be blood gas content (C) or oxygen saturation (S_{O_2}), but not partial pressure (P). Since the arterial blood normally falls on the upper flat portion of the oxygen dissociation curve, the most accurate determination of the ideal-arterial O_2 saturation difference is obtained by first determining the partial pressure difference and then transposing to units of saturation by reference to a standard oxyhemoglobin dissociation curve. Line charts were prepared to simplify this process (Riley *et al.*, 1951).

The way in which the dead space and venous admixture ratios were used to quantify the V/Q abnormality in a patient was described by Riley and Cournand (1949):

> A ratio of dead space to tidal air in excess of 30 per cent indicates that a significant proportion of alveoli are well ventilated but poorly perfused. Venous admixture, when calculated using the "ideal" value for blood leaving the alveolar capillaries, includes a contribution from alveoli with a low ventilation–perfusion ratio. A ratio of venous admixture to cardiac output in excess of 7 per cent indicates that a significant proportion of alveoli are well perfused but poorly ventilated. Analysis of ventilation–perfusion relationships must be done in the normal range of oxygenation, since breathing either a low oxygen mixture or a very high oxygen mixture minimizes the effects under consideration.

When this analysis was introduced, it was not possible to determine the alveolar component of the expired gas (P_E^{ac}) or the alveolar component of the arterial blood (P_a^{ac}, C_a^{ac}), and so calculations were made of the effects of alveolar and anatomic dead space combined and of alveolar and anatomic shunt combined. With the advent of instantaneous gas analyzers, it became possible to estimate P_E^{ac} and thus to separate alveolar dead space from anatomic dead space (Fowler, 1948). With methods to determine blood nitrogen tension, it became possible to estimate C_a^{ac} and hence to separate alveolar shunt from true shunt (Klocke and Rahn, 1961).

More complete analyses of the AaP_{O_2} gradient and of ventilation–perfusion relationships have been presented by Farhi and Rahn (1955) and by Rahn and Farhi (1964).

IV. REFLECTIONS ON A SIMPLER ERA

The beauty of the three-compartment model is its simplicity, yet this is also its weakness. The net effects of myriads of different V/Q ratios in different parts of the lungs can indeed be described in terms of the three-compartment model, but the description changes when the inspired oxygen changes. In 1946 Lilienthal and Riley fell into the trap of assuming that the percentage of venous admixture remained unchanged during low oxygen breathing. Upon this assumption they devised a method for determining the diffusing capacity for oxygen. This was widely accepted and applied for two decades before the fundamental assumption was shown to be simplistic (West, 1965; Riley and Permutt, 1973).

From 1945 to about 1960 the bubble method for determining arterial P_{CO_2} and P_{O_2} provided the only readily available access to the wonders and delights of the three-compartment analysis, and access to the bubble method was almost exclusively through Riley and those trained by him.

This privileged and unfair situation arose because very few people could make the bubble method work without help. Furthermore, few people could even obtain a Roughton–Scholander syringe, other than from Riley's private cache, because glass blowing had declined to the point that James D. Graham was needed to calibrate a capillary tube and join it to a tuberculin syringe with the necessary smoothness and taper. And Mr. Graham asserted the glassblower's prerogative of working when and for whom he saw fit. His personal talent for frustrating a potential buyer was aided by a bona fide shortage of precision-bore capillary tubing of the requisite dimension.

In Andre Cournand's laboratory at Bellevue Hospital, there were a number of people from 1946 to 1948 who developed a modicum of proficiency in performing the bubble method, among whom were Kenneth W. Donald, Giles Filley, Attilio Renzetti, John McClement, and Polly Jones, technician to Dr. Cournand and subsequently to become Mary C. Riley, M.D.

After 1950, bubblers from the Hopkins family and the Baltimore area included Richard H. Shepard, Douglas G. Carroll, Jr., Bruce W. Armstrong, and Jerome E. Cohn. Then came the most apt and evangelical student of all, E. J. Moran Campbell. Moran was proud to belong to the exclusive group with the manipulative finesse to get reproducible results when others could not. He became the leading exponent of simple and sensible applications of three-compartment theory to bedside medicine (Campbell, 1967). John B. L. Howell and Solbert Permutt followed and caught the fever. Word spread that much struggle could be avoided by coming to Baltimore to learn, under direct guidance, how to tame the tiresome bubble. Technicians, fellows, doctors setting up pulmonary function laboratories, all came to Mecca during the fantastic 1950s. Then the faithful stopped coming. The culprit: modern technology.

A reliable P_{O_2} electrode became available well ahead of the P_{CO_2} electrode, but one without the other could not displace the bubble method. When both became available and any technician could turn out rapid accurate analyses, the bubblers' guild was doomed. The art of blood–gas tension analysis became a trade, dominated by salesmen and government grants. Even the old masters hung up their Roughton–Scholanders.

V. NEWER MODELS FOR NEWER TIMES

Briscoe developed a model with two compartments, one of which was poorly ventilated (Briscoe, 1959a). This slow compartment was identified by inert gas studies. Briscoe's model accounts for the hypoxemia in patients with chronic obstructive pulmonary disease better than the venous admixture of the three-compartment model and predicts the effects of oxygen therapy better (Briscoe, 1959b).

West and Dollery introduced a radioactive gas technique that added spatial localization of V/Q abnormalities to the information available from analysis of expired gas and arterial blood (West and Dollery, 1960). Since then techniques for scanning the entire lung for ventilation and perfusion have been developed and widely applied.

Wagner, Saltzman, and West devised a multiple-inert-gas technique that gives the complete distribution of ventilation and of perfusion throughout the lungs (Wagner *et al.*, 1974). This physiological tour de force provides comprehensive information that was undreamed of when the three-compartment model was conceived. It is the culmination, for the present, of years of increasing insight into the question of uneven distribution in the lungs.

REFERENCES

Bateman, J. B. (1945). Factors influencing the composition of alveolar air in normal persons. *Proc. Staff Meet. Mayo Clin.* **20**, 214–224.

Briscoe, W. A. (1959a). A method for dealing with data concerning uneven ventilation of the lung and its effect on blood gas transfer. *J. Appl. Physiol.* **14**, 291–298.

Briscoe, W. A. (1959b). Comparison between alveolar arterial gradient predicted from mixing studies and the observed gradient. *J. Appl. Physiol.* **14**, 299–304.

Campbell, E. J. M. (1967). The J. Burns Amberson Lectures—The management of acute respiratory failure in chronic bronchitis and emphysema. *Am. Rev. Respir. Dis.* **96**, 626–639.

Comroe, J. H., Jr., and Dripps, R. D., Jr. (1944). The oxygen tension of arterial blood and alveolar air in normal human subjects. *Am. J. Physiol.* **142**, 700–720.

Dill, D. B., Edwards, H. T., and Consolazio, W. V. (1937a). Blood as a physiochemical system. XI. Man at rest. *J. Biol. Chem.* **118**, 635–648.

Dill, D. B., Edwards, H. T., and Consolazio, W. V. (1937b). XII. Man at high altitudes. *J. Biol. Chem.* **118**, 649–666.

Enghoff, H. (1938). Volumen inefficax. Bemerkungen zur Frage des schädlichen Raumes. *Upsala Lakarefoeren, Foerh.* **44**, 191.

Farhi, L. E., and Rahn, H. (1955). A theoretical analysis of the alveolar-arterial O_2 difference with special reference to the distribution effect. *J. Appl. Physiol.* **7**, 699–703.

Fenn, W. O., Rahn, H., and Otis, A. B. (1946). A theoretical study of the composition of the alveolar air at altitude. *Am. J. Physiol.* **146**, 637–653.

Fenn, W. O., Otis, A. B., and Rahn, H. (1951). "Studies in Respiratory Physiology," Tech. Rep. No. 6528, p. xii. U.S. Air Force Wright Air Dev. Cent., Dayton, Ohio.

Fowler, W. S. (1948). Lung function studies. II. The respiratory dead space. *Am. J. Physiol.* **154**, 405–416.

Haldane, J. S., and Priestley, J. G. (1935). Investigations of alveolar air. *In* "Respiration," p. 19. Oxford Univ. Press (Clarendon), London.

Houston, C. S., and Riley, R. L. (1947). Respiratory and circulatory changes during acclimatization to high altitude. *Am. J. Physiol.* **149**, 565–588.

Klocke, F. J., and Rahn, H. (1961). The arterial–alveolar inert gas ("N_2") difference in normal and emphysematous subjects, as indicated by the analysis of urine. *J. Clin. Invest.* **40**, 286–294.

Krogh, A. (1908). Some new methods for the tonometric determination of gas tensions in fluids. *Skand. Arch. Physiol.* **20**, 259–278.

Lilienthal, J. L., Jr., Riley, R. L., Proemmel, D. D., and Franke, R. E. (1946). An experimental analysis in man of the oxygen pressure gradient from alveolar air to arterial blood during rest and exercise at sea level and at altitude. *Am. J. Physiol.* **147**, 199–216.

Nielsen, E., and Sonne, C. (1932). Apparatus for fractional analysis of a single expiration. *Acta Med. Scand. Suppl.* **50**, 33–38.

Rahn, H. (1949). A concept of mean alveolar air and the ventilation-blood flow relationships during pulmonary gas exchange. *Am. J. Physiol.* **158**, 21–30.

Rahn, H., and Farhi, L. E. (1964). Ventilation, perfusion, and gas exchange—the $\dot{V}_A/\dot{Q}$ concept. *In* "Handbook of Physiology. Sect. 3: Respiration" (W. O. Fenn and H. Rahn, sect. eds.), Vol. 1, pp. 735–766. Am. Physiol. Soc., Washington, D.C.

Rahn, H., and Fenn, W. O. (1955). "A Graphical Analysis of the Respiratory Gas Exchange." Am. Physiol. Soc., Washington, D.C.

Rahn, H., and Otis, A. B. (1949). Continuous analysis of alveolar gas composition during work, hyperpnea, hypercapnia and anoxia. *J. Appl. Physiol.* **1**, 717–724.

Riley, R. L., and Cournand, A. (1949). "Ideal" alveolar air and the analysis of ventilation–perfusion relationships in the lungs. *J. Appl. Physiol.* **1**, 825–847.

Riley, R. L., and Cournand, A. (1951). Analysis of factors affecting the partial pressures of oxygen and carbon dioxide in gas and blood of lungs: Theory. *J. Appl. Physiol.* **4**, 77–101.

Riley, R. L., and Permutt, S. (1965). The four quadrant diagram for analyzing the distribution of gas and blood in the lung. *In* "Handbook of Physiology. Sec. 3: Respiration" (W. O. Fenn and H. Rahn, sect. eds.), Vol. 2, pp. 1413–1423. Am. Physiol. Soc., Washington, D.C.

Riley, R. L., and Permutt, S. (1973). Venous admixture component of the AaP_{O_2} gradient. *J. Appl. Physiol.* **35**, 430–431.

Riley, R. L., Proemmel, D. D., and Franke, R. E. (1945). A direct method for determination of oxygen and carbon dioxide tensions in blood. *J. Biol. Chem.* **161**, 621–633.

Riley, R. L., Lilienthal, J. L., Proemmel, D. D., and Franke, R. E. (1946). On the determination of the physiologically effective pressures of oxygen and carbon dioxide in alveolar air. *Am. J. Physiol.* **147**, 191–198.

Riley, R. L., Cournand, A., and Donald, K. W. (1951). Analysis of factors affecting the partial pressures of oxygen and carbon dioxide in gas and blood of lung: methods. *J. Appl. Physiol.* **4**, 102–120.

Ross, B. B., and Farhi, L. E. (1960). Dead space ventilation as a determinant in the ventilation–perfusion concept. *J. Appl. Physiol.* **15**, 363–371.

Rossier, P. H., and Blickenstorfer, E. (1946). Espace mort et hyperventilation. *Helv. Med. Acta* **13**, 328.

Rossier, P. H., Buhlmann, A. A., and Wiesinger, K. (1960a). Examination of the blood gases. *In* "Respiration: Physiological Principles and Their Clinical Applications" (transl. by P. C. Luchsinger and K. M. Moser, eds.), p. 167. Mosby, St. Louis, Missouri.

Rossier, P. H., Buhlmann, A. A., and Wiesinger, K. (1960b). Pulmonary ventilatory function. *In* "Respiration: Physiological Principles and Their Clinical Applications" (transl. by P. C. Luchsinger and K. M. Moser, eds.), p. 55. Mosby, St. Louis, Missouri.

Roughton, F. J. W., and Scholander, P. F. (1943). Micro gasometric estimation of the blood gases. I. Oxygen. *J. Biol. Chem.* **148,** 541–550.

Scholander, P. F., and Roughton, F. J. W. (1943). Micro gasometric estimation of the blood gases. II. Carbon monoxide. *J. Biol. Chem.* **148,** 551–563.

Severinghaus, J. W., and Stupfel, M. (1957). Alveolar dead space as an index of distribution of blood flow in pulmonary capillaries. *J. Appl. Physiol.* **10,** 335–348.

Wagner, P. D., Saltzman, H. A., and West, J. B. (1974). Measurement of continuous distributions of ventilation-perfusion ratios: Theory. *J. Appl. Physiol.* **36,** 588–599.

West, J. B. (1965). "Ventilation, Blood Flow and Gas Exchange," p. 103. Blackwell, Oxford.

West, J. B., and Dollery, C. T. (1960). Distribution of blood flow and ventilation–perfusion ratio in the lung, measured with radioactive CO_2. *J. Appl. Physiol.* **15,** 405–410.

West, J. B., Fowler, K. T., Hugh-Jones, P., and O'Donnell, T. V. (1957a). Measurement of the ventilation–perfusion ratio inequality in the lung by the analysis of a single expirate. *Clin. Sci.* **16,** 529–547.

West, J. B., Fowler, K. T., Hugh-Jones, P., and O'Donnell, T. V. (1957b). Measurement of the ventilation–perfusion ratio inequality in the lung by the analysis of a single expirate. *Clin. Sci.* **16,** 549–565.

4

Intrapulmonary Gas Mixing and Stratification

Peter Scheid and Johannes Piiper

PULMONARY GAS EXCHANGE, VOL. I

I. CONCEPTS AND SIGNIFICANCE

A. Stratification and Dead Space

Inspired gas is not expected to achieve direct contact with the surface of the alveolar epithelium because the considerable end-expired volume (functional residual capacity, of about 3 liters) will be interposed. Although this gas volume is spread out as a layer of no more than a few millimeters' thickness, owing to the enormous increase of the cross-sectional area of the airways from the trachea to the alveolar ducts, it may constitute a barrier to exchange of gases between inspired gas and pulmonary capillary blood. The process of overcoming this barrier may be viewed as a mixing process leading to homogenization of lung gas during the respiratory cycle. Although in all simulation studies only diffusion has been considered as the mechanism of intrapulmonary gas mixing, there is now good experimental evidence for convective mixing, in part attributable to the mechanical action of the heartbeat (Engel *et al.*, 1973a,b; Fukuchi *et al.*, 1976; Sikand *et al.*, 1976).

Evidently this intrapulmonary gas mixing is never complete in physiological conditions: even after extremely prolonged breath-holding there is a nonmixing space in proximal airways, the (anatomical or series) dead space. The result of incomplete intrapulmonary gas mixing is generally termed stratification, i.e., persistence of longitudinal concentration differences in lung airways during the respiratory cycle. In this sense, dead space is a stratificational phenomenon, and a very marked one. Stratification proper, however, as conceived by most authors (e.g., Rauwerda, 1946) and by us, means persistence of significant longitudinal concentration (or partial pressure) gradients inside the gas-exchanging airways or alveolar space (Fig. 1).

"Dead space" and "alveolar space" have an anatomical background (conducting airways versus alveolated airways), but are mainly defined functionally (as non-gas-exchanging and gas-exchanging volumes or as nonmixing and well-mixing volumes). The separation line of dead space and alveolar space cannot be regarded as a sharp boundary. Anatomically there is the "transition zone" (Weibel, 1963). Functionally there is a gradual change of expired gas concentration, plotted against time or volume, from inspired to alveolar value, termed "phase 2," flattening smoothly to a more or less sloping alveolar plateau ("phase 3"). Thus a change in the

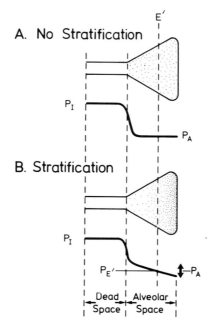

Fig. 1. Schematic representation of stratification. Density of stippling in lung models visualizes partial pressure (or concentration) of a gas (e.g., CO_2). The concentration profile (of a gas with inspired value highest, e.g., O_2) is also shown. E' denotes end-expired gas, and P_I and P_A, partial pressure in inspired and alveolar gas.

transition region of an expirogram between the phases 2 and 3 could be attributed to changes in dead space or to stratification in alveolar space. Furthermore, measures likely to influence stratification, like changes in tidal volume or respiratory frequency, variation of breath-holding time, usually also exert effects on the size of the dead space. Therefore, the problem of a delimitation of stratification in alveolar space from changes in dead space is difficult and in some cases may remain unsolved.

B. Effects on Efficiency of Alveolar Gas Exchange

The important consequence of stratified inhomogeneity is to reduce the efficiency of alveolar gas exchange by giving rise to partial pressure differences for O_2 and CO_2 between end-expired (alveolar) gas and arterial (end-capillary) blood, i.e., alveolar–arterial differences (AaD). Thus the effects of stratification (stratified inhomogeneity) are basically similar to those of unequal distribution of ventilation to perfusion (parallel inhomogeneity).

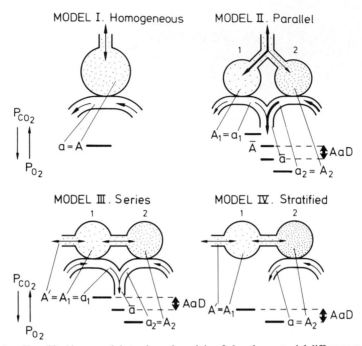

Fig. 2. Simplified lung models to show the origin of alveolar–arterial differences for CO_2 and O_2 (AaD) in steady state. Gas/blood diffusion is assumed to be nonlimiting. Density of stippling marks concentration of CO_2. Model I: Homogeneous lung. $AaD = 0$. Model II: Parallel inhomogeneity or unequal distribution of $\dot{V}_A$ to $\dot{Q}$ (visualized by thickness of arrows for flow). The AaD ($= P_{\bar{A}} - P_{\bar{a}}$) is produced by flow-weighted averaging of A and a. Model III: Series inhomogeneity due to ventilation of compartments in series. The AaD is due to the fact that end-expired gas (A') originates in the proximal compartment (1) only, whereas arterial blood is a mixture. Model IV: Stratified inhomogeneity. Derived from model III by suppressing blood flow to the proximal compartment (1). An AaD arises because end-expired gas (A') is derived from the proximal (1) and arterial blood, from the distal compartment (2).

The mechanism of generating AaD in both kinds of inhomogeneity is visualized in Fig. 2 as simplified two-compartment models. In the case of parallel inhomogeneity (model II) AaD is primarily produced by flow-weighted averaging of P_A and P_a. Model III has been analyzed by West (1971). He considered ventilation, i.e., convection, to be the mechanism of gas transfer between the proximal and distal compartments. However, his results essentially retain their validity if diffusion is involved or even constitutes the only transfer mechanism because diffusion coefficients for CO_2 and O_2 in alveolar gas are similar. AaD in model III is due to the fact that $P_{A'}$ derives from the proximal compartment alone, whereas P_a is due to mixture of arterialized blood originating in both compartments. The simplest two-compartment model to show the effects on gas exchange of stratified inhomogeneity is obtained by suppression of blood flow to the proximal compartment (model IV). In this case, all end-expired (alveolar) gas is derived from the proximal compartment and all arterialized blood from the distal compartment, and AaD reflects directly partial pressure difference between the compartments.

It is of interest to note that model IV generates a pattern of AaD characterized by the ratio AaD_{CO_2}/AaD_{O_2} being close to the gas exchange ratio, R. This pattern is similar to that of alveolar dead space ventilation, which is an extreme case of parallel inhomogeneity (Fig. 3). The other extreme case of parallel inhomogeneity, venous admixture from little-ventilated or unventilated alveoli, can be produced in model III (Fig. 2) by decreasing the (convective or diffusive) gas transfer between the compartments to very low values approaching zero.

This comparison shows that stratified inhomogeneity can produce various patterns of AaD for O_2 and CO_2, particularly of the dead space

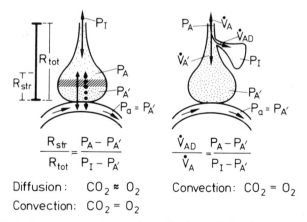

Fig. 3. Similarity between the effects of stratification and alveolar dead space ventilation in respect of alveolar–arterial differences ($P_{\bar{A}} - P_a = P_A - P_{A'}$). (A) Model of stratification. Hatched area: barrier to diffusion (arrow of dots) and to convection (solid arrow). R_{tot}, R_{str}: total resistance and stratificational resistance to O_2 uptake and CO_2 output. (B) Model of alveolar dead space ventilation. The total alveolar ventilation ($\dot{V}_A$) comprises the alveolar ventilation of the normal perfused compartment ($\dot{V}_{A'}$) and the alveolar ventilation of the unperfused compartment ($\dot{V}_{AD}$). Convective transport identical for CO_2 and O_2, diffusive transport nearly equal for both.

type (ratio AaD_{CO_2}/AaD_{O_2} close to unity). It should be of interest to determine what part of AaD is attributable to stratification. However, this may be rather difficult, particularly since there may exist combined or transitional forms of series and parallel inhomogeneity (see also Section VII).

II. DIFFUSION IN GAS PHASE

The physics of diffusion of gases in the gas phase is important for quantitative analysis of gas exchange in all air-filled respiratory organs. It is of interest to point out that diffusion in gas phase is the decisive rate-limiting step of gas transport in various types of gas exchange organs, e.g., in the air capillaries of avian lungs (Scheid, 1978a), in insect tracheoles (Weis-Fogh, 1964), and across the avian egg shell (Wangensteen et al., 1970–1971). The role of intrapulmonary diffusion in limiting gas exchange in mammalian alveolar lungs appears to be less obvious and is investigated in this chapter. The knowledge of the qualitative and quantitative characteristics of diffusion is required both for model calculations and interpretation of experimental data.

A. Diffusion Laws

Two basic differential equations for diffusion (in any medium) have been introduced by Fick (1855). Both equations, and all their integrated forms, contain the diffusion coefficient D as a specific index for diffusivity:

1. First Fick diffusion equation, for steady state (all variables constant with time):

$$J = -D\,(dC/dx) \tag{1}$$

2. Second Fick diffusion equation, for unsteady state (concentration time dependent):

$$(\partial C/\partial t) = D(\partial^2 C/\partial x^2) \tag{2}$$

where D is the diffusion coefficient (length^2/time), J the density of diffusion flux (quantity of gas/length^2 × time); C the concentration (quantity of gas/length^3), x the length, and t the time.

In respiratory physiology, the quantities' fractional concentration F_y and partial pressure P_y are customarily used instead of mass or molar concentration C_y (of gas species y). They can be introduced into diffusion equations by the relationships

$$P_y = C_y/\beta_g \tag{3}$$

$$F_y = C_y/(\beta_g P_{tot}) \tag{4}$$

in which β_g is the "capacitance coefficient" of gases in gas phase [see Piiper *et al.* (1971)] and P_{tot} the total pressure (often equal to atmospheric pressure).

For diffusion in gaseous phase, at constant total pressure, the sum of the partial pressures of the n component gases P_y must be equal to the total pressure P_{tot} (or the sum of fractional concentrations F_y must be equal to unity):

$$\sum_{y=1}^{n} P_y = P_{tot}, \qquad \sum_{y=1}^{n} F_y = 1.0 \tag{5}$$

This important requirement, which is specific for gaseous media, introduces additional complications into the analysis of diffusion in gaseous media (in comparison with diffusion of gases in liquid and solid media) as it imposes a constraint on the components in a multicomponent diffusible system (see Section II,C,1).

For mathematics of diffusion, Jacobs (1935) and Crank (1975) should be consulted, for an introduction to physics of diffusion in gases, and for further references, see Radford (1964) and Reid and Sherwood (1966).

B. Binary Diffusion

In binary (or mutual) diffusion, only two gases are present. The important property of binary diffusion is that the diffusion coefficient, $D_{x/y}$, governing the diffusion of a pair of gases, x and y, is (practically) independent of the fractional concentrations. Thus He in very low concentration diffuses in an SF_6 medium as rapidly as SF_6 in very low concentration in a He medium.

Binary diffusion coefficients of most gases naturally involved in gas exchange or experimentally introduced in lung function studies have been experimentally determined [see Andrussow and Schramm (1969); Worth *et al.* (1978)].

Binary D values can be predicted on the basis of empirical or theoretical relationships:

1. Graham's law is a very simple relationship much used in physiological literature for prediction of relative D values from the molecular mass M of the gases:

$$\frac{D_{x/z}}{D_{y/z}} = \left(\frac{M_y}{M_x}\right)^{1/2} \tag{6}$$

($D_{x/z}$ and $D_{y/z}$ are D for the binary mixtures x with z and y with z, respectively).

This relationship was empirically established by Graham (1832) for pure gases diffusing against atmospheric air through a porous diaphragm out of a vessel that was carefully maintained at atmospheric pressure. Indeed, when the binary D for He, CO, and SF_6 in N_2 or the effective D for these gases in alveolarlike air [from Worth and Piiper (1978a)] are compared, a reasonable agreement with the Graham relationship is obtained (deviations less than 20%). However, when N_2 is replaced by H_2, the agreement deteriorates considerably.

2. Much more accurate predictions may be obtained from an equation based on the Chapman–Enskog theory of gases (Reid and Sherwood, 1966):

$$D_{x/y} = \frac{1.858 \times 10^{-3} T^{3/2} (1/M_x + 1/M_y)^{1/2}}{P_{tot} \sigma_{x/y}^2 \Omega_D} \tag{7}$$

where $D_{x/y}$ is the binary diffusion coefficient (cm²/sec), T the absolute temperature (°K), M_x, M_y the molecular mass of the gas species x and y respectively, P_{tot} the total pressure (atm), $\sigma_{x/y}$ the Lennard–Jones mean collision diameter (Å), and Ω_D the collision integral for diffusion (dimensionless). Values of the variables $\sigma_{x/y}$ and Ω_D have been tabulated (Reid and Sherwood, 1966).

Binary D for gases used in respiratory physiology is in the range 0.07 to 1.7 cm²/sec [at $P_B = 746$ torr, 37°C, dry: CO_2/SF_6, 0.076; O_2/N_2, 0.26; He/H_2, 1.68 cm²/sec, according to Worth et al. (1978)]. Comparison of experimentally determined with predicted D yielded a reasonable agreement, the largest deviations being +17% and −3% (Worth et al., 1978).

Some important inferences may be drawn from the Chapman–Enskog equation:

1. D is inversely proportional to the barometric pressure.
2. In the range 30–40°C, D increases about 0.8%/°C (Ω_D changes little with temperature).
3. D is inversely proportional to the square root of the harmonic mean molecular mass, but not even a relative D value can be derived from the molecular masses alone due to the dependence of D upon the molecular properties σ and Ω_D.

C. Diffusion in Multicomponent Systems

Four gases are normally involved in the diffusion processes in lung airways: N_2, O_2, CO_2, and H_2O (water vapor). Moreover, in lung function testing further test gases may be introduced.

Diffusion in fluid mixtures containing three or more components is obviously more complex than in binary mixtures [see the monograph by Cussler (1976)]. For a quantitative study of diffusion problems in multi-component gas mixtures the Stefan–Maxwell diffusion equations (Stefan, 1871) have to be solved. For this, the values of the binary D for all combinations of the component gases are required. The time course of diffusional equilibration rate of any gas species is eminently dependent upon the concentrations of all the component gases (Chang *et al.*, 1975).

1. Effects of Compensatory Bulk Flow

Even for the case in which in a ternary system the initial concentration of one component is uniform, considerable concentration gradients for this component may arise on account of diffusional flux of the other (two or more) components if their diffusivities are strongly dissimilar (e.g., Modell and Farhi, 1976; Brès and Hatzfeld, 1977). Such "dehomogenization" clearly is outside the scope of binary diffusion.

The following situations characterizing anomalous diffusion have been discerned (Chang *et al.*, 1975): (a) diffusion barrier (no diffusion despite presence of pressure gradient), (b) osmotic diffusion (net gas flux in absence of a concentration gradient), and (c) reverse diffusion (net gas flux against a concentration gradient). These phenomena of anomalous diffusive flux formally require zero, infinite, and negative diffusion coefficient values, respectively.

Qualitatively, these phenomena may be easily explained on the basis of compensatory bulk flow necessitated by unbalanced diffusional fluxes. It must be realized that in a closed system such anomalous diffusion is transitory and ultimately normal diffusion will prevail and bring all concentration differences to zero.

2. Effects of Changing Diffusion Medium

In many cases of diffusion in multicomponent systems it is useful to consider one gas species as diffusing in a medium consisting of the remaining gases. As this medium generally varies with site and time, complex diffusion patterns may develop. Thus Worth and Piiper (1978a), studying the kinetics of equilibration of He and SF_6 in alveolarlike gas mixtures, could explain qualitatively the observed differences in diffusivities when He and SF_6 diffused in the same (codiffusion) or in opposite direction (counterdiffusion) by differences in the effective diffusion medium.

3. Approximation by the Binary Diffusion Model

Solution of multicomponent diffusion problems requires advanced mathematics and costly computation. Therefore it is of practical interest to examine if and to what extent the much simpler binary diffusion model can be applied to studies of intrapulmonary diffusion.

In an experimental investigation of the diffusion of He, CO, and SF_6 in alveolarlike gas mixtures (14% O_2, 6% CO_2, and 80% N_2 or other inert gas) using the subdivided tube technique it was found that with test gas concentrations below 10% the diffusional equilibration of the test gas was practically indistinguishable from the pattern predicted for binary diffusion of the components "test gas" and "background gas mixture" (Worth and Piiper, 1978a). Values for "effective diffusion coefficient" D' calculated by treating the process as binary diffusion were in good agreement with the values predicted on the basis of the following simple formula of Wilke (Fairbanks and Wilke, 1950; Wilke, 1950):

$$\frac{1}{D'_{x/\bar{y}}} = \frac{1}{1 - F_x} \sum_{y=1}^{n} \frac{F_y}{D'_{x/y}} \tag{8}$$

where $D'_{x/\bar{y}}$ is the effective diffusion coefficient of gas x in the background mixture, F_x the fractional concentration of gas x, F_y the fractional concentration of any of the gas species y of the background mixture (excluding x), $D_{x/y}$ the binary diffusion coefficient for x and y, and n the number of gas species of the background mixture.

This useful formula for calculation of effective D' from binary D and fractional composition essentially means that the diffusing properties of a mixture can be approximated by the fraction-weighted *harmonic* mean of binary diffusion coefficients (the fraction-weighted *algebraic* mean of binary diffusion coefficients yields values not in agreement with experimental measurements).

Comparison of effective D values determined in dry and water-vapor-saturated alveolarlike gas mixtures at 37°C showed that the effect water vapor corresponds to that predicted on the basis of the Wilke relationship (Worth and Piiper, 1978a).

In another study using the same technique (Worth and Piiper, 1978b), the diffusional equilibration of O_2 and CO_2 between inspired gas and alveolar gas was simulated by measuring the time course of diffusional mixing between two identical, closed compartments (initially containing 21% O_2 and 79% N_2, H_2, or SF_6, and 14% O_2, 6% CO_2, and 80% N_2, H_2, or SF_6, respectively). With N_2- and SF_6-containing background gas, both CO_2 and O_2 equilibrated as in a binary system. With H_2-containing background, the CO_2 equilibration was of binary diffusion character, but O_2 diffusion was different, being initially faster than later when compared to binary characteristics.

In all cases, except for diffusion of O_2 in H_2-containing gas, the effective diffusion constant was in reasonable agreement with predictions from

Wilke's equation (deviations being less than 7%). For diffusion of O_2 in H_2-containing gas the experimental D' was less than calculated according to Wilke. However, a very good agreement was achieved between experimental results and the approximate solution of the Stefan–Maxwell equations according to a procedure derived by Toor (1964a,b). Also the apparent time dependence of the effective diffusion coefficient, observed particularly at the beginning of the equilibration, was in accordance with the Toor prediction.

It is of interest to point out that in the Toor approach the effects of "changing diffusion medium" are taken into account, but those of "compensatory bulk flow" are not. Therefore, it cannot, without modification, simulate anomalous diffusion (see above).

4. Diffusion in Steady State versus Diffusive Mixing

In pulmonary gas exchange both diffusive mixing (of inspired gas with lung resident gas) and steady state diffusion of CO_2 and O_2 (across a stationary gas layer adjacent to the alveolar surface) are expected to occur. The latter mode is clearly prevalent in gas exchange systems lacking ventilation, e.g., in avian eggs (diffusion through air-filled eggshell pores) and in insects (diffusion in air-filled tracheoles reaching and even penetrating cells). However, for practical reasons, most measurements of diffusivity have been performed, as diffusive mixing, in closed system.

In the case of binary diffusion, the same D value should be valid for both diffusive mixing and steady state. This seems to be true also for all cases of multicomponent diffusion occurring in formal agreement with binary diffusion pattern. In the cases where diffusion in multicomponent systems deviates markedly from binary diffusion characteristics, however, different values for effective D are expected to result from both types of study (H. K. Chang, R. C. Tai, and L. E. Farhi, unpublished observations; Worth and Piiper, 1978b).

5. Conclusions

It follows from theoretical and experimental studies on diffusion that in many cases, and in most physiological and experimental conditions prevailing in lungs, the diffusion of a single gas species may be assumed to follow closely binary diffusion characteristics in spite of the presence of a multicomponent gas system. In particular, binary diffusion characteristic is expected if (1) the fractional concentrations (or concentration differences) of the diffusing gases are small (not exceeding a few percent); and/or (2) the binary D values of the diffusing gases with the individual major components of the background gas are not grossly different.

III. DIFFUSION IN CONVECTIVE FLOW

A tracer that is introduced into a fluid (e.g., a gas stream) flowing in a pipe will be convected down the pipe with the fluid. For a diffusible tracer the net transport rate down the tube may be enhanced by the axial diffusivity of the tracer molecules, and the processes underlying this diffusive mass transport are those discussed in Section II. In this section we review the interactions between convection and diffusion when radial gradients in both fluid velocity and tracer concentration exist within the tube. The underlying theory was first developed by Taylor (1953) and was later refined (Aris, 1956) and applied to gas movements in the lung (Wilson and Lin, 1970).

A. Dispersion in Laminar Flow

Consider a circular tube with a fluid moving under laminar flow conditions, the radial velocity profile across the tube thus being parabolic. In Fig. 4A we assume the position of an observer moving with the mean fluid velocity. We consider the imaginary plane that intersects the parabolic front at the mean fluid velocity. Relative to this plane, there is a central core of the fluid moving from left to right (forward flow), encircled by flow to the left (backward flow); thin arrows mark the radial distribution of the fluid velocity. Consider tracer molecules initially present only to the left of the plane. The molecules will in the central parts be convected through the plane by the forward flow, whereas the peripheral backward flow will not carry any tracer molecules from right to left. There will thus be a net flux of the tracer through the imaginary plane from left to right (in addition to the transport with the bulk flow of the fluid), resulting in its axial dispersion. To the right in Fig. 4 the concentration, averaged over the cross section of the tube, is shown as it appears to the moving observer at Time 0 (concentration step) and some time later.

The case considered by Taylor (1953) is illustrated in Fig. 4B. Diffusion is allowed in radial direction (no axial diffusion), whereby tracer molecules leave the central, forward flow regimes and are carried back behind the plane. Radial diffusion would rapidly diminish the radial gradient if it were not for the convective flows that replenish the radial gradient. This replenishment can, however, only be operative in the region where an axial gradient exists. It is thus apparent that the Taylor mechanism is restricted to the narrow zone around the concentration front.

The effect of radial diffusion of the tracer molecules is to reduce the dispersion produced by the convection (with radially varying velocity). This

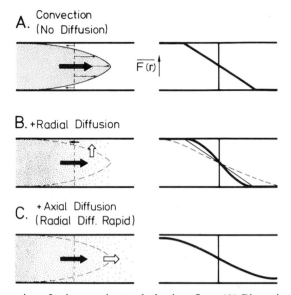

Fig. 4. Dispersion of substance in steady laminar flow. (A) Dispersion by convection alone. (B) Radial diffusion counteracts the convective dispersion (Taylor mechanism). No axial diffusion. (C) Dispersion by axial diffusion, while convective dispersion is abolished by infinitely rapid radial diffusion. Solid arrows, transport by convection; open arrows, by diffusion. The profiles to the right show concentration, averaged over the cross section. Dashed line in the profile of (B) indicates enhancement of axial dispersion in the presence of axial diffusion. For details see text.

is schematically shown in Fig. 4B (to the right), where the thick line represents the dispersion of mean concentration with radial diffusion, and the thin line the dispersion without radial dispersion (Fig. 4A). The Taylor mechanism thus results in lesser dispersion than provided by convection alone, and there exists a "strong tendency for molecular diffusion (in radial direction) to prevent dispersion" (p. 198 of Taylor, 1953). The higher the diffusivity of the tracer, the more pronounced is the antidispersing effect. Hence, although the term "Taylor dispersion" seems thus to be questionable, the term "Taylor diffusion" (Pack *et al.*, 1977; Mazzone *et al.*, 1976) should be avoided since it is not a peculiar type of diffusion but the interaction between convection and diffusion that is responsible for the phenomenon.

Taylor (1953) has shown that for the mean concentration, averaged over any cross section, the dispersion produced by the interaction of convection and radial diffusion is identical to and can thus be treated as diffusion in axial direction with a diffusion coefficient, D', that depends on the mean fluid velocity u, the diameter of the pipe a, and the diffusivity of the tracer D:

$$D' = (ua)^2/192D \qquad (9)$$

This equivalence is particularly useful as it allows the mathematical description of the two-dimensional gas transport (axial and radial dimensions) in terms of a single axial dimension.

It is of importance to identify the limitations to the Taylor mechanism. For very low flow rates, or high diffusivities, the convection will fail to replenish the rapidly abolished radial concentration gradient. The net convective flux of molecules through the moving plane will then be zero (Fig. 4C), and so will be D' of Eq. (9). However, the axial diffusivity, which has been neglected in Fig. 4B and by Taylor (1953), will now become dominant for axial dispersion. Aris (1956) has shown that the Taylor mechanism can be expanded to include this regime of parameters if an effective diffusivity D_{eff} is defined comprising D' of Eq. (9) and the molecular diffusivity, D:

$$D_{eff} = D \left[1 + \frac{1}{192} \left(\frac{ua}{D} \right)^2 \right] \qquad (10)$$

It is apparent from this equation that the axial dispersion dominates Taylor dispersion when $ua/10D \ll 1$ (Wilson and Lin, 1970).

The other extreme, high flow in large tubes with low diffusivity, is of equal importance. Although Eq. (10) would predict no limitation to D_{eff}, the obvious limit for dispersion is that exerted on a nondiffusible tracer by the convective flow, as suggested by Fig. 4A. This is the case in the lung when $a^2u/10LD > 1$ (Wilson and Lin, 1970), where L is the length of the bronchial unit, or when $D_{eff} > uL/20$, which thus constitutes an upper limit to the effective, Taylor diffusivity. Beyond this limit, dispersion cannot simply be described by an equivalent axial diffusivity.

For O_2 during normal breathing, the region in the lung in which the Taylor mechanism should dominate axial dispersion can be estimated from generation 8 to 12 (Wilson and Lin, 1970). Most authors have, however, applied the Taylor mechanism to flow in the upper airways also (e.g., Pack *et al.*, 1977) and have substantially overestimated axial dispersion in this region.

It is worth noting that D_{eff} in Eq. (10) is not a monotonous function of D. Thus the dispersion of two tracers, one with high, the other with low diffusivity, may be similar in given flow, and both may disperse more than a tracer with intermediate diffusivity. The reason is that the dispersion for the highly diffusive tracer is dominated by axial diffusion, while that for the low diffusion tracer is governed by convection. This should be considered when effects of gas dispersion are observed (e.g., Mazzone *et al.*, 1976) whose magnitude does not correspond to the sequence of the molecular weight of the tracers used.

B. Dispersion in Disturbed Flow

The Taylor mechanism considered so far is applicable to the case of steady and fully developed laminar flow in infinitely long tubes. Gas flow in the lung is not steady but variable with time. The flow pattern is highly complex because of the finite length of bronchial tubes and their branching (cf. Pedley, 1977; Pedley *et al.*, 1977). The Taylor theory has later been extended to be applicable to many of these disturbing conditions (Taylor, 1954; Gill *et al.*, 1968; Gill and Sankarasubramanian, 1970, 1971; Flint and Eisenklam, 1970). It has been shown that under these conditions axial dispersion is less than for fully developed laminar flow (Pack *et al.*, 1977). Thus use of D_{eff} from Eq. (10) (in the region where it may be applied) allows us to estimate the maximum effect of Taylor dispersion.

C. Attempts to Measure Taylor Dispersion in Lung Models

Scherer *et al.* (1975) have measured the dispersion of benzene vapor in a glass model representing any six consecutive generations between generations 0 and 13 of the Weibel lung model. They have assumed apparent axial diffusion to be responsible for the observed dispersion and have calculated effective diffusivities that increased linearly with the mean flow velocity. Some comments appear appropriate to their study:

1. Except for the lowest velocities used, the experimental parameters appear to be outside the range where radial diffusion would significantly contribute to the axial dispersion in fully developed laminar flow (see above). Hence it may be questioned if the interpretation of the results in terms of an effective diffusivity is meaningful.
2. The dependence of the dispersion on the diffusivity of the tracer has not been systematically studied by the authors and thus the suggested linear variation of the effective diffusivity with (molecular) diffusivity is doubtful.
3. Even if the critique of (1) and (2) were unjustified, the results of Scherer *et al.* (1975) should not be extended beyond the range of airway generations 0–13 suggested by the authors. Nonetheless, Paiva *et al.* (1976) have used the formulas given by Scherer *et al.* (1975) in their model of the 13 terminal generations.
4. Similar criticism may apply to the results reported in Fig. 2 of Engel and Macklem (1977).

Van Liew and Mazzone (1977) have found less dispersion for gases with high (e.g., He) than with low diffusivity (e.g., SF_6) flowing steadily in a long tube. Their results are qualitatively in agreement with the predictions from the Taylor mechanism, which seems indeed applicable to the experimental conditions of the authors.

D. Significance for Gas Transport in the Lung

The Taylor mechanism qualitatively provides a tool by which gases of different diffusivity are separated, and those with high diffusivity are delayed compared to gases of low diffusivity. However, owing to the complications outlined above, a quantitative appraisal of the effect of the Taylor mechanism on net transport of gases in the lung is difficult. All processes that result in local gas mixing, including cardiogenic mixing (cf. Fukuchi *et al.,* 1976; Sikand *et al.,* 1976), diminish the dispersion provided by the Taylor mechanism. But even the maximum dispersion would yield very little separation of gases as it occurs only over a limited number of airway generations (8–12; see Wilson and Lin, 1970) whose volume is low. Hence, the existing evidence appears to suggest that this appealing mechanism is of little practical relevance to the study of gas transport in the lung (see Section V,B,5).

IV. ANATOMICAL BASIS FOR LUNG MODELS

Some of the morphological details of the lung are important for a quantitative treatment of gas mixing. The first comprehensive account on lung morphometry has been given by Weibel (1963). His model A has been adopted by most authors as a basis for their calculations.

A. Symmetrical Model of Weibel

Weibel's model A constitutes a tree of 24 generations derived in regular dichotomy from the trachea (generation zero). The conductive zone extends to generation 16, the last generation of bronchioles without alveoli (terminal bronchioles). Therefrom originate, in succession, three generations each of respiratory bronchioles and alveolar ducts, and finally the terminal structures, alveolar sacs. For the consideration of gas mixing the following features of this model deserve attention:

1. In this symmetrical model all paths from the trachea into the 2^{23} alveolar sacs are identical. Since the diameter of the individual bronchi de-

creases toward the periphery, it is a reasonable approximation to neglect radial concentration gradients of respired gases; hence, the walls between parallel adjacent units of the same generation can be neglected. With respect to gas mixing the complex lung can thus be approximated by a solid figure, without partitions between parallel adjacent elements.

2. Although both diameter and length of individual branches decrease, the rapid increase in the number of branches results in a tremendous increase in airway volume per generation, particularly in the last few generations. We have plotted in Fig. 5A the equivalent radius against the length of an axisymmetric solid figure having the same distribution of volume to length as the model lung, and have used the same scale for both axes. More than 96% of the volume is contained in the terminal 7 mm (constituting only 2% of the total length), which correspond to the seven last generations. If Fig. 5A is considered, the term "trumpet" appears ill chosen, and a "thumb tack" (La Force and Lewis, 1970) may describe the shape

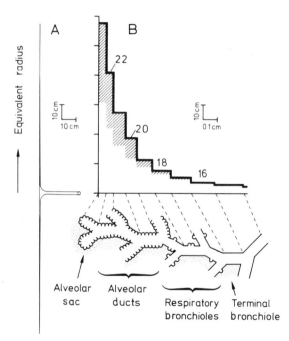

Fig. 5. Lung model of Weibel (1963). (A) The equivalent radius is plotted against axial distance. Same length scale for both axes. (B) The details of the terminal airways (acinus) are resolved by expanding the scale of the abscissa 100-fold, and retaining the ordinate scale. The scheme shows a representative path in the acinus, which originates from one terminal bronchiole: three generations each of respiratory bronchioles and alveolar ducts, which lead into the alveolar sacs.

of the model better. We have resolved the finer details of the terminal airways (Fig. 5B) by expanding the abscissa scale 100-fold while retaining the ordinate scale. It reveals the transitory and respiratory zones, the terminal seven generations, of about 7 mm length.

3. When a tidal volume of 500 ml is delivered at FRC to the lung as a nonmixing bolus at constant flow, its front will rapidly penetrate the proximal airways into the deep lung regions, where the flow velocity will decrease as the thumb tack widens. The tidal front will ultimately reach down to about generations 20 or 21 (first- or second-order alveolar ducts) and will thus be less than 2 mm from the distal end.

B. Alternative Models

The methods used by Gomez and Weibel to derive the symmetrical lung model (Weibel, 1963) were later criticized (Hansen and Ampaya, 1974) and alternative morphometrical models were proposed. A major criticism of Hansen and Ampaya (1974) pertained to the usefulness of thin lung sections for counting numbers of bronchial units, particularly in the periphery of the lung, and for assessing the pattern of branching. In fact, Hansen *et al.* (1975), like most investigators before and after Weibel (see review in Cumming, 1974), observed more variability and irregularity in the bronchial assembly, particularly striking in the region of the alveolar ducts and sacs, than is accounted for by the symmetrical model of Weibel.

Hansen *et al.* (1975) used enlarged positive lung reconstructions and found the branching of the three generations of respiratory bronchioles to be mainly dichotomous, in good agreement with Weibel. However, the number of generations of alveolar ducts arising from a third-order respiratory bronchiole could be up to eight (three in Weibel's model), and frequently a parent branch divided into three or more daughter branches. Alveolar sacs originated from all generations of respiratory bronchioles and ducts, as did alveoli. The number of alveoli per duct was considerably less than in Weibel's model. The principle of space-filling rather than of symmetry appears thus to underly the branching in the periphery.

Two factors in these alternative morphometrical models appear to be of relevance for the discussion of lung gas mixing. First, the larger average number of orders of ducts and the smaller number of alveoli per duct produce an even more abrupt increase of volume with distance in the periphery than is suggested from Fig. 5. Second, there is a considerable variability in the length of individual paths from the trachea to the alveolar sacs. Hence, the representation of the lung by a single solid figure appars to be elusive. Rather, there may be a coexistence of parallel thumb tacks of differing length.

Although these features of irregularity and variability in the lung may be of high significance for the problem of stratification, they have not been identified and described well enough for application in mathematical models, and the complexity of the structure may in fact preclude any such attempt. It must be regarded as the distinctive merit of Weibel to have introduced a morphometrical model that is a good approximation to reality and yet is simple enough for application in mathematical analysis. In fact, all recent theoretical studies on the problem of gas mixing have relied on his model A or on slight modifications thereof. It may, nevertheless, prove crucial for a correct appraisal of lung gas mixing to consider the deviations from Weibel's simplified model (see Section VII).

V. MATHEMATICAL ANALYSIS OF GAS MIXING IN THE LUNG

Several attempts have been made to determine the significance of stratification by calculating gas mixing in lung models resembling the physiological situation as closely as possible in respect of lung morphology and physics of gas transport. However, the immense complexity of the problem has necessitated approximations in the models that preclude a decisive conclusion whether or not stratification has correctly been advocated to explain experimental results (see Section VI).

A. Models Considering Diffusive Mixing Alone

The first calculations were made on the approximating assumption that tidal air is inspired as a nonmixing bolus over an infinitely short period and that gas mixing by diffusion proceeds from the initially sharp front between tidal and lung resident air. Attainment of equilibration within a given time was judged from persisting concentration differences in the model.

1. The Model of Rauwerda

Rauwerda (1946) considered the acinus as the functional terminal lung unit and chose a cone, truncated by two concentric spheres of radius 1 and 8 mm, respectively, closed at either end, to represent the airways therein. Like most later authors, Rauwerda neglected radial concentration differences, and considered the one-dimensional problem of axial diffusion equilibration. He found that an O_2/N_2 concentration step set up 2 mm from the distal end was dissipated to 16% of the initial value after only 0.38 sec, and had disappeared virtually completely after 1 sec.

Rauwerda concluded from these calculations that stratification was unlikely to occur to any significant degree in the alveolar region under normal breathing conditions.

2. The Model of Cumming et al. (1966)

Cumming *et al.* (1966) confirmed the results of Rauwerda, but criticized the boundary conditions in his model, since the closed proximal cone would correspond to the unnatural situation of clamping off the terminal bronchioles, whereas diffusional exchange with proximally adjacent airways would affect gas equilibration in the periphery. The authors have, therefore, used an elongated cone and have thus incorporated into their study of peripheral gas mixing the diffusional exchange with proximal airways (dead space). The truncating spheres were of 0.5- and 2.6-cm radius, the axial length of the cone thus being 2.1 cm, corresponding to the 13 distal generations of Weibel's model A.

A concentration step introduced 2 mm from the distal end resulted after 1 sec in a concentration difference across the seven distal generations of 8% of the initial value. The authors concluded that stratification in the alveolar region was possible under physiological conditions, and retained the hypothesis of Krogh and Lindhard (1914) of stratification being the main reason for the slope in the alveolar plateau in a single-breath N_2 test.

3. The Model of La Force and Lewis

La Force and Lewis (1970) criticized the cone model of Cumming *et al.* (1966) for its poor correlation with lung morphology. This criticism hits Rauwerda less since his short cone is a better representation of the terminal airways (Piiper and Scheid, 1971). La Force and Lewis modeled the terminal 13 generations of Weibel's model A, represented by a solid figure resembling a thumb tack (see Fig. 5A). They used numerical methods to solve the one-dimensional diffusion equation (radial concentration differences were not considered).

A concentration step set at the end of generation 20 was rapidly attenuated as evidenced from the plot of concentration against distance or, even more strikingly, against cumulative airway volume. Adding alveolar volume to the thumb tack model, producing thus an even more abruptly widening thumb tack, resulted in even faster equilibration. The authors concluded that stratification could not persist in the alveolar region for periods of physiological interest.

4. Critique of Models for Diffusive Mixing

The discrepancy in conclusions among the three author groups is partly due to differences in the models chosen, partly to differences in interpretation. Cumming *et al.* (1966) dismissed the study of equilibrium in the more realistic thumb tack model because "the diffusion mixing in such a structure would be slower than in the cone" (p. 69 of Cumming *et al.*, 1966). This contention is opposite to that of La Force and Lewis, and it is of interest to disclose the apparent discrepancy.

We have recalculated in Fig. 6 diffusive gas mixing in a cone with a ratio of distal to proximal cross section of 600, close to that of the thumb tack of La Force and Lewis, and with equal length for both models, both being open at the narrow end. The initial step in concentration was set up at the same distance from the peripheral end in both. Thus the results in the cone can directly be compared with those in the thumb tack [Fig. 5 in La Force and Lewis (1970)].

In Fig. 6A the concentration in both models is plotted against the linear distance for two diffusion periods. It is evident that the concentration gradient is steeper at all locations in the thumb tack than in the cone. Thus, the concentration difference over the terminal 7 mm is 11% in the thumb tack and only 8% in the cone. Since the concentration in the thumb tack is farther from the equilibrium than in the cone, the notion of Cumming *et al.* of slower diffusion mixing in the thumb tack is correct. However, a plot of concentration against cumulative volume (Fig. 6B) reveals that after 1 sec the concentration difference in the distal 80% of volume is less than 1% in the thumb tack compared with 13% in the cone.

The apparent discrepancy is thus caused by the definition of the alveolar region to be considered for stratification. The consideration of cu-

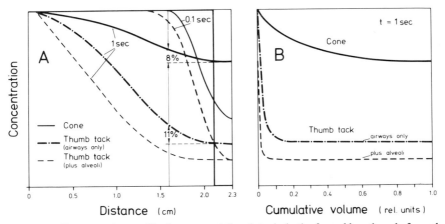

Fig. 6. Concentration profiles in cone and thumb tack, both of equal length and of equal ratio of cross sections at proximal and distal ends. (A) Plot against axial distance, and (B) against cumulative volume. For details see text. Profiles for thumb tack redrawn from La Force and Lewis (1970).

mulative volume for appraisal of stratification is more useful, particularly for comparison with tests like the single-breath maneuver. To generalize, the time course of equilibration in any (one-dimensional) system depends on both diffusion resistance (e.g., axial length) and capacitance (e.g., volume). For equilibration in the entire system (dead space plus alveolar region), the fastest time course will be realized with homogeneous distribution of capacitance to resistance, i.e., in a cylinder. If, on the other hand, only the alveolar region is considered and dead space neglected, then equilibration is fastest with most of the resistance in proximal and most of the capacitance in distal regions, like in the thumb tack.

These considerations have some important implications: (1) the shape of the model is important for stratification and hence the cylindrical and conical models must be dismissed in these studies; (2) morphology suggests distinction of a proximal part, reflecting resistance to gas mixing in the system, from a distal part, providing a gas capacity; (3) although stratification is mainly influenced by the axial distance in the peripheral part, the capacitance, the volume of the proximal, resistive part, determines mainly the dead space (Baker et al., 1974); (4) the dead space and its variation with time is a poor measure for stratification because it reflects the events in proximal regions, which can largely differ from those in the periphery.

B. Models Considering Convection and Diffusion

La Force and Lewis (1970) contended that convection would be of only small effect on gas mixing since the inspired tidal front would rapidly come to a halt because of the shape of the trumpet. However, his results, like those in the cone, show that the initial concentration front is not only rapidly blunted but also retreats very rapidly proximally. This suggests that neglect of axial diffusion during convection is not warranted. Pedley (1970) and Wilson and Lin (1970) have proposed equations to treat simultaneous convection and diffusion, and independently, Cumming et al. (1971), Paiva (1972a,b) and Scherer et al. (1972) have considered both transport mechanisms in models on stratification.

1. The Model of Cumming et al. (1971)

Calculations were based on Weibel's model A. Convection and diffusion were treated as independent phenomena occurring successively in small increments. Thus, $\frac{1}{10}$ of V_T were admitted to the lung without diffusion, followed by a period of $\frac{1}{10}$ of inspired time during which diffusion occurred without convection. Ten such steps for inspiration were followed by another 10 for expiration.

The authors analyzed their data in terms of dead-space volume; however, this may be inappropriate as suggested above. A plot of expired N_2 against cumulative volume, resulting from the simulation of a single-breath test, showed a concentration difference of 1.1% of the inspired–alveolar difference between 750 and 1250 ml of expired volume. The authors conclude that stratification is well possible in normal breathing although the boundary conditions are not yet accurately enough defined "so that any firm statement about the completeness or otherwise of gas mixing is not at the moment possible" (p. 341 of Cumming et al., 1971). Although the figure of 1.1% was later quoted as evidencing stratification in this model (Paiva, 1973), the original Fig. 12 suggests a perfectly flat alveolar plateau beyond 900 ml expired. Hence, we hesitate to interpret the results of Cumming et al. (1971) as revealing stratification.

Paiva (1973) has criticized some aspects of the mathematical analysis in the model of Cumming et al. However, the results of Cumming et al. are in good qualitative agreement with all subsequent investigations, and the basic features are discussed below.

2. The Model of Paiva

Paiva (1973) considered mass transport in the lung by the simultaneous action of convection and diffusion and applied numerical methods to solve the underlying mass transport equation. His model is based on the 13 last generations of Weibel's model A. Although he accounted for variability in length of the bronchial branches, he considered only one representative path, treating thus the bronchial tree as a solid figure with smoothed wall at the transitions between generations. He assumed a flat flow profile and neglected radial concentration gradients, within airways and alveoli. He did not allow for tidal changes in lung volume.

Paiva considered the alveolar walls by reducing the cross section for axial diffusion and convection to that of the airways, neglecting both diffusion and convection in axial direction within the alveoli, a procedure that was later justified (Paiva, 1974).

The differential equation derived for this model is written as

$$\frac{\partial F}{\partial t} = \frac{s}{S} \left[\frac{1}{s} \frac{\partial}{\partial x} \left(Ds \frac{\partial F}{\partial x} \right) - \frac{\dot{V}}{s} \frac{\partial F}{\partial x} \right] \tag{11}$$

where $F = F(x, t)$ is the concentration of the inspired test gas at distance x from the distal end at time t; S and s are total cross section of the model with and without alveoli, and both vary with x but not with t; D is the diffusion coefficient; $\dot{V}$ is the ventilatory flow rate. Except for consideration of the alveolar walls, this equation is similar to that already proposed by Pedley (1970) and used by later authors.

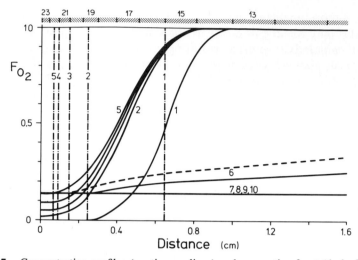

Fig. 7. Concentration profiles (continuous lines) and convective front (dashed–dotted lines) at various times during inspiration (1–5) and expiration (6–10). Linear abscissa scale for distance from the terminal end of the bronchial tree. Extension of generations shown on upper abscissa. Dashed line labeled 6 calculated assuming no diffusion on expiration. (Modified from Paiva, 1973.)

The main results of Paiva (1973) are qualitatively similar to those of Cumming *et al.* (1971) and of all later studies (Fig. 7):

a. During inspiration, the concentration front (e.g., location of the point where $F = 0.5$) lags far behind the tidal volume front, finally reaching, with a tidal volume of 500 ml, a depth corresponding to only about 150 ml (dead space).

b. For the major part of inspiration the concentration front is practically stationary, indicating that convective advancement is balanced by its retreat due to diffusive loss into the periphery.

c. Stratification is present in the alveolar region during most of inspiration. In the results of Paiva, reported in Fig. 7, there is at end-inspiration a concentration difference of 3% (of the initial inspired–alveolar concentration difference) over the terminal three generations, and even of 30% over the terminal six generations, much more than predicted by La Force and Lewis (1970).

d. On expiration, all intrapulmonary concentration gradients are rapidly convected out of the lung, partly because of the shape of the thumb tack but aided by diffusion (compare dashed and continuous curves labeled 6). Correspondingly, the alveolar plateau for expired N_2 should show no significant slope in its latter parts.

Paiva obtained similar results with sinusoidally varying tidal flow and when imposing a moderate degree of inhomogeneity, and concluded that "the role played by gas diffusion can be shown in the growth front of the single-breath test [phase II] but not in the alveolar plateau" (p. 408 of Paiva, 1973).

Paiva has made a number of simplifying assumptions, among which are the following: (a) the model does not change its volume with respiration; (b) no gas exchange takes place across the alveolar walls; (c) radial concentration and flow velocity gradients are neglected; and (d) the finer details in shape of the alveolar region are neglected as is axial mass transport inside the alveoli. Many of these parameters have been investigated in more recent studies. However, the conclusions of Paiva do not appear to be invalidated by these assumptions.

3. The Model of Scherer et al.

Scherer *et al.* (1972) used a model similar to that of Paiva but allowed for tidal changes in the alveolar volume. Their equation is very similar to Eq. (11) except that $\dot{V}$, which is constant in Paiva's calculations, decreases with the distance into the periphery as the flow is exhausted into the alveoli, and vice versa during expiration.

The results of a single-breath maneuver are in full agreement with those of Paiva: (a) concentration gradients, which exist during most of inspiration, vanish rapidly during expiration, (b) beyond about 500 ml of expired air there is no detectable slope in the alveolar plateau.

4. The Model of Davidson and Fitz-Gerald

So far all models have neglected the finer details of the lung, particularly in its terminal, alveolated region. Gas equilibration in radial direction was assumed to be infinitely fast, and any axial transport inside the alveoli was neglected. Paiva (1974) addressed the problem of radial and axial diffusion in an alveolar duct, represented by airways and apposed alveoli. The time course of gas equilibration in this model, evidenced by mean concentration in alveoli and ducts, was very similar to that obtained by considering no radial concentration gradients and allowing axial diffusion in the ducts only. Chang *et al.* (1973) investigated the same problem and found that the shape of the alveolar partitions was of importance.

A more comprehensive account to this question was provided by Davidson and Fitz-Gerald (1974), who considered convection and diffusion in a model of the terminal five generations. The physical model, based on Weibel's model A, consists of a cylinder with radial baffles at the transitions between generations, branching being accounted for by reducing the flux at these transitions. This detailed model was fitted to a trumpet model of the upper airways (Pedley, 1970) in which convection and (axial) diffusion were both considered. Allowance was made for gas exchange across the alveolar walls and for tidal changes of alveolar volume.

The authors focused attention on the O_2 uptake rates in the presence or absence of convective mass transport in the alveolar region and found significant differences under most conditions. Their curves reveal significant concentration gradients in the terminal lung regions during inspiration, even when both convection and diffusion are operative.

Davidson and Fitz-Gerald considered inspiration only and Davidson (1975) has complemented the analysis including expiration. Plots of expired concentration versus expired volume in a single-breath test reveal attainment of a horizontal alveolar plateau. Comparison with similar curves of Paiva (1973) and Scherer *et al.* (1972) appears to us to reveal a somewhat more gradual rise to the alveolar plateau (phase II) and thus possible differences in the predicted dead-space values. However, the calculations do not lend support to stratification as a major contributor to the sloping alveolar plateau.

5. The model of Pack et al.

The main objection of Pack *et al.* (1977) against all earlier analyses was that the upper airways had been neglected, in which dispersion by convection and the Taylor mechanism should exert its largest effect on mass transport. These authors solved the one-dimensional mass transport equation [Eq. (11)] by assuming for the axial diffusivity the effective value suggested for the Taylor mechanism in fully developed laminar flow. The results were then compared with those in which the effective diffusivity equaled the (axial) molecular diffusivity, which allowed appraisal of the Taylor mechanism on gas mixing.

The results showed a somewhat more rapid gas transport through the upper airways when the Taylor mechanism was operative. The net gain in gas transport by the Taylor mechanism was, however, negligibly small since the volume contained in the upper airways is small. Hence, when the concentration front reaches the rapidly widening parts of the thumb tack, all effects are virtually abolished. The authors concluded that the Taylor mechanism had no important influence on stratification. As discussed in Section III,A, the authors may have overestimated the effect of the Taylor mechanism, particularly in the most proximal airways.

C. Conclusions

Differences in the details of the results are present among the model analyses on account of differences in the boundary conditions and mathematical procedures employed. However, no model appears to contradict the following statements: (1) Stratification does exist in the alveolar region during most of the breath. (2) However, this stratification is unlikely to contribute significantly to the slope of the alveolar plateau. (3) The Taylor mechanism of axial gas dispersion is insignificant for overall gas transport in the lung.

VI. EXPERIMENTAL APPROACHES TO IDENTIFICATION OF STRATIFIED INHOMOGENEITY

In this section earlier work is only summarily reported because it has been repeatedly reviewed in recent years (Farhi, 1969; Piiper and Scheid, 1971; Cumming, 1974; Engel and Macklem, 1977). A more detailed account is given of the attempts at quantitative measurement of gas mixing kinetics and their interpretation [reviewed in Piiper (1979)].

A. Experimental Methods

1. Sloping Alveolar Plateau

A sloping alveolar plateau is generally considered as a criterion of stratification in model studies (see Section V), but in real lungs *in vivo* it can be produced by processes unrelated to stratification:

a. Continuing respiratory gas exchange not only produces sloping CO_2 and O_2 plateaus in steady state breathing, but also contributes to the slope of N_2 concentration in expired gas after a single breath of pure O_2 owing to a progressive fall in the gas exchange ratio, R.

b. Regional (parallel) inhomogeneities, if bound to differences in expiration pattern (sequential emptying), can generate sloping alveolar plateaus. Unequal distribution of ventilation ($\dot{V}_A$) to perfusion ($\dot{Q}$) with low $\dot{V}_A/\dot{Q}$ regions expiring last may be made responsible for sloping CO_2 and O_2 plateaus in steady state. In experiments involving single-breath inspiration of insoluble inert gases, the same effect would be produced by unequal distribution of $\dot{V}_A$ to volume (V_A) in such a manner that regions of low $\dot{V}_A/V_A$ expire last.

On account of these alternative explanations, experimental evidence for sloping alveolar plateaus must be considered with much reservation. The best evidence, but not entirely conclusive [see Piiper and Scheid (1971)], is provided by the study of the sum and the ratio of Ar and N_2 in the expirate after a single-breath inspiration of argon-containing gas (Sikand *et al.*, 1966).

2. Variation of Diffusivity

As diffusion has generally been considered to be the main mechanism of intrapulmonary gas mixing (destratification), numerous studies involving simultaneous application of (practically) insoluble test gases of different diffusivity have been performed since Georg et al. (1965) and Cumming et al. (1967). In all of these studies some separation of gases has been found in accordance with the expectations based on stratification: the gases of higher molecular weight and, therefore, of lower diffusivity, showed alveolar plateaus of higher slope or displayed slower kinetics in wash-out or single-breath equilibration experiments. In some experiments a quantitative evaluation of the data was attempted (see below).

The application of intravenously infused soluble test gases in steady state for study of stratification (Adaro and Farhi, 1971; Adaro, 1972) deserves particular attention. In experiments on anesthetized dogs, they administered simultaneously acetylene and freon 22, two gases of considerably different diffusivity, but of identical solubility. Since the effects of a given $\dot{V}_A/\dot{Q}$ inhomogeneity on gas exchange are identical for inert gases of equal solubility (or blood/gas partition coefficient) (Farhi and Yokoyama, 1967) these gases should display exactly the same clearance (same $P_a/P_{\bar{v}}$). The authors found less clearance (higher $P_a/P_{\bar{v}}$) for the less diffusible gas freon 22, as should be expected if stratification had imposed a higher gas exchange resistance to the less diffusible gas. The important advantage of this procedure is that soluble gases are better "models" for respiratory gases O_2 and CO_2 than insoluble gases. Moreover, the method is expected to be insensitive to unequal ventilation/volume distribution.

Another technique to achieve controlled variation of diffusivity is to change the diffusion medium by changing either the gas composition of lung gas (replacing N_2 by heavier or lighter gases) or the total pressure (hyperbaric conditions). The measured parameters have mostly been alveolar–arterial differences (AaD) for O_2 or CO_2 and diffusing capacity for CO (D_{CO}). In many cases a "paradoxical" behavior was found: increase of AaD or decrease of D_{CO} with the heavier background gas [reviewed in Worth et al. (1976)]. In such cases the so-called Taylor dispersion (see Section III) has been invoked as a basis of explanation of the experimental data (e.g., Johnson and Van Liew, 1974; Kvale et al., 1975). However, more recent theoretical and experimental studies have not been able to confirm the importance of the Taylor dispersion mechanism for alveolar gas exchange efficiency (Pack et al., 1977; Worth et al., 1977). At least a part of the paradoxical results of experiments with changing background gas seems to be due to changes in parallel distribution resulting from the mechanical properties of the gases involved (Worth et al., 1976).

3. Breath-Holding

As gas mixing in the lung is a transient phenomenon, effects are expected from varying the time available to mixing. Thus experiments involving varying breath-holding time should yield useful information on stratification. This is particularly true for experimental tests involving insoluble inert gas tracers (Rauwerda, 1946; Kjellmer *et al.*, 1959; Sikand *et al.*, 1966; Cumming *et al.*, 1967; Power, 1969) since under these conditions continuing gas exchange does not interfere with the process under investigation. It must be realized, however, that mixing observed under these conditions reflects in part exchange between alveolar and dead space regions and that with extended breath-holding times, e.g., in isolated lung lobes, exchange of gases between closely adjacent parallel lung units may become important (see Section VII).

B. Attempts at Quantification

In a number of studies, starting with Georg *et al.* (1965) and Cumming *et al.* (1967), a separation of simultaneously administered insoluble inert gases in the lung during respiratory maneuvers has been demonstrated, and stratification has been invoked as the mechanism by Krogh and Linhard (1914, 1917) and by others. Although these results appeared to prove the presence of stratification in lungs, the important question remained: To what extent does stratification limit gas exchange? Our group in Göttingen set out to assess quantitatively intrapulmonary gas mixing by the simultaneous use of two or three insoluble test gases (He, Ar, SF_6).

1. Lung Model

To arrive at quantitative evaluation without the prejudice of using any particular morphometrical lung models, an extremely simplified lung model of "lumped parameter" type was employed. In the model, all resistance to intrapulmonary mixing was concentrated into a uniform "gas-filled membrane" dividing the alveolar space into a proximal and a distal compartment. The permeability of the barrier was characterized by a conductance, which had the same dimension as pulmonary diffusing capacity D_L, i.e., (amount of gas) $\times$ (time)$^{-1}$ $\times$ (partial pressure)$^{-1}$. This conductance was at first termed "stratificational diffusing capacity." However, since convective mixing mechanisms appear to be involved, it is preferable to refer to it as "conductance of mixing," G_{mix}.

Since G_{mix} and D_L have the same dimension they can be directly compared. Moreover, since mixing in airways and gas/blood diffusion may be regarded as serially arranged step processes, their reciprocal conductances may be considered as additive to a compound reciprocal conductance ($1/G_c$):

$$\frac{1}{G_c} = \frac{1}{G_{mix}} + \frac{1}{D_L} \tag{12}$$

It is somewhat difficult to decide if the pulmonary diffusing capacity obtained in routine physiological experiments includes or excludes the mixing conductance. In the cases to be considered below we believe that, owing to the particular procedures used, the measured diffusing capacity did not effectively comprise G_{mix}, i.e., was close to D_L. However, since in most cases G_{mix} turned out to be considerably higher than D_L, this argument is of minor importance.

2. Experimental Results and Calculations

    a. Simultaneous Washout of He and SF$_6$ in Excised Dog Lung (Okubo and Piiper, 1974). The mixing conductance G_{mix} was calculated from a comparison of the wash-out rate constants of He (faster) and SF$_6$ (slower) with measured values of ventilation frequency, effective tidal volume, and lung volume, using a modified wash-out equation that was extended by a diffusional term. Determination of G_{mix} for wash-out with varied tidal volumes, but at constant end-inspired volume, was considered as testing of diffusing conditions at various levels of lung airways. A comparison of the resulting data with the morphometrical human lung model of Weibel (1963) revealed a reasonable agreement between the relative values of G_{mix} and total cross-sectional area of airways at the level calculated to be reached by the tidal volume.

    G_{mix} for O_2, interpolated according to diffusivity from the G_{mix} for SF$_6$ and He, was compared to $D_{L_{O_2}}$ previously determined in excised dog lung lobes of similar size. The ratio $(D_L/G_{mix})_{O_2}$ came out about 0.1–0.2, indicating that the resistance to mixing in airways was about 10–20% of the total gas/blood resistance to O_2 transfer.

    b. Simultaneous Equilibration of He, Ar, and SF$_6$ between Inspired and Lung Gas in Man (Sikand *et al.*, 1976). From functional residual capacity, 1 liter of a gas mixture containing He, Ar, and SF$_6$ was inspired, and expired after breath-holding of varied duration. An essential feature was calculation of the mean test gas concentration in the lung resident gas from volume and concentrations of inspired and expired gas and the end-expiratory lung volume. From the decrease of the test gas concentration difference between end-expired gas and lung resident gas with progressing breath-holding time, a value of G_{mix} was obtained for each test gas. The G_{mix} value obtained by interpolation for O_2 was on the average 78 ml/min/torr.

According to Comroe *et al.* (1962) $D_{L_{O_2}}$ in normal man is about 26 ml/min/torr. However, if a special rebreathing technique with $^{18}O_2$ as test gas in tracer concentration is used, a much higher $D_{L_{O_2}}$, averaging 48 ml/min/torr, was obtained in healthy subjects (Piiper and Meyer, 1978). Thus the ratio $(D_L/G_{mix})_{O_2}$ can be estimated at 0.3 (with high $D_{L_{O_2}}$) or 0.6 (with low $D_{L_{O_2}}$), meaning that about 20 or 40%, respectively, of the total resistance to O_2 uptake from gas inspired into the alveolar space into pulmonary capillary blood is attributable to incomplete gas mixing (stratification).

c. Simultaneous Wash-out of He and SF₆ in Man (Kawashiro *et al.*, 1976). In this study the different wash-out time courses of He and SF_6 were characterized by a "separation index" from which an average $G_{mix\,O_2}$ of 80 ml/min/torr was calculated. It follows from the design of the evaluation procedure that this value does not include the contribution made by convective mixing. Introduction of the convective mixing conductance value estimated by Sikand *et al.* increased the total $G_{mix\,O_2}$ to 160 ml/min/torr. If the above-mentioned values of D_L for man are used, the resulting ratios $(D_L/G_{mix})_{O_2}$ are in the range 0.2–0.6, in remarkable agreement with the values calculated from the experimental data of Sikand *et al.* (1976).

3. Some Critical Remarks

1. In all the experimental series some difficulties arose from delimiting the effects of stratification proper (i.e., in the alveolar space) from those of dead space. In the wash-out experiments of Kawashiro *et al.* (1976) the separation of He and SF_6 could in part be attributed to the larger single-breath dead space for SF_6. The remaining part of separation (about one-half of the "separation index") was explained on the basis of stratification, and a G_{mix} value was obtained therefrom. From their data it can be calculated that the G_{mix} value for O_2 would have been underestimated by a factor of 3 had the dead space effect not been taken into account. In the experiments of Okubo and Piiper the whole separation of He and SF_6 was ascribed to stratification, thereby possibly overestimating its limiting role and underestimating G_{mix}. From the design of the breath-holding experiments of Sikand *et al.* (1976), the effects of dead space are expected to be smaller than in the wash-out experiments.

2. The choice of the site for separation of the two alveolar compartments was somewhat arbitrary. Both Okubo and Piiper and Kawashiro *et*

al. set the boundary at the tidal/resident gas interface, whereas Sikand *et al.* preferred a boundary situated at a deeper level so that the proximal and distal alveolar compartments were close to equal. The latter authors showed, however, that the effects of changes in the compartment volume ratio on G_{mix} were relatively minor. There is a remarkable agreement between G_{mix} obtained by Okubo and Piiper for varied inspiration depths and the relative cross-sectional area of Weibel's lung model. This may mean not more than that the changes in tidal volume were accompanied by changes in G_{mix} in accordance with the overall lung morphometry in terms of the relationship between increase of airway cross-sectional area and increase in cumulative lung volume per length of airway.

3. The results of Sikand *et al.* (1976) could be best explained by assuming an important contribution of convective processes to intrapulmonary mixing: for O_2 the convective conductance was calculated to be considerably higher than the diffusive conductance. By basing their method of evaluation on the separation of He and SF_6, and not on the absolute value of their wash-out kinetics, Okubo and Piiper and Kawashiro *et al.* measured probably only the diffusive component of mixing. In the isolated, unperfused lung lobes investigated by Okubo and Piiper this may have been permissible since the cardiac mixing action was absent. Kawashiro *et al.* evaluated their data both on the basis of no convective mixing and of contribution of convective mixing according to the results of Sikand *et al.*, the resulting $G_{mix\,O_2}$ differing between both cases by a factor of 2.

4. Quantitative assessment of G_{mix} was based on a simplified model consisting of only a small number of compartments, while the stratificational resistance is in fact more or less continuously distributed along the airway path. Also regional variation in stratified inhomogeneity was neglected. Although the disadvantage to such simplification is obvious, it permits an at least approximating estimation of the effects of stratification. The situation is similar to dealing with parallel inhomogeneities by using the three-compartment model of Riley.

5. It was assumed that G_{mix} for O_2 can be calculated from G_{mix} for inert gas equilibration and that $G_{mix\,O_2}$ thus obtained can be compared with $D_{L_{O_2}}$ on the basis of Eq. (12). This assumption is based on a model in which only the distal compartment is perfused and all O_2 transport is hence through the mixing resistance estimated from inert gases. In fact, perfusion to the proximal compartment would render the mixing resistance for O_2 less than for inert gases (cf. West *et al.*, 1969; Scheid, 1978a). However, since alveolation and probably perfusion are highest in the terminal air spaces where the stratification is probably least, the errors involved may be small.

6. Various technical problems were manifest and considerable scatter of individual measurements was apparent.

These critical observations are meant to show that the results of these studies and their interpretation must be considered with reservations. However, as a whole they appear to indicate that stratification exerts a measurable limitation on alveolar gas exchange.

VII. CONCLUSIONS

Experimental evidence seems to support existence of stratification. In particular, the differences in mixing observed with gases of different diffusivity in single-breath and wash-out maneuvers and the effects of breath-holding are easiest explained by stratification. On the other hand, theoretical analyses of gas mixing in lung models arrive at the opposite conclusions that gas mixing in terminal air spaces is complete and that stratification cannot be the mechanism for the experimental observations. Hence, the models used in the theoretical analyses appear to be inappropriate to explain the experimental data, whose validity cannot be seriously questioned. We would like to propose two refined, alternative models that may prove useful in an attempt at resolving the discrepancy. Both are based on the existence of parallel inhomogeneity with peripheral gas mixing.

A. Parallel Distribution of Stratified Inhomogeneity

Morphometrical evidence suggests variation in the length of distal airways (see Section IV), and modeling this complex system by one representative path into one thumb tack may be doubtful. Rather, there should be a parallel distribution of lung portions of different rise of volume with distance. Thus thumb tacks (abrupt rises) may coexist with trumpets (gradual rises) (Fig. 8A). While gas mixing in the terminal air spaces of the

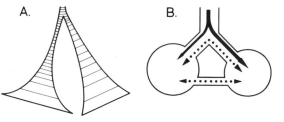

Fig. 8.   Alternative models to explain experimental observations. See text.

thumb tack may be complete (no stratification), the trumpet may give rise to significant stratification. This model could explain the experimental observations.

B. Gas Mixing between Parallel Lung Regions

Both stratification (longitudinal incomplete mixing) and regional "parallel" inhomogeneity (unequal distribution of ventilation and perfusion to parallel lung units) lead to differences in gas concentration among terminal airways. Given enough time, all these inhomogenities are bound to disappear. It is generally assumed that stratified inhomogeneities disappear at a faster rate, owing to the smaller distances involved, than do regional inhomogeneities. Hence, effects of breath-holding are usually attributed to diminishing stratification only, while regional inhomogeneities persist. There is every reason to believe this to be true for the parallel inhomogeneity due to gravity, since here long distances (centimeters to decimeters) are involved. But even in normal lungs, and more so in diseased lungs, functional inhomogeneities of the parallel type may exist, independent of gravity, on a much smaller scale. Therefore, part of the fast mixing processes may in fact derive from (convective or diffusive) mixing between closely adjacent lung units with parallel inhomogeneity.

A schematic model is shown in Fig. 8B. The mixing path may comprise (peripheral) bronchial connections or other collateral channels like the pores of Kohn. Hogg *et al.* (1972) have in fact used this model to explain their observations of a significant slope in the alveolar plateau, and its time dependence, after occlusion of small airways in the excised dog lung by beads.

These models may prove useful also to study gas exchange in diseased lungs. Particularly in emphysematous lungs, modifications in the shape of the terminal airways may be expected giving rise to the situation of Fig. 8A.

In the real lung, both models may coexist, and the situation may be more complex when possible differences in the distribution of ventilation and perfusion of the individual compartments are considered. In this case it is important to realize that results of insoluble inert gas equilibration studies (influenced by $\dot{V}_A/V_A$ distribution) cannot easily be applied to predict effects on steady state gas exchange (influenced by $\dot{V}_A/\dot{Q}$ distribution) unless both distributions are positively correlated to one another [see Piiper and Scheid (1971)].

To our knowledge, neither model has yet been utilized in an attempt to explain experimental data quantitatively. Yu (1975) has considered the possibility of the model of Fig. 8A. He regarded the coexistence of different paths in the lung as a mechanism to produce axial dispersion within an average, representative path, and quantified this dispersion by an effective diffusivity, comparable to the Taylor diffusivity (see Section III). However, this equivalence appears to us to be dubious, as this "diffusivity" would be identical for all gases.

In conclusion, it must be admitted that the quantitative significance of stratification in overall pulmonary gas exchange has not yet been adequately clarified.

VIII. APPENDIX: STRATIFICATION IN NONMAMMALIAN VERTEBRATES

Stratification, meaning concentration gradients of respired gases at the gas exchange epithelium, has been identified particularly in birds and in fish. In this section we present the problem of stratification in both animal groups and show that the effects stratification exerts on gas exchange are largely dependent on structural features of the gas exchange systems. The comparative aspects of gas exchange in vertebrates have recently been reviewed by Piiper and Scheid (1977) and by Scheid (1980).

A. Avian Parabronchial Lungs

1. Morphological Basis

The functional unit for gas exchange in the avian lung is the parabronchus, which is a long (some centimeters), narrow (<1 mm) tube, open at both ends. The parabronchus joins two types of conducting bronchi, the medioventral and mediodorsal secondary bronchi. Ventilatory gas flows through the parabronchus during both inspiration and expiration in the same direction, from its mediodorsal toward medioventral end. From the lumen of the parabronchus depart narrow (some micrometers) air capillaries that form a dense meshwork around the parabronchus, where they meet equally fine blood capillaries for gas exchange contact. Each blood capillary traverses this periparabronchial tissue in a more or less straight path from the periphery toward the parabronchial lumen, where the blood is drained by larger venules. Thus the contact site of each blood capillary constitutes a small fraction of the parabronchial length.

2. Series Ventilation in the Parabronchus

As air flows through the parabronchus, O_2 is taken up from and CO_2 is excreted into the air all along the parabronchus (Fig. 9). Hence, the gas

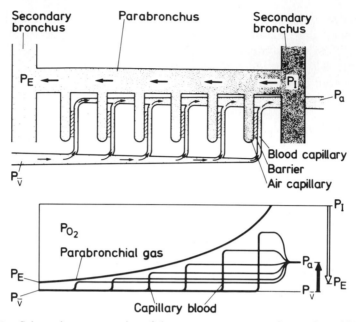

Fig. 9. Schematic representation of the crosscurrent system for parabronchial gas exchange. Gas flowing from right to left through parabronchus is depleted of O_2 (density of stippling) as O_2 is taken up by the blood capillaries. P_{O_2} profiles in parabronchial gas and capillary blood shown below. Arterial P_{O_2}, P_a, derived as a mixture from all capillaries; this value can exceed end-parabronchial P_{O_2}, P_E.

concentrations vary within the gas exchange region on account of the serial arrangement of parabronchial subelements, consisting of fractions of the parabronchus with their blood capillaries. The term stratification may thus be invoked to describe the apparent inhomogeneity. Figure 10A shows, however, that the series ventilation does in general result in an improvement of gas exchange as evidenced from the fact that arterial P_{O_2} can exceed end-parabronchial (end-expired) P_{O_2}, and likewise for CO_2. In contrary, the reciprocating series ventilation of alveolar lungs (Fig. 10B) shows impairment of gas exchange, as it produces positive values of the AaD_{O_2}. The reason for the negative end-parabronchial-to-arterial P_{O_2} differences is that arterial blood constitutes a mixtures of well-arterialized blood in initial-parabronchial and poorly arterialized blood in end-parabronchial capillaries, while end-parabronchial gas displays the lowest P_{O_2} and highest P_{CO_2}. It has been shown that the gas exchange efficacy of this serial-multicapillary or crosscurrent system (Scheid and Piiper, 1972) is superior to that of the alveolar system (Piiper and Scheid, 1975).

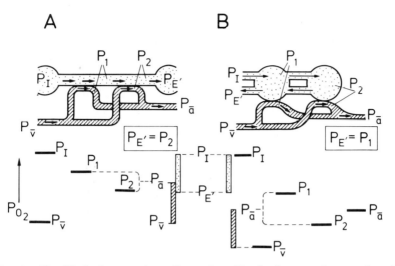

Fig. 10. Simplified schema to show effects of stratification in gas exchange region of (A) avian and (B) mammalian lungs. In the avian flow-through system, expired gas partial pressure $P_{E'}$ reflects that of the distal compartment, P_2; in the mammalian reciprocating system, $P_{E'} = P_1$.

3. Stratification along the Air Capillaries

Diffusion is the only mechanism by which respired gases are transported within the air capillaries between the parabronchial lumen and the gas/blood separating membrane (Fig. 11). The anatomical situation may be compared with the radial diffusion of gases from the conducting airways into the alveoli of the alveolar lung, except for the generally longer pathways into the air capillaries. Analysis of gas exchange between blood capillaries and air capillaries (Scheid, 1978a) shows that significant concentration gradients exist along the gas phase of the air capillaries. However, the effect of this stratified resistance is restricted, owing to the arrangement of capillary blood flow in the air capillary from peripheral to proximal. In fact, in this countercurrent-like arrangement (Scheid, 1978a) gas can exchange with blood at proximal parts of the air capillary; thus, the (stratified) diffusion resistance offered by the air capillaries does not have to be passed by all gas exchanged with the blood.

The avian air capillary thus provides a stratificational resistance that is not in series with other resistances in the gas transport chain (e.g., gas/blood separating membrane). Hence, the effect of this resistance to mixing of an insoluble tracer gas in the lung air spaces will in general differ from the effect imposed on a gas species that is exchanged with the blood. Similarly, as blood capillaries contact alveoli of all generations in the res-

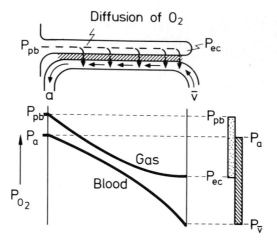

Fig. 11. Stratification in the air capillary of avian parabronchi. Considerable drop in P_{O_2} from value in parabronchial lumen P_{pb} to that at the end of the air capillary P_{ec}. The peculiar arrangement of blood flow past the air capillary (countercurrentlike system) results in only moderate impairment of gas exchange by stratified inhomogeneity.

piratory zone of the alveolar lung, the stratificational resistance derived from insoluble inert gas equilibration studies may in general overestimate that for gases that are exchanged with the blood, e.g., O_2 and CO_2 (see Section VI,B,3).

4. Cardiogenic Mixing in the Parabronchial Lung

The close vicinity of the heart and lungs in the avian thorax results in cardiac tapping of the lung, and gas movement in phase with the heart beat has in fact been measured in the bronchial system of birds (Scheid and Piiper, 1971a). Measurements of Scheid *et al.* (1977) and calculations of Scheid (1978b) suggest that the cardiogenic agitation effects convective mixing between gas in the parabronchi and in adjacent air spaces and results in an increase of the (relatively small) parabronchial gas volume.

B. Fish Gills

1. Series Ventilation

In fish gills respired water flows through narrow spaces bounded by the secondary lamellae (Fig. 12). The direction of water flow in the interlamellar space and of blood flow in the lamella oppose each other (countercurrent system). Although serial concentration gradients in the respiratory medium (water) occur that formally appear to constitute a stratified

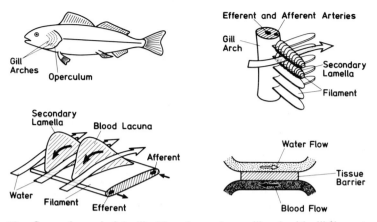

Fig. 12. Gas exchange in fish gills. The scheme shows gill arch with gill filaments, which carry second lamellae. Blood, from afferent arteries, flows through blood lacunae in the secondary lamella, and is drained by efferent arteries. Two adjacent secondary lamellae form the water-perfused interlamellar space. Blood and water flow in opposite directions (countercurrent system).

inhomogeneity, the arterial P_{O_2} can be substantially higher than expired P_{O_2} on account of the mutual arrangement of water and blood in the countercurrent system (Piiper and Scheid, 1975). Hence, as in the crosscurrent model of avian lungs, the structural peculiarities of the system allow negative expired-arterial P_{O_2} differences to occur despite stratification. In fact, the gas exchange efficiency of the countercurrent can even exceed that of the avian crosscurrent system.

2. Diffusion Limitation in Gill Water

It is reasonable to assume that water flow past the secondary lamellae is laminar. Thus diffusion is the only mechanism for transport of respired gases between the central parts of the interlamellar water and the lamellar membrane. Since diffusion coefficients are about 10^5 times smaller in water than in air, radial concentration gradients within the interlamellar water are likely to exist and to limit gas exchange in the gills. In fact, a theoretical analysis and its application to experimental data suggests that the diffusion resistance inside the water is comparable with that of the water/blood barrier (Scheid and Piiper, 1971b, 1976). This diffusion resistance in water should be regarded as a stratificational resistance as it is located in the gas exchange region and constitutes a series resistance to gas transfer with the blood. Scheid and Piiper (1971b) have in fact assessed its effect by an analog model of a resting water layer apposed to the lamellar membrane.

REFERENCES

Adaro, F. (1972). Separation of stratification effects from unequal distribution effects by study of inert gas exchange. *Bull. Physio-Pathol. Respir.* **8,** 164–165.

Adaro, F., and Farhi, L. E. (1971). Effects of intralobular gas diffusion on alveolar gas exchange. *Fed. Proc., Fed. Am. Soc. Exp. Biol.* **30,** 437.

Andrussow, L., and Schramm, B. (1969). Transportphänomene I (Viscosität und Diffusion). *In* "Landolt-Börnstein, Zahlenwerte und Funktionen aus Physik, Chemie, Astronomie, Geophysik und Technik" (H. Borchers, H. Hansen, K. H. Hellwege, K. Schäfer, and E. Schmidt, eds.). Springer-Verlag, Berlin and New York.

Aris, R. (1956). On the dispersion of a solute in a fluid flowing through a tube. *Proc. R. Soc. London, Ser. A* **235,** 67–77.

Baker, L. G., Ultman, J. S., and Rhoades, R. A. (1974). Simultaneous gas flow and diffusion in a symmetric air-way system: a mathematical model. *Respir. Physiol.* **21,** 119–138.

Brès, M., and Hatzfeld, C. (1977). Three-gas diffusion experimental and theoretical study. *Pflügers Arch.* **371,** 227–233.

Chang, H. K., Cheng, R. T., and Farhi, L. E. (1973). A model study of gas diffusion in alveolar sacs. *Respir. Physiol.* **18,** 386–397.

Chang, H. K., Tai, R. C., and Farhi, L. E. (1975). Some implications of ternary diffusion in the lung. *Respir. Physiol.* **23,** 109–120.

Comroe, J. H., Forster, R. E., Dubois, A. B., Briscoe, W. A., and Carlsen, E. (1962). "The Lung," 2nd ed. Yearbook Publ., Chicago, Illinois.

Crank, J. (1975). "The Mathematics of Diffusion," 2nd ed. Oxford Univ. Press (Clarendon), London and New York.

Cumming, G. (1974). Alveolar ventilation: recent model analysis. *In* "Physiology Series One. Vol. 2: Respiratory Physiology" (J. G. Widdicombe, ed.), pp. 139–166. Butterworth, London.

Cumming, G., Crank, J., Horsfield, K., and Parker, I. (1966). Gaseous diffusion in the airways of the human lung. *Respir. Physiol.* **1,** 58–74.

Cumming, G., Horsfield, K., Jones, J. G., and Muir, D. C. F. (1967). The influence of gaseous diffusion on the alveolar plateau at different lung volumes. *Respir. Physiol.* **2,** 386–398.

Cumming, G., Horsfield, K., and Preston, S. (1971). Diffusion equilibrium in the lungs examined by nodal analysis. *Respir. Physiol.* **12,** 329–345.

Cussler, E. L. (1976). "Multicomponent Diffusion." Elsevier, Amsterdam.

Davidson, M. R. (1975). Lung gas mixing during expiration following an inspiration of air. *Bull. Math. Biol.* **37,** 113–126.

Davidson, M. R., and Fitz-Gerald, J. M. (1974). Transport of O_2 along a model pathway through the respiratory region of the lung. *Bull. Math. Biol.* **36,** 275–303.

Engel, L. A., and Macklem, P. T. (1977). Gas mixing and distribution in the lung. *In* "International Review of Physiology. Series II: Respiratory Physiology" (J. G. Widdicombe, ed.), Vol. 14, pp. 37–82. Univ. Park Press, Baltimore, Maryland.

Engel, L. A., Menkes, H., Wood, L. D. H., Utz, G., Joubert, J., and Macklem, P. T. (1973a). Gas mixing during breath holding studied by intrapulmonary gas sampling. *J. Appl. Physiol.* **35,** 9–17.

Engel, L. A., Wood, L. D. H., Utz, G., and Macklem, P. T. (1973b). Gas mixing during inspiration. *J. Appl. Physiol.* **35,** 18–24.

Fairbanks, D. F., and Wilke, C. R. (1950). Diffusion coefficients in multicomponent gas mixtures. *Ind. Eng. Chem.* **42,** 471–475.

Farhi, L. E. (1969). Diffusive and convective movement of gas in the lung. *In* "Circulatory and Respiratory Mass Transport'' (G. E. W. Wolstenholme and J. Knight, eds.), pp. 277–297. Churchill, London.

Farhi, L. E., and Yokoyama, T. (1967). Effects of ventilation–perfusion inequality on elimination of inert gases. *Respir. Physiol.* **3,** 12–20.

Fick, A. (1855). Über Diffusion. *Poggendorfs Ann.* **94,** 59–86.

Flint, L. F., and Eisenklam, P. (1970). Dispersion of matter in transitional flow through straight tubes. *Proc. R. Soc. London, Ser. A* **315,** 519–533.

Fukuchi, Y., Roussos, C. S., Macklem, P. T., and Engel, L. A. (1976). Convection, diffusion and cardiogenic mixing of inspired gas in the lung; an experimental approach. *Respir. Physiol.* **26,** 77–90.

Georg, J., Lassen, N. A., Mellemgaard, K., and Vinther, A. (1965). Diffusion in the gas phase of the lungs in normal and emphysematous subjects. *Clin. Sci.* **29,** 525–532.

Gill, W. N., and Sankarasubramanian, R. (1970). Exact analysis of unsteady convective diffusion. *Proc. R. Soc. London, Ser. A* **316,** 341–350.

Gill, W. N., and Sankarasubramanian, R. (1971). Dispersion of a non-uniform slug in time-dependent flow. *Proc. R. Soc. London, Ser. A* **322,** 101–117.

Gill, W. N., Ananthakrishnan, V., and Nunge, R. J. (1968). Dispersion in developing velocity fields. *AIChEJ.* **14,** 939–946.

Graham, T. (1832). On the law of diffusion of gases. *Philos. Mag.* **2,** 175–190, 269–276, 351–358.

Hansen, J. E., and Ampaya, E. P. (1974). Lung morphometry: A fallacy in the use of the counting principle. *J. Appl. Physiol.* **37,** 951–954.

Hansen, J. E., Ampaya, E. P., Bryant, G. H., and Navin, J. J. (1975). Branching pattern of airways and air spaces of a single human terminal bronchiole. *J. Appl. Physiol.* **38,** 983–989.

Hogg, W., Brunton, F., Kryger, M., Brown, R., and Macklem, P. (1972). Gas diffusion across collateral channels. *F. Appl. Physiol.* **38,** 568–575.

Jacobs, M. H. (1935). Diffusion processes. *Ergeb. Biol.* **12,** 1–160. (Reprinted as monograph "Diffusion Processes." Springer-Verlag, Berlin and New York, 1967.)

Johnson, L. R., and Van Liew, H. D. (1974). Use of arterial P_{O_2} to study convective and diffusive gas mixing in the lungs. *J. Appl. Physiol.* **36,** 91–97.

Kawashiro, T., Sikand, R. S., Adaro, F., Takahashi, H., and Piiper, J. (1976). Study of intrapulmonary gas mixing in man by simultaneous wash-out of helium and sulfur hexafluoride. *Respir. Physiol.* **28,** 261–275.

Kjellmer, I., Sandqvist, L., and Berlund, E. (1959). "Alveolar plateau" of the single breath nitrogen elimination curve in normal subjects. *J. Appl. Physiol.* **14,** 105–108.

Krogh, A., and Lindhard, J. (1914). On the average composition of the alveolar air and its variation during the respiratory cycle. *J. Physiol. (London)* **47,** 431–445.

Krogh, A., and Lindhard, J. (1917). The volume of the dead space in breathing and the mixing of gases in the lungs of man. *J. Physiol. (London)* **51,** 59–90.

Kvale, P. A., Davis, J., and Schroter, R. C. (1975). Effect of gas density and ventilatory pattern on steady state CO uptake by the lung. *Respir. Physiol.* **24,** 385–398.

La Force, R. C., and Lewis, B. M. (1970). Diffusional transport in the human lung. *J. Appl. Physiol.* **28,** 291–298.

Mazzone, R. W., Modell, H. I., and Farhi, L. E. (1976). Interaction of convection and diffusion in pulmonary gas transport. *Respir. Physiol.* **28,** 217–225.

Modell, A. I., and Farhi, L. E. (1976). Ternary gas diffusion—*in vitro* studies. *Respir. Physiol.* **27,** 65–71.

Okubo, T., and Piiper, J. (1974). Intrapulmonary gas mixing in excised dog lung lobes studied by simultaneous wash-out of two inert gases. *Respir. Physiol.* **21,** 223–239.

Pack, A., Hooper, M. B., Nixon, W., and Taylor, J. C. (1977). A computational model of pulmonary gas transport incorpoating effective diffusion. *Respir. Physiol.* **29**, 101–124.

Paiva, M. (1972a). Stochastic simulation of the gas diffusion in the air phase of the human lung. *Bull. Math. Biophys.* **34**, 457–466.

Paiva, M. (1972b). Computation of the boundary conditions for diffusion in the human lung. *Comput. Biomed. Res.* **5**, 585–595.

Paiva, M. (1973). Gas transport in the human lung. *J. Appl. Physiol.* **35**, 401–410.

Paiva, M. (1974). Gaseous diffusion in an alveolar duct simulated by a digital computer. *Comput. Biomed. Res.* **7**, 533–543.

Paiva, M., Lacquet, L. M., and Van der Linden, L. P. (1976). Gas transport in a model derived from Hansen–Ampaya anatomical data of the human lung. *J. Appl. Physiol.* **41**, 115–119.

Pedley, T. J. (1970). A theory for gas mixing in a simple model of the lung. *AGARD Conf. Proc.* **65**.

Pedley, T. J. (1977). Pulmonary fluid dynamics. *Annu. Rev. Fluid Mech.* **9**, 229–274.

Pedley, T. J., Schroter, R. C., and Sudlow, M. F. (1977). Gas flow and mixing in the airways. *In* "Bioengineering Aspects of the Lung" (J. B. West, ed.), pp. 163–265. Dekker, New York.

Piiper, J. (1979). Series ventilation, diffusion in airways and stratified inhomogeneity. *Fed. Proc., Fed. Am. Soc. Exp. Biol.* **38**, 17–21.

Piiper, J., and Meyer, M. (1978). Pulmonary diffusing capacity for CO and O_2 measured simultaneously by a rebreathing technique. *Fed. Proc., Fed. Am. Soc. Exp. Biol.* **37**, 905.

Piiper, J., and Scheid, P. (1971). Respiration: Alveolar gas exchange. *Annu. Rev. Physiol.* **33**, 131–154.

Piiper, J., and Scheid, P. (1975). Gas transport efficacy of gills, lungs and skin: Theory and experimental data. *Respir. Physiol.* **23**, 209–221.

Piiper, J., and Scheid, P. (1977). Comparative physiology of respiration: Functional analysis of gas exchange organs in vertebrates. *In* "International Review of Physiology. Series II: Respiratory Physiology" (J. G. Widdicombe, ed.), Vol. 14, pp. 219–253. Univ. Park Press, Baltimore, Maryland.

Piiper, J., Dejours, P., Haab, P., and Rahn, H. (1971). Concepts and basic quantities in gas exchange physiology. *Respir. Physiol.* **13**, 292–304.

Power, G. G. (1969). Gaseous diffusion between airways and alveoli in the human lung. *J. Appl. Physiol.* **27**, 701–709.

Radford, E. P. (1964). The physics of gases. *In* "Handbook of Physiology. Sect. 3: Respiration" (W. O. Fenn and H. Rahn, ed.), Vol. 1, pp. 125–152. Am. Physiol. Soc., Washington, D.C.

Rauwerda, P. E. (1946). Unequal ventilation of different parts of the lung and the determination of cardiac output. Ph.D. Thesis, State Univ. of Groningen, Groningen, The Netherlands.

Reid, R. C., and Sherwood, T. K. (1966). "The Properties of Gases and Liquids," 2nd ed. McGraw-Hill, New York.

Scheid, P. (1978a). Analysis of gas exchange between air capillaries and blood capillaries in avian lungs. *Respir. Physiol.* **32**, 27–49.

Scheid, P. (1978b). Estimation of effective parabronchial gas volume during intermittent ventilatory flow: theory and application in the duck. *Respir. Physiol.* **32**, 1–14.

Scheid, P. (1979). Mechanisms of gas exchange in bird lungs. *Rev. Physiol. Biochem. Pharmacol.* **86**, 137–186.

Scheid, P., and Piiper, J. (1971a). Direct measurement of the pathway of respired gas in duck lungs. *Respir. Physiol.* **11,** 308–314.

Scheid, P., and Piiper, J. (1971b). Theoretical analysis of respiratory gas equilibration in water passing through fish gills. *Respir. Physiol.* **13,** 305–318.

Scheid, P., and Piiper, J. (1972). Cross-current gas exchange in avian lungs: Effects of reversed parabronchial air flow in ducks. *Respir. Physiol.* **16,** 304–312.

Scheid, P., and Piiper, J. (1976). Quantitative functional analysis of branchial gas transfer: Theory and application to *Scyliorhinus stellaris (Elasmobranchii). In* "Respiration of Amphibious Vertebrates" (G. M. Hughes, ed.), pp. 17–38. Academic Press, New York.

Scheid, P., Worth, H., Holle, J. P., and Meyer, M. (1977). Effects of oscillating and intermittent ventilatory flow on efficacy of pulmonary O_2 transfer in the duck. *Respir. Physiol.* **31,** 251–258.

Scherer, P. W., Shendalman, L. H., and Greene, N. M. (1972). Simultaneous diffusion and convection in single breath lung washout. *Bull. Math. Biophys.* **34,** 393–412.

Scherer, P. W., Shendalman, L. H., Greene, N. M., and Bouhuys, A. (1975). Measurement of axial diffusivities in a model of the bronchial airways. *J. Appl. Physiol.* **38,** 719–723.

Sikand, R. S., Cerretelli, P., and Farhi, L. E. (1966). Effects of $\dot{V}_A$ and $\dot{V}_A/\dot{Q}$ distribution and of time on the alveolar plateau. *J. Appl. Physiol.* **21,** 1331–1337.

Sikand, R. S., Magnussen, H., Scheid, P., and Piiper, J. (1976). Convective and diffusive gas mixing in human lungs: Experiments and model analysis. *J. Appl. Physiol.* **40,** 362–371.

Stefan, J. (1871). Über das Gleichgewicht und die Bewegung, insbesondere die Diffusion von Gasmengen. *Sitzungsber. Akad. Wiss. Wien, Abt. 2* **63,** 63–124.

Taylor, G. I. (1953). Dispersion of soluble matter in solvent flowing slowly through a tube. *Proc. R. Soc. London, Ser. A* **219,** 186–203.

Taylor, G. I. (1954). The dispersion of matter in turbulent flow through a pipe. *Proc. R. Soc. London, Ser. A* **223,** 446–468.

Toor, H. L. (1964a). Solution of the linearized equations of multicomponent mass transfer: I. *AIChE J.* **10,** 448–455.

Toor, H. L. (1964b). Solution of the linearized equations of multicomponent mass transfer: II. Matrix methods. *AIChE J.* **10,** 460–465.

Van Liew, H. D., and Mazzone, R. W. (1977). Mixing in flowing gas. *Respir. Physiol.* **30,** 27–34.

Wangensteen, O. D., Wilson, D., and Rahn, H. (1970–1971). Diffusion of gases across the shell of the hen's egg. *Respir. Physiol.* **11,** 16–30.

Weibel, E. R. (1963). "Morphometry of the Human Lung." Springer-Verlag, Berlin and New York.

Weis-Fogh, T. (1964). Diffusion in insect wing muscle, the most active tissue known. *J. Exp. Biol.* **41,** 229–256.

West, J. B., Glazier, J. B., Hughes, J. M. B., and Maloney, J. E. (1969). Pulmonary capillary *siol.* **30,** 479–487.

West, J. B., Blazier, J. B., Hughes, J. M. B., and Maloney, J. E. (1969). Pulmonary capillary flow, diffusion, ventilation and gas exchange. *In* "Circulatory and Respiratory Mass Transport" (G. E. W. Wolstenholme and J. Knight, eds.), pp. 256–272. Churchill, London.

Wilke, C. R. (1950). Diffusional properties of multicomponent gases. *Chem. Eng. Prog.* **46,** 95–104.

Wilson, T. A., and Lin, K.-H. (1970). Convection and diffusion in the airways and the design of the bronchial tree. *In* "Airway Dynamics" (A. Bouhuys, ed.), pp. 5–19. Thomas, Springfield, Illinois.

Worth, H., and Piiper, J. (1978a). Diffusion of helium, carbon monoxide and sulfur hexafluoride in gas mixtures similar to alveolar gas. *Respir. Physiol.* **32**, 155–166.

Worth, H., and Piiper, J. (1978b). Model experiments on diffusional equilibration of oxygen and carbon dioxide between inspired and alveolar gas. *Respir. Physiol.* **35**, 1–7.

Worth, H., Takahashi, H., Willmer, H., and Piiper, J. (1976). Pulmonary gas exchange in dogs ventilated with mixtures of oxygen with various inert gases. *Respir. Physiol.* **28**, 1–15.

Worth, H., Adaro, F., and Piiper, J. (1977). Penetration of inhaled He and SF_6 into alveolar space at low tidal volumes. *J. Appl. Physiol.* **43**, 403–408.

Worth, H., Nüsse, W., and Piiper, J. (1978). Determination of binary diffusion coefficients of various gas species used in respiratory physiology. *Respir. Physiol.* **32**, 15–26.

Yu, C. P. (1975). On equation of gas transport in the lung. *Respir. Physiol.* **23**, 257–266.

5

Blood–Gas Equilibration in Lungs

Johannes Piiper and Peter Scheid

PULMONARY GAS EXCHANGE, VOL. I
Copyright © 1980 by Academic Press, Inc.
All rights of reproduction in any form reserved.
ISBN 0-12-744501-3

I. EQUILIBRIUM CONDITION

A. Concepts

It is generally accepted that diffusion is the mechanism by which gases are transported across the alveolar membrane. The transfer rate of a gas species is thus determined, both in direction and in magnitude, by the difference in its partial pressure between alveolar gas and capillary blood. With finite exchange rate, partial pressures in alveolar gas and in capillary blood will approach each other. This equilibration process is discussed in Section II. Distinct from the equilibration of end-capillary blood and alveolar gas is the situation when the net transfer of a gas species is zero. This implies partial pressure equilibrium between pulmonary capillary blood and alveolar gas all along the contact length.

It should thus be possible to measure, by noninvasive techniques, mixed-venous partial pressure of gas as its alveolar partial pressure when its net exchange is abolished. The principle of using the lung in this way as an aerotonometer (Pflüger) dates back to Wolffberg (1871), but technical problems have precluded its reliable application until recently. The main interest has centered around measurement of $P_{\bar{v}_{O_2}}$ and $P_{\bar{v}_{CO_2}}$ for use with the (indirect) Fick principle in calculating cardiac output (cf. Hamilton, 1962; Butler, 1965).

B. Methods for Determining Lung Gas Equilibrium

To attain blood–gas equilibrium, the alveolar space must be functionally closed and time must be allowed for the equilibrium to establish. The time required depends among other factors on the diffusive and perfusive conductances of the gas under study (see Section II); it must not exceed the recirculation time, 10–20 sec, as from then on $P_{\bar{v}}$ will change with time. Basically two methods have been used to realize gas–blood equilibrium directly or by extrapolation in man.

With the *breath-holding methods* (Christiansen *et al.,* 1914) an appropriate mixture is inspired, the breath is held, and an expired sample is analyzed for the gas composition. Many variations of this procedure have been developed that allow estimation of $P_{\bar{v}}$ even when equilibrium is not complete (Fenn and Dejours, 1954; Kim *et al.*, 1966; cf. Farhi and Haab, 1967).

More widely used have been *rebreathing methods,* introduced by Plesch (1909) and utilized in many variations to date to estimate $P_{\bar{v}}$. The subject breathes in and out of a bag, in an attempt to establish gas concentration equality between lung and bag, the gas composition of which can be measured. This method has become particularly successful with the development of rapid, continuous gas analyzers (e.g., respiratory mass spectrometers). Attainment of gas–blood equilibrium during rebreathing is recognized by a "rebreathing plateau," i.e., $dP_A/dt = 0$. During this period, it may be assumed that $P_A = P_{\bar{v}} \,(=P_a)$. Most widely practiced have been the plateau method of Collier (1956) and the slope method of Defares (1958; see Jernérus *et al.*, 1963; Dension *et al.*, 1969).

C. Interactions among Gases during Equilibrium

Presence of the "background" gases impose certain constraints that have to be observed for exact analysis of the equilibrium of any gas.

1. Interaction between CO_2 and O_2

When breath-holding or rebreathing is performed with O_2-rich mixtures, CO_2 may closely approach equilibrium. However, the equilibrium condition of zero net CO_2 transport and partial pressure equalization between gas and blood cannot simultaneously be attained in this case owing to the Haldane effect. Two cases may be discerned (Fig. 1).

a. $\dot{M}_{CO_2} > 0$ but $P_{\bar{v}_{CO_2}} = P_{A_{CO_2}} = P_{C'_{CO_2}}$. This is the case when the respiratory exchange ratio $R = \dot{M}_{CO_2}/\dot{M}_{O_2}$ equals the Haldane factor (CO_2 con-

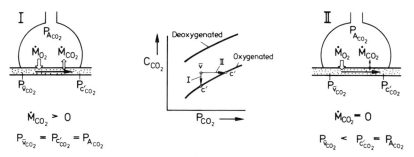

Fig. 1. Action of the Haldane effect on CO_2 equilibrium during breath-holding or rebreathing when there is O_2 uptake from alveolar space into blood. For details, see the text.

centration change in blood per change in chemically bound O_2 at constant P_{CO_2}, approximately 0.32 for human blood). In this case, the rate at which CO_2 is released from hemoglobin upon oxygenation in pulmonary capillaries balances the transport rate of CO_2 into the alveolar space (Kim et al., 1966; Meyer et al., 1976).

b. $\dot{M}_{CO_2} = 0$, *but* $P_{\bar{v}_{CO_2}} < P_{c'_{CO_2}} = P_{A_{CO_2}}$. In this case, CO_2 content in capillary blood, C_{CO_2}, does not change, but P_{CO_2} in blood increases with oxygenation. $P_{c'_{CO_2}}$ for this case is called "oxygenated mixed venous P_{CO_2}" in distinction from the actual value of $P_{\bar{v}_{CO_2}}$ ("true mixed venous P_{CO_2}"). In most rebreathing experiments oxygenated $P_{\bar{v}_{CO_2}}$ has been determined.

O_2 equilibrium is similarly affected by CO_2 transfer. It is evident that for either gas a true equilibrium can only be attained when the other gas is in equilibrium at the same time (Cerretelli et al., 1966).

2. Volume Shrinkage

It can be stated quite generally that true equilibrium conditions for one gas can only be attained in the presence of equilibrium for all the remaining gases. This, however, is impossible in alveolar lungs since the sum of partial pressures of all gases in venous blood is considerably below atmospheric pressure, mainly because of the steeper CO_2 than O_2 dissociation curve (and to a lesser extent to $R < 1.0$).

A detailed analysis by Piiper (1965) shows that a steady state of "constant composition" will be reached in a closed lung "pocket" in which $dP_A/dt = 0$, yet $P_A > P_{\bar{v}}$ for all gases. There is a finite gas uptake in this case, which is accompanied by volume shrinkage, $dV/dt < 0$. The discrepancy between P_A and $P_{\bar{v}}$ for the individual gases depends on the relative conductances (see below) and is more marked for O_2 than for CO_2. When a gas of low solubility (e.g., N_2) constitutes the main background component, $P_A \approx P_{\bar{v}}$ for O_2 and CO_2 and $dV/dt \approx 0$. When the lung is open, lung shrinkage is prevented by fresh gas drawn into the alveolar space.

D. CO_2 Equilibrium

Partial pressure equilibrium at conditions of no net gas transfer had been the presupposition when methods for bloodless measurement of $P_{\bar{v}}$ were developed. A direct proof for O_2 and CO_2 became possible only recently with the development of direct techniques for measurement of P_{O_2} and P_{CO_2} in blood. For O_2, equality between alveolar and blood partial pressures at zero uptake was observed (Denison et al., 1969; Jones et al., 1969; Cerretelli et al., 1970; see, however, Yu et al., 1973). For CO_2, however, several authors found the gas partial pressure to exceed the blood value in conditions when equality (e.g., rebreathing plateau) or a higher blood than gas P_{CO_2} (e.g., in steady gas exchange) were expected (Piiper and Scheid, 1971; Forster and Crandall, 1976). During rebreathing with no net gas transfer, small positive gas–blood P_{CO_2} differences may be expected from H^+ disequilibrium and from slow reaction kinetics of CO_2/HCO_3^- in blood; however, in steady state with net CO_2 elimination from blood to alveolar gas, these mechanisms are unable to explain positive gas–blood P_{CO_2} differences (Hill et al., 1973; Forster and Crandall, 1975; Bidani and Crandall, 1978).

Some authors have derived empirical correction factors for using the rebreathing P_{CO_2} in the indirect (CO_2) Fick method for cardiac output (Dension et al., 1969; Jones et al., 1969). However, of greater significance are the consequences of equilibrium P_{CO_2} differences, if they exist in steady state, for the analysis of alveolar gas exchange. In fact, in their presence, the ideal alveolar P_{O_2} concept (see below) would lead to errors in determining alveolar dead space ventilation, shuntlike effects of inhomogeneities, and pulmonary diffusing capacity for O_2 and CO_2 (cf. Piiper and Scheid, 1971). We thus briefly review the evidence for and against existence of positive gas-to-blood P_{CO_2} differences (ΔP_{CO_2}).

1. Rebreathing Experiments

A number of authors have reported positive, alveolar-to-mixed venous, $(A - \bar{v})_{CO_2}$, or alveolar-to-arterial P_{CO_2} differences, $(A - a)_{CO_2}$, in rebreathing conditions when CO_2 exchange was abolished. Such results have been reported in anesthetized dogs (Gurtner et al., 1969; Guyatt et al., 1973; Yu et al., 1973), in normal subjects at rest and during exercise, and in patients (Jones et al., 1967, 1969, 1972; Clark, 1968; Denison et al., 1969, 1971; Field et al., 1971; Laszlo et al., 1971). In many cases, positive ΔP_{CO_2} were not seen at rest but only in exercise. In some cases, prolonged rebreathing apparently abolished ΔP_{CO_2}. In other studies, positive ΔP_{CO_2} under similar experimental conditions were not observed (Collier, 1956; Cain and Otis, 1960; Clausen et al., 1970; McEvoy et al., 1973; Scheid et al., 1972).

Scheid et al. (1972) performed experiments in dogs under well-controlled conditions similar to those of other authors who had observed positive ΔP_{CO_2}. The four experimental methods used are illustrated in Fig. 2. The striking result was that with none of the methods significant gas–blood P_{CO_2} differences were found, even under conditions when theories (Gurtner et al., 1969) would predict enhancement of positive differences (e.g., high pulmonary blood flow, high P_{CO_2}, and low pH in mixed venous blood).

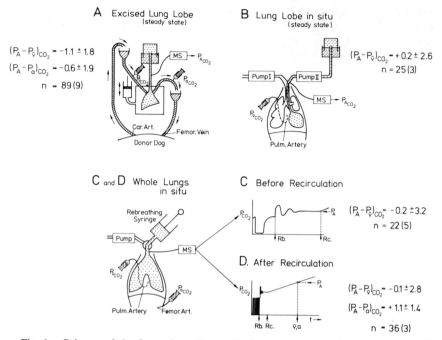

Fig. 2. Scheme of the four rebreathing methods used in the study of blood–gas CO_2 equilibrium in dog lungs. Average results ($\pm$ SD; n, number of measurements; in brackets, number of dogs) are indicated for P_{CO_2} differences between alveolar gas and (mixed venous or arterial) blood. (Modified from Scheid *et al.*, 1972.)

2. Measurements in Steady State

a. Experiments in Man. Under resting conditions most authors found end-expired (or calculated alveolar) P_{CO_2} to be close to arterial P_{CO_2}, or slightly below (Ulmer and Reichel, 1961; Larson and Severinghaus, 1962; West, 1962; Clausen *et al.*, 1970). However, Jones *et al.* (1966) and Whipp and Wasserman (1969) observed positive gas–blood differences under these conditions. Particularly at high CO_2 output, they may be caused by the fluctuations in alveolar P_{CO_2} [cf. Matell (1963); Piiper and Scheid (1971); see Section IV,D].

b. Experiments on Dogs. Jennings and Chen (1975) found in resting conscious dogs in acute or chronic hypercapnia (inhaling 5–10% CO_2) higher P_{CO_2} in mixed-expired gas than in arterial blood. With 10% inspired CO_2, mixed-expired P_{CO_2} was even higher than mixed venous P_{CO_2}. These results were not confirmed by Scheid *et al.* (1979a), who found blood P_{CO_2} to be above or equal to alveolar P_{CO_2} under similar conditions in anesthetized dogs.

c. Experiments in Chickens. Davies and Dutton (1975) found in the chicken in steady state conditions that end-expired P_{CO_2} exceeded not only arterial P_{CO_2} [this is explained by the crosscurrent model for avian lungs according to Scheid and Piiper (1970, 1972)], but also mixed venous P_{CO_2}. Meyer *et al.* (1976) reproduced the finding of positive end expired-to-mixed venous P_{CO_2} differences in the chicken, but concluded from rebreathing experiments and theoretical considerations that the positive $(P_{E'} - P_{\bar{v}})_{CO_2}$ during steady state is caused by a particular action of the Haldane effect in a crosscurrent gas exchange system, without a positive gas–blood P_{CO_2} difference across the blood–gas membrane occurring anywhere in the lung.

d. Multiple Inert-Gas Infusion Experiments. Robertson and Hlastala (1977) compared the pulmonary clearance of CO_2 in anesthetized dogs with that of five inert gases of different solubilities, infused intravenously. They found the excretion of CO_2 to be higher than predicted from the behavior of the inert gases. The results were best explained by assuming a negative arterial-to-alveolar P_{CO_2} difference of 5 torr.

3. Conclusions

The present experimental evidence for positive gas–blood P_{CO_2} differences in lungs is conflicting. The theories invoked for their explanation are in part not easy to accept (cf. Piiper and Scheid, 1971; Effros, 1972). Further experimentation is required in which particular care must be directed to a number of experimental parameters, neglect of which can produce apparent positive gas–blood P_{CO_2} differences. Clarification of this issue is mandatory for the understanding of pulmonary gas exchange [recently reviewed by Piiper (1979) and Scheid and Piiper (1980)].

II. DIFFUSION LIMITATION: CONCEPT AND GENERAL MODEL

The large alveolar–capillary surface area and the minute thickness of the tissue layers separating blood from alveolar air create conditions that allow efficient diffusive equilibration between blood and alveolar gas with respect to O_2 and CO_2. However, the diffusive conductance (i.e., diffusing capacity) of lungs is finite and is thus expected to limit O_2 transfer, particularly under critical conditions (reduced atmospheric P_{O_2}, increased O_2 demand in heavy exercise, diseased lungs).

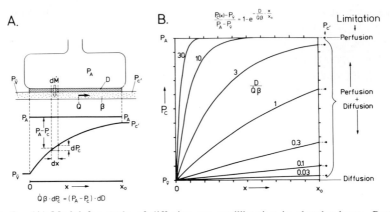

Fig. 3. (A) Model for study of diffusive gas equilibration in alveolar lungs. Partial-pressure equilibration in blood from mixed venous ($P_{\bar{v}}$) toward alveolar (P_A) value. $P_{c'}$, partial pressure in end-capillary blood; $d\dot{M}$, gas transfer rate through membrane elements of diffusing capacity, dD, into blood in element of capillary length dx, giving rise to increase dP_c of blood partial pressure (see equation below); β, β_g, capacitance coefficients in blood and gas. (B) Equilibration profiles for various values of parameter $D/(\dot{Q}\beta)$ as determined by equation at top. x, contact length of capillary with alveolar space, from 0 to x_0. High values of this parameter, perfusion limitation; low values, diffusion limitation (to the right).

A. Model

A very simple model, shown in Fig. 3, will be used to establish the basic principles of diffusive gas equilibration. This model consists of a blood stream (pulmonary capillary blood) that is separated from a homogeneous gas space (alveolar gas) by a membrane (tissue layer) representing a resistance to diffusion. (The composite nature of this "membrane," which functionally may include diffusion and reaction in blood, is discussed in Section IV,A.)

Fick's second law of diffusion may be used to describe gas transfer across the membrane. The differential equation relating blood flow ($\dot{Q}$), "capacitance coefficient" [β, see Piiper *et al.* (1971b)], and diffusing capacity (D) to the alveolar (P_A) and blood (P_c) partial pressures is shown in Fig. 3A. Its integration yields the relationship shown in Fig. 3B for P_c at a distance x from the venous end of the capillary. Its plot in Fig. 3B reveals the decisive influence of the variable $D/(\dot{Q}\beta)$ upon the course of equilibration. The equilibration reached in the end-capillary blood ($x = x_0$, $P_c = P_{c'}$) is shown to the right in Fig. 3B. The total transfer rate $\dot{M}$ may be obtained from this relationship and the mass balance in in-flowing and out-flowing blood:

$$\dot{M} = (P_A - P_v)\dot{Q}\beta(1 - e^{-D/(\dot{Q}\beta)}) \tag{1}$$

The (total) conductance G for gas exchange between alveolar air and capillary blood may be defined as transfer rate divided by the total effective partial pressure difference $(P_A - P_{\bar{v}})$,

$$G = \dot{Q}\beta(1 - e^{-D/(\dot{Q}\beta)}) \tag{2}$$

B. Limitation by Diffusion and Perfusion

If D is large so that $D \gg \dot{Q}\beta$, gas transfer is limited by perfusion only; in this case, the (perfusive) conductance

$$G = \dot{Q}\beta \tag{3}$$

The relative difference between the conductance without diffusion limitation and the actual conductance is an index for diffusion limitation, L_{diff} (see Fig. 4).

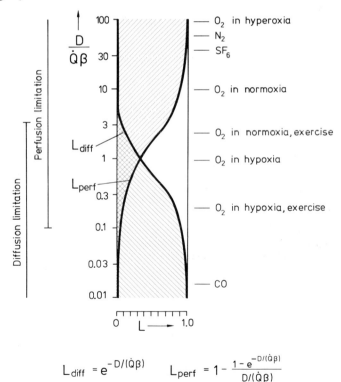

$$L_{\text{diff}} = e^{-D/(\dot{Q}\beta)} \qquad L_{\text{perf}} = 1 - \frac{1 - e^{-D/(\dot{Q}\beta)}}{D/(\dot{Q}\beta)}$$

Fig. 4. Dependence of limitation by diffusion, L_{diff}, and by perfusion, L_{perf}, (abscissa) upon $D/(\dot{Q}\beta)$ (ordinate, logarithmic). The lines to the left extend over the respective ranges in which $L > 5\%$. Approximate ranges for some gases in different experimental situations are shown to the right.

Similarly, if $\dot{Q}\beta$ is large so that $\dot{Q}\beta \gg D$, transfer rate is limited by diffusion only. In this case, the (diffusive) conductance

$$G = D \tag{4}$$

The relative difference between the conductance without perfusion limitation and the actual conductance is an index for perfusion limitation L_{perf} (see Fig. 4). The role of diffusion and perfusion limitation is determined by the quotient $D/(\dot{Q}\beta)$, i.e., by the relative magnitudes of diffusive conductance (D) and perfusive conductance ($\dot{Q}\beta$).

The relationships are illustrated in Figs. 3 and 4. When $0.1 < D/(\dot{Q}\beta) < 3$, transfer is both diffusion and perfusion limited. Outside this range, only diffusion ($D/(\dot{Q}\beta) < 0.1$) or perfusion ($D/(\dot{Q}\beta) > 3$) limits gas exchange significantly ($>5\%$). Other authors have expressed diffusion limitation by use of "apparent" values for β (Gong et al., 1972b) or $\dot{Q}$ (Hyde et al., 1968), which may be derived from Eqs. (2) and (3).

C. Physical Properties of Gases

The diffusing capacity for a tissue membrane comprises a number of factors:

$$D = d\alpha F/\ell \tag{5}$$

in which d is the diffusion coefficient, α the solubility coefficient, F the surface area of the barrier, and ℓ the thickness of the barrier. Substitution of Eq. (5) into the $D/(\dot{Q}\beta)$ ratio reveals that the following physical properties of gases are of importance: (1) diffusivity in the barrier (d), and (2) blood/barrier solubility ratio (β/α).

The solubility ratio for inert gases, independent of their solubilities, is close to unity. For gases chemically bound in blood, O_2, CO, and CO_2, the β/α ratio is much greater than unity. The variation of the β/α ratio among different gas species encompasses a much wider range than that of the diffusion coefficient d.

The $D/(\dot{Q}\beta)$ values for transfer of O_2, CO_2, CO, and some inert gases in normal human lungs are indicated in Fig. 4: (1) All inert gases of potential use in respiratory physiology, even SF_6, are not diffusion limited. (2) CO transfer is practically exclusively diffusion limited (very high β/α ratio); only in lung regions with very low $\dot{Q}$ may perfusion limitation become perceptible. (3) O_2 is perfusion limited in hyperoxia and also in normoxia (except in regions with elevated $\dot{Q}$, and at heavy exercise), but in hypoxia diffusion limitation is present and particularly so during heavy exercise.

III. LUNG MODELS AND EXPERIMENTAL DESIGNS FOR DETERMINATION OF PULMONARY DIFFUSING CAPACITY

For a quantitative experimental study of alveolar–capillary diffusion, steady state or non-steady state methods may be used.

A. Steady State Methods

The relationship that describes lung gas equilibration (Fig. 3B) may be applied to O_2 and solved for D (use being made of the mass balance in blood):

$$D_{O_2} = \frac{\dot{M}_{O_2}}{(P_{c'} - P_{\bar{v}})_{O_2}} \ln \left(\frac{P_A - P_{\bar{v}}}{P_A - P_{c'}} \right) \tag{6}$$

This equation allows calculation of D_{O_2} from measured values for P_{O_2} and O_2 uptake. Equation (6) is valid for β_{O_2} = const, i.e., for an O_2 dissociation curve that is linear in the range between P_v and $P_{c'}$. Such an approximately linear range can be assumed for human and dog blood between P_{O_2} = 40 and 15 torr. In this range, β_{O_2} is maximal and hence the ratio $D/(\dot{Q}\beta)$ is minimal. Diffusion limitation is thus most pronounced so that estimation of D becomes technically feasible. If the condition β_{O_2} = const cannot be met accurately enough, D may be obtained by the Bohr integration technique, which has been improved and simplified by Farhi and Riley (1957), Briehl and Fishman (1960), and King and Briscoe (1967).

There is evidence that O_2 transfer is partly reaction limited, particularly with increasing S_{O_2} (Staub et al., 1962; Thews, 1963). To take this into account, an appropriate effective (dynamic) O_2 dissociation curve may be used. According to Thews (1968) this dynamic curve for normoxic conditions is close to a straight-line relationship between $P_{\bar{v}_{O_2}}$ and $P_{A_{O_2}}$.

For CO, whose transfer is practically purely diffusion limited, $P_{c'} - P_{\bar{v}} = 0$, Eq. (6) simplifies to

$$D_{CO} = \dot{M}_{CO}/(P_A - P_{\bar{v}})_{CO} \tag{7}$$

The equation is further simplified if $P_{\bar{v}}$ can be assumed to be zero (nonsmokers, no preceding exposure to CO).

B. Unsteady State Methods: General Features

In these methods an existing equilibrium for gas exchange is disturbed in a stepwise manner and the approach to a new steady state is observed (usually by measuring P_A). The kinetics of this approach is determined by several variables, notably by conductances (diffusive, convective) and capacitances (volumes).

The simplest lung model may be represented by a constant conductance and a single capacitance (volume compartment), the time course of approach of P_A to $P_{\bar{v}}$ being monoexponential in this case. This model (model I, Fig. 5) is commonly used for breath-holding experiments. Model II (Fig. 5) depicts the situation realized in rebreathing between an alveolar compartment and a bag. In this case, the time course of changing P_A toward $P_{\bar{v}}$ is biexponential. Distinct from these "closed" methods (breath-holding, rebreathing) is an "open" method in which a sudden step change, e.g., of inspired gas composition, is imposed during open-circuit breathing (Fig. 5, model III).

The differential equations governing mass transport in the alveolar lung are presented for each of the three models in Fig. 5. An apparently straight portion is seen in the semilog plots of the difference of P_A and its asymptotic value, after completion of initial mixing and before recircula-

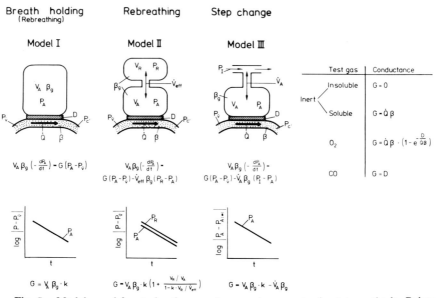

Fig. 5. Models used for study of gas exchange using non-steady state methods. Below each model, differential equation determining the rate of change of alveolar partial pressure. Semilogarithmic plots (schematic) for each model, displaying linear range before recirculation, from which rate constants k may be determined. For each model, the relationship between conductance G and k is depicted below. To the right, conductance for various test gases [cf. Eqs. (2)–(4)]. For details, see the text.

tion. This may be used to extract the rate constant k, which is related to the model parameters as shown in Fig. 5. The total conductance G, which determines alveolar–capillary transfer (see Section II) is different for different test gases used, inert (soluble or insoluble) gases, O_2, or CO (tabulated in Fig. 5). In practice, k is determined and used to calculate D (O_2, CO) or $\dot{Q}$ (soluble inert gases) with the other parameters known or measured. The relationships used for this calculation are tabulated in Fig. 6. They follow from the expressions given for k of the various models in conjunction with G for the various gases.

The continuous change of alveolar partial pressure is superimposed on changes in capillary partial pressure taking place within a capillary blood transit [0.5–1 sec (Johnson *et al.*, 1960)]. Since the equilibration of alveolar gas is slow compared with the capillary contact time, the partial pressure changes in a capillary may be considered as equilibration to a constant alveolar gas [the inherent small error is discussed in Hyde *et al.* (1966)].

C. Breath-Holding (Single-Breath) Methods (Model I)

In the well-known single-breath D_{CO} method a mixture containing about 0.3% CO is inspired (from RV to TLC) and expired after 10 sec of breath-holding (Forster *et al.*, 1954; Ogilvie *et al.*, 1957). Then k is computed from the breath-holding time t and the alveolar P_{CO} at the beginning $[P_A(0)]$ and at the end of breath-holding $P_A(t)$ considering, if necessary, P_{CO} in blood (P_b, back pressure). The single-breath curve may also be analyzed using several values of P_A along a slow continuous expiration (Newth *et al.*, 1977).

Hyde *et al.* (1966) have elaborated an experimental procedure for determination of single-breath D_{O_2} with isotopic O_2 in tracer concentration (0.2% $^{18}O-^{16}O$), which was later used by Cross *et al.* (1969), Garman *et al.* (1970), and Gong *et al.* (1972b). In our terminology, $\dot{Q}$ is calculated from the rate constant k for C_2H_2 equilibration, and D_{O_2} from k for isotopic O_2 equilibration, using $\dot{Q}$ and V_A (determined from dilution of neon). Important is that prior to the breath-holding maneuver, the subject rebreathes to bring alveolar P_{CO_2} and P_{O_2} close to their mixed venous values, which creates conditions allowing a simple evaluation of the equilibration of isotopic O_2 (see below).

When breath-holding is applied to a soluble inert gas such as C_2H_2 (perfusion limitation), $k_{C_2H_2}$ allows calculation of $\dot{Q}$. For V_A, the equivalent diluting space for C_2H_2 (V_A') comprising lung tissue volume must be used (see below).

	Breath holding	Rebreathing	Step change
Insoluble gas $\quad V_A$	$V_I \dfrac{P_I}{P_A}$	$V_R \dfrac{P_{R(0)} - P_{A(\infty)}}{P_{A(\infty)}}$	$V_E \dfrac{P_E - P_{I(2)}}{P_{I(1)} - P_{I(2)}}$
$\dot{V}$	—	$\dfrac{k}{1/V_R + 1/V_A}$	kV_A
Soluble inert gas $\quad \dot{Q}$	$\dfrac{kV'_A\beta_g}{\beta}$	$\dfrac{kV'_A\beta_g}{\beta}\left(1 + \dfrac{V_R/V_A}{1 - kV_R/\dot{V}_{\text{eff}}}\right)$	$\dfrac{kV'_A\beta_g}{\beta}\left(1 - \dfrac{\dot{V}_A}{kV_A}\right)$
Oxygen $\quad D_{O_2}$	$\dot{Q}\beta \ln\left(\dfrac{1}{1 - k\dfrac{V_A\beta_g}{\dot{Q}\beta}}\right)$	$\dot{Q}\beta \ln\left[\dfrac{1}{1 - k\dfrac{V_A\beta_g}{\dot{Q}\beta}\left(1 + \dfrac{V_R/V_A}{1 - kV_R/V_{\text{eff}}}\right)}\right]$	$\dot{Q}\beta \ln\left[\dfrac{1}{1 - k\dfrac{V_A\beta_g}{\dot{Q}\beta}\left(1 - \dfrac{\dot{V}_A}{kV_A}\right)}\right]$
Carbon monoxide $\quad D_{CO}$	$V_A\beta_g k$	$V_A\beta_g k\left(1 + \dfrac{V_R/V_A}{1 - kV_R/V_{\text{eff}}}\right)$	$V_A\beta_g k\left(1 - \dfrac{\dot{V}_A}{kV_A}\right)$

Fig. 6. Equations for calculating model parameters (V_A, $\dot{V}$, $\dot{Q}$, D) from rate constants of various gases in non-steady state methods. Compare with Fig. 5.

D. Rebreathing methods (Models I and II)

When effective ventilation approaches infinity during rebreathing, model I may be used. However, in practice, this condition is not met (ventilation limitation), and model II is more appropriate for analysis of rebreathing kinetics.

Determination of D_{CO} by a rebreathing procedure has been initiated by Kruhøffer (1954; Kjerulf-Jensen and Kruhøffer, 1954). In these studies, ^{14}CO uptake was analyzed from multiple gas samples withdrawn during rebreathing. The method was further applied by Lewis *et al.* (1959), Lawson (1970), and Gong *et al.* (1972a), who utilized infrared CO analyzers with continuous recording or spot sampling.

An important improvement was the introduction of the stable CO isotope, $C^{18}O$ (see below). Rebreathing with isotopic CO ($C^{18}O$, ^{13}CO, or $^{13}C^{18}O$) was applied by Sackner *et al.* (1975) and Miller and Camporcsi (1977). These authors utilized model I for their analysis. The more correct

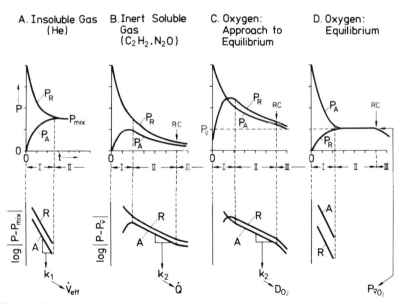

Fig. 7.   Pattern of partial pressure in bag (P_R) and lung (P_A) of various test gases during rebreathing. For gases of low solubility (A) both P_A and P_R approach an equilibrium, P_{mix}. For soluble inert gas (B) and O_2 (C) the initial mixing phase (I) is followed by a phase (II), the kinetics of which is mainly determined by $\dot{Q}$ (B) or D and $\dot{Q}$ (C). Onset of recirculation (RC) delimits phases III and II. The rate constant of phase I, k, for the insoluble gas may be used to calculate $\dot{V}_{eff}(A)$. The rate constant k_2 for the soluble inert gas (B) yields $\dot{Q}$; k_2 for O_2 (C) may be used with $\dot{Q}$ to calculate D_{O_2}. In D, equilibrium is reached for O_2 during phase II between blood and gas, $P_A = P_R = P_{\bar{v}}$.

model II was used by Sølvsteen (1964, 1965a,b), who contributed a systematic theoretical analysis, and by our group (Adaro et al., 1976; Piiper and Meyer, 1978; Meyer, 1979).

For D_{O_2}, the method was progressively developed from a rebreathing method for determination of mixed venous blood P_{O_2} and P_{CO_2} (Cerretelli et al., 1966, 1970). In the first studies, $\dot{Q}$ was determined from rebreathing $P_{\bar{v}_{O_2}}$ and steady state O_2 uptake (Piiper et al., 1971a) or by direct Fick (Adaro et al., 1973; Scheid et al., 1973). Later, after checking against the direct and indirect Fick (Teichmann et al., 1974), $\dot{Q}$ was determined from a soluble inert gas added to the rebreathing mixture (Cerretelli et al., 1974). In animal experiments, the mixed venous P_{O_2} (required for determination of k) was measured directly in blood samples (Adaro et al., 1973; Scheid et al., 1973); in man, $P_{\bar{v}_{O_2}}$ was mostly determined by a separate rebreathing maneuver, or by an extrapolation technique (Veicsteinas et al., 1976), which, however, was later abandoned as not sufficiently accurate. In order to lower normoxic alveolar P_{O_2} close to $P_{\bar{v}_{O_2}}$ rapidly, one or two priming oxygen-free breaths may be administered (Veicsteinas et al., 1976; Piiper and Meyer, 1978).

The behavior of test gases during a rebreathing maneuver for determination of D_{O_2} is schematically illustrated in Fig. 7.

For the volumes V_A and V_R, the mean values between end-inspiration and end-expiration should be used. The total (apparatus + lung) dead space may be obtained from the difference between total and effective ventilation. Functionally, it is part of the (non-gas-exchanging) V_R. The diluting volume for a soluble gas (V'_A) is larger than for an insoluble gas (V_A) by the lung tissue volume equilibrating with inert gas (V_{tis}) times the tissue/gas partition coefficient (β_{tis}/β_g). V_{tis} may be determined by the back-extrapolation procedure of Cander and Forster (1959).

E. Step Change of Inspired Gas (Model III)

This principle was introduced by Burrows and Harper (1958). After a step change of inspired gas from room air to 0.1–0.2% CO in air (or vice versa) was imposed, the wash-in and wash-out of CO were recorded and compared to N_2 wash-out. Thews and co-workers performed experiments in which the inspired fractions of three gases were changed simultaneously: O_2, CO_2, and He or Ar (Thews and Vogel, 1968; Vogel and Thews, 1968; Thews et al., 1971; Schmidt et al., 1972). Both in normal subjects and in patients with lung disease, two compartments with different $\dot{V}_A/\dot{Q}$ and $D/\dot{Q}$ ratios could be discerned (Vogel et al., 1968; Schmidt et al., 1972).

F. Use of Isotopes

Gases containing radioactive isotopes are widely applied in physiological experiments and clinical lung function tests owing to two important advantages: (1) continuous measurement by radiation detectors is relatively easy; (2) local measurement over restricted lung areas is possible. Using short-lived radioactive isotopes of CO_2, O_2, and CO, West and co-workers have worked out the regional distribution of ventilation, diffusing capacity, and perfusion in the human lung (West and Dollery, 1960; Dollery et al., 1960; West et al., 1962).

In rebreathing and breath-holding experiments for determination of D, stable, naturally occurring, but rare isotopes of C and O have proven to be useful for different reasons. The isotopes $C^{18}O$ (Wagner et al., 1971) and ^{13}CO are useful because mass spectrometers built for continuous recording of respired gases do not possess the mass resolving power necessary for distinguishing $^{12}C^{16}O$ from $^{14}N^{14}N$ (both with mass number 28). Another advantage is that in smokers $P_{\bar{v}}$ for $^{12}C^{16}O$ unlike for other isotopes may be high enough to produce significant errors when not accounted for.

Of particular interest is the use of rare O_2 isotopes ($^{18}O-^{16}O$, $^{18}O-^{18}O$), introduced by Hyde et al. (1966), because it offers important advantages: (1) Mixed venous P for the isotopes can be assumed to be zero, which eliminates the important source of error produced by an erroneous determination of the asymptote for O_2 equilibration (Cerretelli et al., 1974). (2) In breath-holding or rebreathing, when there is an equilibrium of the abundant isotope ($^{32}O_2$), the gas–blood transfer of a rare isotope ($^{34}O_2$ or $^{36}O_2$) occurs in accordance with a constant $\beta = C_{\bar{v}_{O_2}}/P_{\bar{v}_{O_2}}$, provided the P_{O_2} for the rare isotope is small compared with that of the abundant isotope (Piiper and Meyer, 1978; Scheid et al., 1979b). This holds true only if there is an equilibrium of the abundant isotope(s). This requirement was met in the studies of Hyde and associates (Hyde et al., 1966; Cross et al., 1969; Gong et al., 1972b; Garman et al., 1970) using breath-holding and of Piiper and Meyer (1978) applying rebreathing techniques.

IV. PROBLEMS IN APPLICATION OF MODELS TO REAL LUNGS

The models used to define diffusion limitation and diffusing capacity have the advantages of simplicity and versatility. However, their application to conditions in real lungs raises a number of problems (Wagner, 1977), the more fundamental of which are considered in this section.

A. Composite Nature of the Diffusing Capacity

In the models the gas–blood barrier is assumed to be uniform and homogeneous, but in real lungs it is composed of multiple layers of irregular thickness (alveolar epithelium, interstitium, and endothelium). Furthermore, blood plasma, red cell membrane, and red cell interior constitute resistances to diffusion, although gas transport in plasma and within red cells may be facilitated by convective mixing (Miyamoto and Moll, 1971; Zander and Schmid-Schönbein, 1973). Finally, there are chemical reactions and, in case of CO_2, ion transfer processes between red cells and plasma that may limit the overall gas transfer rate. The relative importance of these individual steps in limiting the rate of CO_2, O_2, and CO transfer has not yet been identified in detail despite remarkable recent progress (see this volume, Chapter 6). On the other hand, incomplete gas mixing in the alveolar space may add a resistance to gas uptake (see this volume, Chapter 4).

What is measured as "diffusing capacity" D is an overall conductance resulting from a combination of all these single diffusion, reaction, and ionic transfer processes. A relatively simple analysis is possible when the various steps can be considered to be arranged in series and the chemical reactions involved to be of first-order kinetics (Moll, 1962). In the widely accepted analysis of CO uptake by Roughton and Forster (1957) the processes involved are grouped into extraerythrocyte and intraerythrocyte processes (see Section VI,B).

Gurtner, Burns, and co-workers (see this volume, Chapter 8) claim the existence of a specific carrier mechanism mediating facilitated O_2 and CO transfer in the lung (Burns and Gurtner, 1973; Gurtner *et al.*, 1975; Burns *et al.*, 1975, 1976, 1977; Mendoza *et al.*, 1977; Sybert *et al.*, 1978; Ayash *et al.*, 1978).

The evidence is based on (1) decrease of D_{CO} with increasing pulmonary P_{CO}, suggesting saturation kinetics; (2) drug-induced changes in D_{CO}, which indicate that the mixed-function oxidase cytochrome P-450 or a related compound is the carrier; (3) induction of large specific changes of $(A - a)_{O_2}$ differences in isolated perfused lungs by drugs known to bind and thereby inactivate P-450 [$(A - a)$ for CO_2 and inert gases remaining constant].

The evidence (1) was not confirmed in human lungs by Meyer (1979), who showed rebreathing D_{CO} to be constant in the concentration range where marked P_{CO} dependence had been obtained using the steady state technique by Mendoza *et al.* (1977) in dog and by Ayash *et al.* (1978) in man. Also, Power and Bradford (1969) observed no P_{CO} dependence of single-breath D_{CO} in man.

Therefore, the hypothesis of a specific facilitated transfer of O_2 and CO remains an open issue awaiting reinvestigation.

B. Capacitance Coefficient

The capacitance coefficient of blood, β, is a decisive factor for diffusion limitation in models of alveolar–capillary gas transfer. Its role in real lungs imposes several problems.

1. O_2–CO_2 Interaction

Owing to the Bohr–Haldane effect, the O_2 dissociation curve along which oxygenation proceeds in the pulmonary capillary depends on the distribution of CO_2 transfer along the capillary and vice versa. Thus the exchange for both gases is coupled, and CO_2 is thus effectively slowed by O_2 despite the high CO_2 diffusivity (see Section VI). Moreover, recent evidence suggests that equilibration of H^+ and HCO_3^- between red cells and plasma is considerably delayed (see Section VI and this volume, Chapter 6).

2. Pulmonary Capillary Hematocrit

The hematocrit in pulmonary vessels seems to be lower than the hematocrit in large vessels because of faster transit through the pulmonary vascular system of red blood cells as compared to plasma (e.g., Rapaport et al., 1956; Cosentino et al., 1961). Implications for gas exchange may, however, be limited since the decisive parameter is flow of plasma and erythrocytes, which is the same in pulmonary capillaries as in large vessels. However, the reduced contact time for the red cells may cause problems on account of intraerythrocyte diffusion–reaction limitation. In dogs, D_{O_2} and D_{CO} were found to be proportional to the hematocrit (Mochizuki et al., 1958; Piiper, 1962a,b; Burrows and Niden, 1963). This result was interpreted to indicate that either the "membrane" diffusion resistance played a minor role against the intraerythrocyte processes or that D_M was proportional to hematocrit (only areas of membrane adjacent to red cells being utilized for O_2 and CO transfer).

3. Unequal Distribution of Hematocrit

Variabilities and changes in diameter of pulmonary capillaries due to transmural pressure (Glazier et al., 1969; Warrell et al., 1972) could result in regional variation in hematocrit and thus in β. This would result in similar variations in $D/(\dot{Q}\beta)$, the impact of which is identical to $D/\dot{Q}$ inhomogeneity (see Section V). The potential effects of differences in hematocrit on gas–blood equilibration have been experimentally verified by King and Mazal (1976).

C. Pulsatility of Pulmonary Capillary Blood Flow

The assumption of continuous and constant pulmonary capillary blood flow in analysis of alveolar gas exchange is in disagreement with experimental data on uptake of N_2O (Lee and DuBois, 1955), CO (Menkes *et al.,* 1970), and O_2 and CO_2 (Bosman *et al.,* 1965). The effects of pulsatile changes of $\dot{Q}$ and/or Q_c on alveolar gas exchange have been examined on lung models (Crandall and Flumerfelt, 1967; Graeser *et al.,* 1969; Hlastala, 1972; Wagner and West, 1972; Lin and Cumming, 1973; Bidani *et al.,* 1978). The general conclusion of these studies is that an impairment of alveolar gas exchange efficiency is produced by pulsatile changes of $\dot{Q}$ and, to a lesser degree, of Q_c, but that the effects are insignificant in hypoxia. Moreover, simultaneous pulsations in capillary volume and flow, likely to occur *in vivo,* have practically no effect (Bidani *et al.,* 1978). Therefore, the use of models with constant pulmonary capillary blood flow seems to be justified under most physiological conditions.

D. Variations of Alveolar Gas and Arterial Blood Composition during a Respiratory Cycle

Effects of variations in time of alveolar and arterial blood gases on gas exchange are similar to regional variations. The latter result from functional inhomogeneities that are considered, for their importance, in Section V.

The classical studies of respiratory cyclic variations of alveolar P_{CO_2} and P_{O_2} by DuBois and co-workers (DuBois, 1952; DuBois *et al.,* 1952) have been complemented and validated by a number of computer calculations on lung models (Nye, 1970; Suwa and Bendixen, 1972; Hlastala, 1972; Lin and Cumming, 1973). At least under resting conditions the effects of variations in analysis of gas exchange do not seem to be very important if the alveolar gas is sampled at about four-fifths of the gas volume along a normal expiration to obtain a mean value (Rahn, 1954). However, end-expired P_{CO_2} may be markedly above (mean) alveolar P_{CO_2}, particularly in exercise, and may thus create apparent positive alveolar-to-arterial P_{CO_2} differences (see Section I,D).

A sloping alveolar plateau can be produced, aside from the "breath-holding effect" considered here, by other factors like delayed wash-out of dead space, stratification, and $\dot{V}_A/\dot{Q}$ inhomogeneity coupled with sequential emptying [see Piiper and Scheid (1971)]. More specific for the "breath-holding effect" are experimentally recorded oscillations of P_{O_2} (Purves, 1966; Folgering *et al.*, 1978) and P_{CO_2} (Plaas-Link *et al.*, 1977; Carruthers *et al.*, 1978) in arterial blood. These results stress the importance of extending arterial blood sampling to at least one whole respiratory cycle if mean arterial P_{CO_2} and P_{O_2} are desired.

E. Tidal versus Continuous Ventilation

In the models for rebreathing and for step change of inspired gas the effective ventilation was assumed to be continuous, not tidal, for simplicity of calculations. For rebreathing, the errors introduced by this assumption appear to be small (Sølvsteen, 1965a).

F. Technical Problems

Aside from the accuracy required for measurement in blood and gas, special attention should be directed to temperature and water vapor.

An accurate continuous measurement of deep body temperature is required, particularly for methods based on comparison of gas and blood values, In dogs, rectal temperature is not satisfactory; a good site for temperature measurement is the aortic arch [see Haab *et al.* (1974)].

Several studies have shown that expired gas is not saturated with water vapor at deep body temperature (e.g., Liese *et al.*, 1974). On the other hand, measurement of the partial pressure of H_2O is difficult. With mass spectrometers the electronic compensation circuit of Scheid *et al.* (1971; cf. Slama and Scheid, 1975) yields fractional concentrations that may easily be converted to partial pressures at alveolar conditions.

V. GAS–BLOOD EQUILIBRATION IN FUNCTIONALLY INHOMOGENEOUS LUNGS

A. General Features

Normal, and particularly diseased, lungs are known to be functionally inhomogeneous. Experimental evidence has notably been obtained in experiments with radioactive gases in which regional differences in $\dot{V}_A/V_A$, $\dot{Q}/V_A$ have been observed (West and Dollery, 1960; Dollery *et al.*, 1960; West *et al.*, 1962; Michaelson *et al.*, 1973; Pande *et al.*, 1975). Regional differences in these functional parameters are likely to be present even between smaller subunits of the lung, too small to be demonstrable by methods using radioactive gases. These inhomogeneities create serious problems in assessing the diffusion aspect, because both diffusion limitation within a homogeneous lung compartment, and inhomogeneity contribute to inefficiency of alveolar gas transfer, but discrimination of their contributions is a difficult task. On the other hand, the different methods designed, and the gases used, for study of diffusion limitation (determination of D) display differences in their sensitivities to inhomogeneities (Johnson and Miller, 1968) and may thus be utilized to provide valuable information on the kind and extent of inhomogeneity.

Inhomogeneity is produced by unequal allotment of the parameters $\dot{V}_A$, $\dot{Q}$, D, and V_A to the different functional lung units, expressed as local variation of their ratios. In the presence of unaccounted functional inhomogeneities, diffusion limitation is, in general, overestimated and the diffusing capacity D is thus underestimated. The extent of this underestimation is determined by several factors, notably by (1) the kind and extent of inhomogeneity, (2) the method used, and (3) the test gas used (O_2 or CO). Table I provides an overview of the various inhomogeneities leading to underestimation of D. The following features are apparent:

1. As gas transfer in steady state models is independent of lung volume, inhomogeneity in V_A does not affect steady state D_{O_2} or D_{CO}.
2. Since CO transfer is virtually exclusively diffusion limited, inhomogeneity in $\dot{Q}$ does not affect D_{CO} either in steady state or in unsteady state methods (with the exception of very small $\dot{Q}$ or very high alveolar P_{CO}; see below).
3. Unsteady-state O_2 methods are influenced by all possible kinds of inhomogeneity, whereas steady state D_{CO} should be affected only by $\dot{V}_A/D$ variance.

B. Steady State D_{O_2}

The alveolar–endcapillary P_{O_2} difference $(A - c')_{O_2}$ constitutes the decisive parameter for calculating steady-state D_{O_2}. In practice, it is estimated from the alveolar–arterial P_{O_2} difference $(A - a)_{O_2}$, which is commonly considered to derive from three factors (Riley and Cournand, 1951): (1) shunt or venous admixture, (2) unequal distribution of $\dot{V}_A$ to $\dot{Q}$, and (3) diffusion limitation.

The simplest model to use for calculation of D is that underlying the ideal–alveolar air concept (Rahn, 1949; Riley and Cournand, 1949). Shunt may be estimated in hyperoxia and hence $P_{c'_{O_2}}$ calculated from $P_{a_{O_2}}$. Ideal–alveolar P_{O_2}, $(P_{Ai})_{O_2}$, is determined as the P_{O_2} value on the gas R line at arterial P_{CO_2} (more correctly, the shunt effect on CO_2 should be

TABLE I

Effects of Functional Inhomogeneities on Determination of D_{O_2} and D_{CO}

	$\dot{V}_A$	$\dot{Q}$	D	V_A
Steady state				
O_2	+	+	+	o
CO	+	(o)	+	o
Non-steady state				
O_2	+	+	+	+
CO	+	(o)	+	+

considered, particularly in hypoxia). The $(Ai - c')_{O_2}$ difference is then used to calculate D_{O_2} according to Eq. (6).

The problem with this approach is that it attributes, after correcting for "true shunt," all inhomogeneity to alveolar dead space ventilation. Other types of inhomogeneity with finite $\dot{V}_A/\dot{Q}$ ratios give rise to a relatively larger $(A - a)_{O_2}$ than $(a - A)_{CO_2}$ and thus produce a "shuntlike" effect (i.e., predominantly O_2 affected) aside from an "alveolar–dead-space-like effect" (i.e., both O_2 and CO_2 affected in relation to R) (Riley and Cournand, 1949, 1951). The shuntlike effect is difficult to assess, because its size varies greatly with alveolar P_{O_2} (Farhi and Rahn, 1955; Riley and Permutt, 1973). Attribution of all $\dot{V}_A/\dot{Q}$ inhomogeneity effect to alveolar dead space leads thus to an underestimation of D_{O_2} (Haab et al., 1964).

More complex models incorporating a log-normal $\dot{V}_A/\dot{Q}$ distribution type have been found particularly attractive for many (practical and theoretical) reasons (Rahn, 1949; Farhi and Rahn, 1955; West, 1969). Experimental results for both man (Lenfant and Okubo, 1968) and dog (Wagner et al., 1975) are in fact in reasonable agreement with this distributional pattern.

Chinet et al. (1971) have calculated O_2 (and CO) exchange parameters in lung models with known D_{O_2}, displaying a log-normal $\dot{V}_A/\dot{Q}$ distribution, and calculated D_{O_2} according to Eq. (6). With both (mean) end-expired and ideal–alveolar P_{O_2}, D_{O_2} was underestimated, to a lesser degree with $P_{Ai_{O_2}}$. In applying the model to experimental data obtained in anesthetized dogs, Geiser et al. (1979) calculated the D_{O_2} based on log-normal $\dot{V}_A/\dot{Q}$ distribution [the extent of which was estimated from $(a - A)_{CO_2}$] to be 60% higher than D_{O_2} after $P_{Ai_{O_2}}$.

Piiper et al. (1961) attributed the $(A - c')_{O_2}$ difference in dog experiments to diffusion limitation and used a model with unequal distribution of D to $\dot{Q}$ to evaluate the data (Piiper, 1961a). However, since $(a - A)_{CO_2}$ was not measured, no correction for alveolar dead-space ventilation could be applied, resulting thus in an underestimation of D_{O_2}. Generally, both

$\dot{V}_A/\dot{Q}$ and $D/\dot{Q}$ inhomogeneities are likely to be present in real lungs. Their combined effects have been analyzed in theory (Piiper, 1961b), but a quantitative evaluation of their component effects from experimental gas exchange data in steady state appears to be extremely difficult and has not been attempted yet.

C. Steady State D_{CO}

The ideal–alveolar air approach has been applied by Filley *et al.* (1954) to the measurement of steady state D_{CO} and is now widely used. However, aside from the fact that this approach is correct only with inhomogeneity of alveolar–dead-space type, a special problem arises with CO. Since CO transfer is predominantly diffusion limited (Table I), it should be only slightly affected by $\dot{V}_A/\dot{Q}$ inhomogeneities. Hence, the use of CO_2 in estimating P_{Ai} for CO may result in serious overestimation of D_{CO} (Chinet *et al.*, 1971). In fact, it is mainly the unequal distribution of D to $\dot{V}_A$ that exerts effects on D_{CO} in steady state. Therefore, the Filley method should not be applied uncritically.

Since perfusion and its unequal distribution affects CO transfer much less than O_2 transfer, apparent D_{CO} in inhomogeneous lung models has been shown to be larger than apparent D_{O_2} (with comparable true values of both) (Chinet *et al.*, 1971). This has been experimentally verified (Haab *et al.*, 1968, 1970).

D. D_{CO} by Unsteady State Methods

1. Breath-Holding D_{CO}

Since with this method the absorption kinetics of CO is determined by $D_{CO}/(V_A\beta_g)$ (Fig. 5), inhomogeneity with respect to this parameter should influence the experimental values. In fact, D_{CO} is underestimated in lung models with unequal distribution of D to alveolar volume V_A (Forster, 1957; Piiper and Sikand, 1966). The presence of such inhomogeneity is revealed by nonmonoexponential decay of alveolar P_{CO} with time of breath-holding, as has frequently been observed (Sikand and Piiper, 1966). In this case the value for D_{CO} depends on the time interval chosen for analysis.

Also, the variation of inspired volume to alveolar volume ratio $\dot{V}_A/V_A$ is expected to influence unsteady state D_{CO}, but when present alone will not produce an apparent nonmonoexponential CO absorption pattern. It will only produce underestimation of D_{CO} in proportion to underestimation of V_A from insoluble gas dilution (Piiper and Sikand, 1966).

At high alveolar CO concentrations perfusion limitation may become observable owing to reduction in β_{CO} at higher CO saturation. Hyde *et al.* (1971) found single-breath D_{CO} in man to be 14% lower with inhalation of 4% CO as compared to D_{CO} measured with the usual inspired CO concentration of 0.2%. From this result the pattern of unequal $D/\dot{Q}$ was estimated.

2. D_{CO} by Step Change of Inspired Gas

A detailed model analysis of the "equilibration method" involving wash-in and wash-out of CO and an insoluble gas was performed by Burrows *et al.* (1960a). The effective inhomogeneity variables are again $\dot{V}_A/V_A$ and D/V_A. Nonuniformity with respect to these parameters was demonstrated in lungs of normal humans and patients (Mittman and Burrows, 1959; Burrows *et al.*, 1960b).

E. D_{O_2} by Unsteady State Methods

1. Breath-Holding D_{O_2}

The method is in principle influenced by all types of inhomogeneity considered in Table I. In all studies in which D_{O_2} and D_{CO} were determined simultaneously (see Sections V,C and VI,B), the ratio D_{O_2}/D_{CO} was lower than unity and much lower than the values predicted from diffusion coefficient, solubility, and reaction kinetics with hemoglobin of both gases. The low experimental ratio was attributed to the $D/\dot{Q}$ inequality, which would reduce D_{O_2}, but have no (or little) effect on D_{CO}.

2. Rebreathing D_{O_2}

During rebreathing all local intrapulmonary gas composition differences are expected to be reduced by mixing. This probably constitutes an important advantage of using rebreathing methods in lungs with any kind of inhomogeneity. If effective ventilation could be increased sufficiently to abolish all ventilation limitation and thus to homogenize lung gas composition, the primarily inhomogeneous lung would behave as a homogeneous lung. However, in markedly underventilated lung regions this goal probably cannot be achieved in practice. The effects of unequal distribution of $\dot{V}_A$, D, $\dot{Q}$, and V_A have been studied in models by Scheid *et al.* (1973).

3. D_{O_2} by Step Change of Inspired Gas

The method of Thews and Vogel (1968) is strongly influenced by inequalities with respect to $\dot{V}_A/V_A$, $\dot{V}_A/\dot{Q}$, and $D/\dot{Q}$. Indeed, the method was devised with the aim of elaborating the pattern of distribution of these variables from the wash-in–wash-out kinetics of insoluble gas, CO_2, and O_2. The authors could identify two compartments in the lungs of both healthy young subjects and patients with obstructive lung disease (Thews et al., 1971).

VI. PULMONARY DIFFUSING CAPACITY

A. D_{CO} and D_{O_2} Determined by Different Methods

1. Diffusing Capacity for CO

D_{CO} has been measured in a great number of studies. A view of physiological literature yields the following overall mean values ($\pm$ SD) for normal humans in resting conditions:

Breath-holding D_{CO} = 34 ± 8 ml/min/torr   (45 references)

Steady-state D_{CO} = 21 ± 4 ml/min/torr   (34 references)

The reasons for the significantly larger D_{CO} value obtained with breath-holding techniques have not been established, but the following factors may be involved. (1) Single-breath D_{CO} is routinely measured at total lung capacity, steady state D_{CO} at normal lung volumes. D_{CO} has been shown to increase with breath-holding lung volumes (e.g., Gurtner and Fowler, 1971; Ogilvie et al., 1957; Adaro et al., 1976). (2) The effects of inhomogeneities influence the D_{CO} by both methods (see above), but this overall effect may be less on the single-breath D_{CO}. A comparative model study has not been performed. (3) The actual functional inhomogeneity may be less with a maximal inspiration from residual volume than normal inspiration from FRC, particularly in older subjects with increased closing volume.

The average

rebreathing D_{CO} = 29 ± 4 ml/min/torr   (8 references)

is close to the average single-breath D_{CO}. However, a comparison of rebreathing D_{CO} with single-breath D_{CO} at the same lung volume revealed rebreathing D_{CO} to be about 30% higher at the same (mean) lung volumes (Adaro et al., 1976). This may be an effect of the homogenization of lung gas by rebreathing. Furthermore, it should be considered that alveolar P_{O_2} is considerably lower, and alveolar P_{CO_2} higher, in rebreathing conditions as compared to breath-holding after an inspiration of room air to vital capacity (with CO), and that both hypoxia and hypercapnia have been shown to increase single breath D_{CO} (Forster, 1964).

The wash-out method of Burrows and co-workers yields D_{CO} values in agreement with the single-breath method (Mittman and Burrows, 1959).

2. Diffusing Capacity for O_2

The value for D_{O_2} (in ml/min/torr) in normal man at rest is controversial. Recent estimates for steady state D_{O_2} by Turino *et al.* (1963) and by Kreuzer and Van Lookeren Campagne (1965) yield values of about 26. By contrast, Haab *et al.* (1965) report a value of 47 for young man in supine position. With breath-holding methods, using stable O_2 isotopes, the average D_{O_2} values found at total lung capacity range from 25 to 33 (Hyde *et al.*, 1966; Garman *et al.*, 1970; Gong *et al.*, 1972b; Cross *et al.*, 1973) and are thus in the range of steady state D_{O_2} values. The range for re-breathing D_{O_2} in normal subjects is rather wide: 22 (Gong *et al.*, 1972a), 31 (Cerretelli *et al.*, 1974), 30 (Veicsteinas *et al.*, 1976), 41–53 (Micheli and Haab, 1970), 48 (Meyer and Piiper, 1978). Using the step change of inspired gas method, Schmidt *et al.* (1972) report a mean D_{O_2} value of 31.

The generally higher rebreathing D_{O_2} should again be attributed to better mixing of alveolar gas by rebreathing, which diminishes the effects of inhomogeneities.

B. Relationship between D_{O_2} and D_{CO}

1. Theoretical Predictions

Roughton and Forster (1957) introduced the partitioning of the diffusing capacity of the lung (D_L in their terminology) into the diffusing capacity of the gas–blood barrier or membrane (D_M) and the gas uptake capacity of pulmonary capillary blood, which is given by the specific gas uptake capacity per unit blood volume (θ) multiplied by the pulmonary capillary blood volume (Q_c):

$$\frac{1}{D} = \frac{1}{D_M} + \frac{1}{Q_c\theta} \tag{8}$$

The formula was at first applied to analysis of single-breath D_{CO} at different levels of alveolar P_{O_2}. Thereby θ is varied and both D_M and Q_c can be obtained from measurements of D_{CO}. Its use has been validated by morphometric determination of Q_c (Vreim and Staub, 1973). The formula was later extended to O_2 (Staub *et al.*, 1962) and to CO_2 (Hyde *et al.*, 1968).

It is generally agreed that the ratio $D_{M_{O_2}}/D_{M_{C}}$ is equal to the ratio of Krogh's diffusion constants for O_2 and CO in water or tissue ($= 1.23$). Assuming equal capillary volumes, the remaining problematic factor is the ratio θ_{O_2}/θ_{CO}. The values of θ_{O_2} available from the literature (in ml O_2/min/torr/ml of blood) vary from 2.7 (Staub *et al.*, 1962) through 1.5 (Holland *et al.*, 1977) to 1.0 (Mochizuki, 1966). The θ_{CO} value (in same units) is about 0.9 (Roughton and Forster, 1957; Holland, 1969). This θ_{CO} value is valid for the replacement of O_2 by CO in oxyhemoglobin in red cells. The θ_{CO} value for the association reaction of CO with free hemoglobin in red cells is expected to be higher by an unknown factor.

Thus, the θ_{CO} values are applicable only in hyperoxic conditions, where S_{O_2} in pulmonary capillary blood is expected to reach full saturation in the initial segment of the capillary. But in normoxia, and particularly in hypoxia, when sizable O_2 unsaturation is present along the entire pulmonary capillary (or at least a large fraction of it) effective θ_{CO} could be appreciably larger than 0.9. Therefore, particularly in experimental studies in which D_{CO} has been determined simultaneously with D_{O_2} in hypoxia, all that can be stated on the expected relationship θ_{O_2}/θ_{CO} is that it should be smaller than 3 ($= 2.7/0.9$) or smaller than 1.1 (1.0/0.9), depending on which θ values are used, but a lower limit for the θ_{O_2}/θ_{CO} ratio cannot be fixed.

2. Experimental Results

In simultaneous determinations of D_{O_2} and D_{CO} in man, Shepard *et al.* (1958) and Turino *et al.* (1963) found D_{O_2}/D_{CO} ratios that were well above 1.0, and increased with intensity of exercise (to about 2 and 1.7, respectively). In the experiments of Kreuzer and Van Lookeren Campagne (1965), however, the ratio was 0.86 (at rest). Quite a different pattern was found in breath-holding studies with (isotopic) O_2 and CO (Hyde *et al.*, 1966, 1967; Garman *et al.*, 1970; Gong *et al.*, 1972b; Cross *et al.*, 1973), the D_{O_2}/D_{CO} ratio ranging from 0.56 to 0.78 at rest, from 0.68 to 0.89 at exercise. The relatively low D_{O_2} was attributed to unequal distribution of D to $\dot{Q}$. Since the D_{O_2}/D_{CO} ratio remained low in rebreathing (0.58 at rest, 0.71 at exercise), it was concluded that $D/\dot{Q}$ inequalities were present within smaller lung regions, which did not correspond to regional topographical or gravitational variations (Gong *et al.*, 1972a).

A reinvestigation by simultaneous determination of D_{O_2} and D_{CO} in man at rest and during exercise in our laboratory (Piiper and Meyer, 1978; Meyer and Piiper, 1978) gave a rather different result: the ratio D_{O_2}/D_{CO} averaged 1.14 at rest and 1.25 at exercise. As this ratio is very close to the ratio of Krogh diffusion constants, one might interpret this result as indicative of the dominant role of diffusion processes as compared to chemical reaction in uptake of O_2 and CO in lungs. However, since the effective θ_{O_2}/θ_{CO} ratio is not known (and may be in the same range), such a conclusion would be at least premature. A reason for the marked discrepancy from the results of preceding studies using similar breath-holding and rebreathing techniques remains obscure.

A remarkable experimental approach has recently been devised by Burns and Shepard (1979). They perfused excised dog lung lobes with blood containing dithionite, thereby reducing P_{O_2} of pulmonary capillary blood everywhere to zero, and determined simultaneously D_{O_2} (which in these conditions should represent $D_{M_{O_2}}$) and D_{CO} by a rebreathing technique. Definitive results have not yet been published.

C. Diffusing Capacity for CO_2

In conventional analysis of alveolar gas exchange it is assumed that CO_2 equilibration between end-capillary blood and alveolar gas is practically complete, because of the high physical solubility of CO_2 in tissue and of the high Krogh diffusion constant resulting therefrom (20 times higher than for O_2). In fact, D_{CO_2} values obtained in humans with breath-holding using the stable isotope $^{13}CO_2$ were not significantly different from infinity (Hyde et al., 1968). Similarly, rebreathing $^{13}CO_2$ yielded D_{CO_2} values (ml/min/torr) in three normal subjects of 150–190 at rest and 250–320 at moderate exercise (M. Meyer, P. Scheid, and J. Piiper, unpublished observations). Simultaneous values of D_{O_2} averaged 45 and 60, respectively.

A D_{CO_2}/D_{O_2} ratio lower than expected from the Krogh diffusion constant ratio (20) may be due to several factors: (1) The effect of functional inhomogeneities in reducing apparent D is the greater the higher the D value (see above). (2) The complex processes involved in CO_2 kinetics and distribution in blood (see this volume, Chapter 6) are expected to diminish the overall efficiency of blood–alveolar CO_2 transfer. (3) The technical problems in determining D_{CO_2} are considerable. In particular, the large effective dilution volume of $^{13}CO_2$ is a problem (Hyde et al., 1968).

Calculations based on the parameter $D/(\dot{Q}\beta)$ (see above) reveal that in resting conditions CO_2 exchange is very slightly diffusion limited, $(P_{c'} - P_A)_{CO_2}$ being about 0.2 torr. But in heavy exercise a more marked diffusion limitation is expected. These calculations are in agreement with the conclusions of Wagner and West (1972) that owing to the high β value for CO_2 compared with that for O_2, CO_2 exchange may be equally or even more impaired than O_2 exchange when D is reduced or metabolism increased.

D. Diffusing Capacity at Exercise

A number of factors are known to influence D [see Forster (1964)]. Of particular interest is the adjustment of D to the increased O_2 uptake and CO_2 output in physical exercise.

The literature values for D_{CO} with breath-holding and steady state methods exhibit a wide scatter in respect of both the absolute values and the changes observed with exercise. But the overall mean values ($\pm$ SD) for both methods are closer than in resting conditions:

Single-breath $D_{CO} = 47 \pm 7$ ml/min/torr   (12 references)

Steady-state $D_{CO} = 40 \pm 13$ ml/min/torr   (27 references)

Also, the mean rebreathing D_{CO} are similar to these values:

Rebreathing $D_{CO} = 46$ ml/min/torr

(Gong *et al.*, 1972a; Sackner *et al.*, 1975; Adaro *et al.*, 1976; Meyer and Piiper, 1978).

There exist much less data on determination of D_{O_2} during heavy exercise. With several modifications of the steady state method mean maximum D_{O_2} values (in ml/min/torr) range from 57 to 92 (Riley *et al.*, 1954; Shepard *et al.*, 1958; Turino *et al.*, 1963; Haab *et al.*, 1965). The D_{O_2} values found with the breath-holding isotopic O_2 method are much lower, in the range 40–43 (Gong *et al.*, 1970; Garman *et al.*, 1970; Cross *et al.*, 1973), and with the rebreathing technique, very variable D_{O_2} values at exercise have been reported: 43 (Gong *et al.*, 1972a), 107 (Veicsteinas *et al.*, 1976), 62 (Meyer and Piiper, 1978).

The question whether D rises steadily with severity of exercise or ultimately reaches a maximum has been frequently discussed, but the experimental data appear to be insufficient for settling this issue.

The increase of D during exercise is considered to be caused by an increase in the effective gas–blood contact area. Two mechanisms are discerned: (1) increase of the diameter of capillary vessels by increased transmural pressure, and (2) recruitment of capillaries not perfused in resting conditions. However, a distinction between these two possibilities is largely hypothetical.

Two other mechanisms, however, leading to an *apparent* increase of D must also be considered: (1) The functional inhomogeneity of the lung may be decreased at exercise, whereby D would be less underestimated during exercise than during resting conditions. In particular, the unequal vertical distribution of perfusion due to gravity is equalized by increase in the mean pressure in pulmonary vessels (West, 1965). (2) The effects of inhomogeneity on the measurement of steady state D_{O_2} (and possibly on D_{O_2} determined by other methods) are relatively reduced with higher O_2 uptake, despite the extent of inhomogeneity itself remaining constant (Piiper, 1969).

Therefore, the D values measured at exercise are of greater interest than the resting values for two reasons: (1) they are better approximations to the diffusing capacity and (2) they characterize the maximum capacity of the lungs for diffusive gas–blood gas exchange.

E. Physiological versus Morphometrical Diffusing Capacity

In the last two decades a new access to study of lung function, and particularly of alveolar gas exchange, has been opened by the quantitative morphological (morphometrical) approach initiated and steadily furthered by Weibel and his associates (Weibel, 1963, 1973).

According to the latest morphometrical analysis of normal human lungs (Gehr *et al.*, 1978), the effective ("available") D_{O_2} is estimated as lying between a maximum estimate of 130–190 and a minimum estimate of 62–91 ml/min/torr. This lower limit of morphometrical D_{O_2} is about identical with the maximuum D_{O_2} measured at exercise (see above).

It is of interest to note that previous morphometrical estimates of D_{O_2} were considerably higher and that for other animals, particularly the dog, there is still a considerable discrepancy between the high morphometric D_{O_2} and the much lower D_{O_2} determined from studies of gas exchange function (e.g., Geiser *et al.*, 1979). The following reasons may contribute to the discrepancies between morphometrical and physiological estimates of D: (1) The lung structure may be affected by the histological techniques. (2) In particular, the alveolar surface lining layer may in part be removed (Mazzone *et al.*, 1978), resulting in overestimation of D by morphometrical techniques. (3) The model underlying calculation of D from morphometrical data may be too simple (see Section IV,A). (4) The physical properties (Krogh's diffusion constant; rate of association, θ) used in this model are not known with certainty.

It may be of interest to remark that in other gas exchange organs, in which diffusion limitation of gas transfer is much more prominent, a much better accordance between morphometrical and physiological diffusing capacity has been found, for example, dogfish gills (Scheid and Piiper, 1976) and salamander skin (Piiper *et al.*, 1976).

REFERENCES

Adaro, F., Scheid, P., Teichmann, J., and Piiper, J. (1973). A rebreathing method for estimating pulmonary D_{O_2}: Theory and measurements in dog lungs. *Respir. Physiol.* **18,** 43–63.
Adaro, F., Meyer, M., and Sikand, R. S. (1976). Rebreathing and single breath pulmonary

CO diffusing capacity in man at rest and exercise studied by $C^{18}O$ isotope. *Bull. Eur. Physiopathol. Resp.* **12**, 747–756.

Ayash, R., Sybert, A., and Gurtner, G. H. (1978). Saturation kinetics for steady state pulmonary CO transfer in man. *Am. Rev. Respir. Dis.* **117**, 310.

Bidani, A., and Crandall, E. D. (1978). Analysis of P_{CO_2} differences during rebreathing due to slow pH equilibration in blood. *J. Appl. Physiol.* **45**, 666–673.

Bidani, A., Flumerfelt, R. W., and Crandall, E. D. (1978). Analysis of the effects of pulsatile capillary blood flow and volume on gas exchange. *Respir. Physiol.* **35**, 27–42.

Bosman, A. R., Lee, G. de J., and Marshall, R. (1965). The effect of pulsatile capillary blood flow upon gas exchange within the lungs of man. *Clin. Sci.* **28**, 295–309.

Briehl, R. W., and Fishman, A. P. (1960). Principles of the Bohr integration procedure and their application to measurement of diffusing capacity of the lung for oxygen. *J. Appl. Physiol.* **15**, 337–348.

Burns, B., and Gurtner, G. H. (1973). A specific carrier for oxygen and carbon monoxide in the lung and placenta. *Drug Metab. Dispos.* **1**, 374–377.

Burns, B., and Shepard, R. H. (1979). DL_{O_2} in excised lungs perfused with blood containing sodium dithionite $(Na_2S_2O_4)$. *J. Appl. Physiol.* **46**, 100–110.

Burns, B., Gurtner, G. H., Peavy, H., and Cha, Y. N. (1975). A specific carrier for oxygen and carbon monoxide in the lung. *In* "Lung Metabolism" (A. Junod and R. De Haller, eds.), pp. 159–184. Academic Press, New York.

Burns, B., Cha, Y. N., and Purcell, J. M. (1976). A specific carrier for O_2 and CO in the lung: Effects of volatile anesthetics on gas transfer and drug metabolism. *Chest* **69**, 316–321.

Burns, B., Lacis, A., Freeland, H., and Rabold, R. (1977). Enhanced facilitated diffusion of CO in the lung: parallel induction of cytochrome P-450 by methoxyflurane pretreatment. *Fed. Proc., Fed. Am. Soc. Exp. Biol.* **36**, 591.

Burrows, B., and Harper, P. V., Jr. (1958). Determination of pulmonary diffusing capacity from carbon monoxide equilibration curves. *J. Appl. Physiol.* **12**, 283–291.

Burrows, B., and Niden, A. H. (1963). Effects of anemia and hemorrhagic shock on pulmonary diffusion in the dog lung. *J. Appl. Physiol.* **18**, 123–128.

Burrows, B., Niden, A. H., Harper, P. V., Jr., and Barclay, W. R. (1960a). Non-uniform pulmonary diffusion as demonstrated by the carbon monoxide equilibration technique: Mathematical considerations. *J. Clin. Invest.* **39**, 795–801.

Burrows, B., Niden, A. H., Mittman, C., Talley, R. C., and Barclay, W. R. (1960b). Non-uniform pulmonary diffusion as demonstrated by the carbon monoxide equilibration technique: Experimental results in man. *J. Clin. Invest.* **39**, 943–951.

Butler, J. (1965). Measurement of cardiac output using soluble gases. *In* "Handbook of Physiology" Section 3, Respiration, Vol. II, (W. O. Fenn and H. Rahn, eds.), pp. 1489–1503. Am. Physiol. Soc., Washington, D.C.

Cain, S. M., and Otis, A. B. (1960). Effect of carbonic anhydrase inhibition on mixed venous CO_2 tension in anesthetized dogs. *J. Appl. Physiol.* **15**, 390–392.

Cander, L., and Forster, R. E. (1959). Determination of pulmonary parenchymal tissue volume and pulmonary capillary flow in man. *J. Appl. Physiol.* **14**, 541–551.

Carruthers, B., Ponti, J., and Purves, M. J. (1978). Observations on the partial pressure of CO_2 in carotid arterial blood in cats. *J. Physiol. (London)* **284**, 166P–167P.

Cerretelli, P., Cruz, J. C., Farhi, L. E., and Rahn, H. (1966). Determination of mixed venous O_2 and CO_2 tensions and cardiac output by a rebreathing method. *Respir. Physiol.* **1**, 258–264.

Cerretelli, P., Di Prampero, P. E., and Rennie, D. W. (1970). Measurement of mixed venous oxygen tension by a modified rebreathing procedure. *J. Appl. Physiol.* **28**, 707–711.

Cerretelli, P., Veicsteinas, A., Teichmann, J., Magnussen, H., and Piiper, J. (1974). Estimation by a rebreathing method of pulmonary O_2 diffusing capacity in man. *J. Appl. Physiol.* **37**, 526–532.

Chinet, A., Micheli, J. L., and Haab, P. (1971). Inhomogeneity effects on O_2 and CO pulmonary diffusing capacity estimates by steady-state methods. Theory. *Respir. Physiol.* **13**, 1–22.

Christiansen, J., Douglas, C. G., and Haldane, J. S. (1914). The absorption and dissociation of carbon dioxide by human blood. *J. Physiol. (London)* **48**, 244–271.

Clark, T. J. H. (1968). The ventilatory response to CO_2 in chronic airway obstruction measured by a rebreathing method. *Clin. Sci.* **34**, 559–568.

Clausen, J. P., Larsen, O. A., and Trap-Jensen, J. (1970). Cardiac output in middle-aged patients determined with CO_2 rebreathing method. *J. Appl. Physiol.* **28**, 337–342.

Collier, C. R. (1956). Determination of mixed venous CO_2 tension by rebreathing. *J. Appl. Physiol.* **9**, 25–29.

Cosentino, A., Storey, W., and Staub, N. C. (1961). Small vessel hematocrit in lungs. *Fed. Proc., Fed. Am. Soc. Exp. Biol.* **20**, 426.

Crandall, E. D., and Flumerfelt, R. W. (1967). Effects of time-varying blood flow on oxygen uptake in pulmonary capillaries. *J. Appl. Physiol.* **23**, 944–953.

Cross, C. E., Meyer, D. H., and Gillespie, J. R. (1969). A comparison of the lung uptakes of isotopic tracer $^{18}O_2$, CO and C_2H_2. *Physiologist* **12**, 203.

Cross, C. E., Gong, H., Jr., Kurpershoek, C. J., Gillespie, J. R., and Hyde, R. W. (1973). Alterations in distribution of blood flow to the lung's diffusion surfaces during exercise. *J. Clin. Invest.* **52**, 414–421.

Davies, D. G., and Dutton, R. E. (1975). Gas–blood P_{CO_2} gradients during avian gas exchange. *J. Appl. Physiol.* **39**, 405–410.

Defares, J. G. (1958). Determination of $P\bar{v}_{CO_2}$ from the exponential CO_2 rise during rebreathing. *J. Appl. Physiol.* **13**, 159–164.

Denison, D., Edwards, R. H. T., Jones, G., and Pope, H. (1969). Direct and rebreathing estimates of the O_2 and CO_2 pressures in mixed venous blood. *Respir. Physiol.* **7**, 326–334.

Denison, D., Edwards, R. H. T., Jones, G., and Pope, H. (1971). Estimates of the CO_2 pressures in systemic arterial blood during rebreathing on exercise. *Respir. Physiol.* **11**, 186–196.

Dollery, C. T., Dyson, N. A., and Sinclair, J. D. (1960). Regional variations in uptake of radioactive CO in the normal lung. *J. Appl. Physiol.* **15**, 411–417.

DuBois, A. B. (1952). Alveolar CO_2 and O_2 during breath holding, expiration, and inspiration. *J. Appl. Physiol.* **5**, 1–12.

DuBois, A. B., Brett, A. G., and Fenn, W. O. (1952). Alveolar CO_2 during the respiratory cycle. *J. Appl. Physiol.* **4**, 535–548.

Effros, R. M. (1972). Pulmonary capillary carbon dioxide gradients and the Wien effect. *J. Appl. Physiol.* **32**, 221–222.

Farhi, L. E., and Haab, P. (1967). Mixed venous blood gas tensions and cardiac output by "bloodless" methods: Recent developments and appraisal. *Respir. Physiol.* **2**, 225–232.

Farhi, L. E., and Rahn, H. (1955). A theoretical analysis of the alveolar–arterial O_2 difference with special reference to the distribution effect. *J. Appl. Physiol.* **7**, 699–703.

Farhi, L. E., and Riley, R. L. (1957). Graphic analysis of moment-to-moment changes in blood passing through the pulmonary capillary, including a demonstration of three graphic methods for estimating the mean alveolar–capillary diffusion gradient (Bohr integration). *J. Appl. Physiol.* **10**, 179–190.

Fenn, W. O., and Dejours, P. (1954). Composition of alveolar air during breath holding with and without prior inhalation of oxygen and carbon dioxide. *J. Appl. Physiol.* **7,** 313–319.

Field, G. B., Jones, G., and McFadden, E. R., Jr. (1971). Alveolar–arterial P_{CO_2} differences during rebreathing in chronic-airways obstruction. *J. Appl. Physiol.* **31,** 490–496.

Filley, G. F., Macintosh, D. J., and Wright, G. W. (1954). Carbon monoxide uptake and pulmonary diffusing capacity in normal subjects at rest and during exercise. *J. Clin. Invest.* **33,** 530–539.

Folgering, H., Smolders, F. D. J., and Kreuzer, F. (1978). Respiratory oscillations of the arterial P_{O_2} and their effects on the ventilatory controlling system in the cat. *Pfluegers Arch.* **375,** 1–7.

Forster, R. E. (1957). Exchange of gases between alveolar air and pulmonary capillary blood: pulmonary diffusing capacity. *Physiol. Rev.* **37,** 391–452.

Forster, R. E. (1964). Diffusion of gases. *In* "Handbook of Physiology. Sect. 3: Respiration" (W. O. Fenn and H. Rahn, eds.), Vol. 1, pp. 839–872. Am. Physiol. Soc., Washington, D.C.

Forster, R. E., and Crandall, E. D. (1975). Time course of exchanges between red cells and extracellular fluid during CO_2 uptake. *J. Appl. Physiol.* **38,** 710–718.

Forster, R. E., and Crandall, E. D. (1976). Pulmonary gas exchange. *Annu. Rev. Physiol.* **38,** 69–93.

Forster, R. E., Fowler, W. S., Bates, D. V., and Van Lingen, B. (1954). The absorption of carbon monoxide by the lungs during breathholding. *J. Clin. Invest.* **33,** 1135–1145.

Garman, R. F., Hyde, R. W., Fisher, A. B., and Forster, R. E. (1970). The single breath O_2 diffusing capacity (DL_{O_2}) at rest and exercise; its use in determining pulmonary diffusion/perfusion relationships. *Physiologist* **13,** 200.

Gehr, P., Bachofen, M., and Weibel, E. R. (1978). The normal human lung: Ultrastructure and morphometric estimation of diffusing capacity. *Respir. Physiol.* **32,** 121–140.

Geiser, J., Chinet, A., and Haab, P. (1979). Pulmonary O_2 diffusing capacity estimates from assumed log-normal $\dot{V}_A/\dot{Q}$ distributions. *Respir. Physiol.* **36,** 31–44.

Glazier, J. B., Hughes, J. M. B., Maloney, J. E., and West, J. B. (1969). Measurement of capillary dimensions and blood volume in rapidly frozen lungs. *J. Appl. Physiol.* **26,** 65–76.

Gong, H., Meyer, D., Hyde, R., Gillespie, J., and Cross, C. (1970). $^{18}O_2$ diffusing capacity at rest and during exercise in normal man. *Clin. Res.* **18,** 484.

Gong, H., Kurpershoek, C., and Cross, C. E. (1972a). $^{18}O_2$ diffusing capacity measured by a rebreathing method in normal man. *Clin. Res.* **20,** 195.

Gong, H., Jr., Kurpershoek, C. J., Meyer, D. B., and Cross, C. E. (1972b). Effects of cardiac output on $^{18}O_2$ lung diffusion in normal resting man. *Respir. Physiol.* **16,** 313–326.

Graeser, H. J., Kim, Y. G., and Crandall, E. D. (1969). The effects of time-varying blood flow on diffusional resistance to oxygen transfer in the pulmonary capillaries. *Biophys. J.* **9,** 1100–1114.

Gurtner, G. H., and Fowler, W. S. (1971). Interrelationships of factors affecting pulmonary diffusing capacity. *J. Appl. Physiol.* **30,** 619–624.

Gurtner, G. H., Song, S. H., and Farhi, L. E. (1969). Alveolar to mixed venous P_{CO_2} difference under conditions of no gas exchange. *Respir. Physiol.* **7,** 173–187.

Gurtner, G., Peavy, H., Summer, W., and Burns, B. (1975). Physiological evidence for the presence of a specific O_2, CO carrier in the lung and placenta. *Prog. Respir. Res.* **8,** 166–176.

Guyatt, A. R., Yu, C. J., Lutherer, B., and Otis, A. B. (1973). Studies of alveolar-mixed venous CO_2 and O_2 gradients in the rebreathing dog lung. *Respir. Physiol.* **17,** 178–294.

Haab, P., Duc, G., Stucki, R., and Piiper, J. (1964). Les échanges gazeux en hypoxie et la capacité de diffusion pour l'oxygène chez le chien narcotisé. *Helv. Physiol. Acta* **22,** 203–227.

Haab, P., Perret, C., and Piiper, J. (1965). La capacité de diffusion pulmonaire pour l'oxygène chez l'homme normal jeune. *Helv. Physiol. Acta* **23,** C23–C25.

Haab, P., Robert, M., and Piiper, J. (1968). Comparaison de la capacité de diffusion pulmonaire du chien narcotisé mesurée simultanément par l'oxygène et le monoxyde de carbone. *J. Physiol. (Paris)* **60,** Suppl. 2, 455–456.

Haab, P., Robert, M., and Piiper, J. (1970). Comparative measurements of $D_L CO$ and $D_L O_2$ in the dog. *Experientia* **26,** 680.

Hamilton, W. F. (1962). Measurement of the cardiac output. *In* "Handbook of Physiology. Sect. 2: Circulation" (W. F. Hamilton and P. Dow, eds.), Vol. 1, pp. 551–584. Am. Physiol. Soc., Washington, D.C.

Hill, E. P., Power, G. G., and Longo, L. D. (1973). Mathematical simulation of pulmonary O_2 and CO_2 exchange. *Am. J. Physiol.* **224,** 904–917.

Hlastala, M. P. (1972). A model of fluctuating alveolar gas exchange during the respiratory cycle. *Respir. Physiol.* **15,** 214–232.

Holland, R. A. B. (1969). Rate at which CO replaces O_2 from $O_2 Hb$ in red cells of different species. *Respir. Physiol.* **7,** 43–63.

Holland, R. A. B., Van Hezewijk, W., and Zubzanda, J. (1977). Velocity of oxygen uptake by partly saturated adult and fetal human red cells. *Respir. Physiol.* **29,** 303–314.

Hyde, R. W., Forster, R. E., Power, G. G., Nairn, J., and Rynes, R. (1966). Measurement of O_2 diffusing capacity of the lungs with a stable O_2 isotope. *J. Clin. Invest.* **45,** 1178–1193.

Hyde, R. W., Rynes, R., Power, G. G., and Nairn, J. (1967). Determination of distribution of diffusing capacity in relation to blood flow in the human lung. *J. Clin. Invest.* **46,** 463–474.

Hyde, R. W., Puy, R. J. M., Raub, W. F., and Forster, R. E. (1968). Rate of disappearance of labeled carbon dioxide from the lungs of humans during breath holding: A method for studying the dynamics of pulmonary CO_2 exchange. *J. Clin. Invest.* **47,** 1535–1552.

Hyde, R. W., Marin, M. G., Rynes, R. J., Karreman, G., and Forster, R. E. (1971). Measurement of uneven distribution of pulmonary blood flow to CO diffusing capacity. *J. Appl. Physiol.* **31,** 605–612.

Jennings, D. B., and Chen, C. C. (1975). Negative arterial-mixed expired P_{CO_2} gradient during acute and chronic hypercapnia. *J. Appl. Physiol.* **38,** 382–388.

Jernérus, R., Lundin, G., and Thomson, D. (1963). Cardiac output in healthy subjects determined with a CO_2 rebreathing method. *Acta Physiol. Scand.* **59,** 390–399.

Johnson, R. L., Jr., and Miller, J. M. (1968). Distribution of ventilation, blood flow, and gas transfer coefficients in the lung. *J. Appl. Physiol.* **25,** 1–15.

Johnson, R. L., Jr., Spicer, W. S., Bishop, J. M., and Forster, R. E. (1960). Pulmonary capillary blood volume, flow and diffusing capacity during exercise. *J. Appl. Physiol.* **15,** 893–902.

Jones, N. L., McHardy, G. J. R., Naimark, N., and Campbell, E. J. M. (1966). Physiological dead space and alveolar–arterial gas pressure differences during exercise. *Clin. Sci.* **31,** 19–29.

Jones, N. L., Campbell, E. J. M., McHardy, G. J. R., Higgs, B. R., and Clode, M. (1967). The estimation of carbon dioxide pressure of mixed venous blood during exercise. *Clin. Sci.* **32,** 311–327.

Jones, N. L., Campbell, E. J. M., Edwards, R. H. T., and Wilkoff, W. G. (1969). Alveolar-to-blood P_{CO_2} difference during rebreathing in exercise. *J. Appl. Physiol.* **27,** 356–360.

Jones, N. L., Robertson, D. G., Kane, J. W., and Campbell, E. J. M. (1972). Effect of P_{CO_2} level on alveolar–arterial P_{CO_2} difference during rebreathing. *J. Appl. Physiol.* **32**, 782–787.

Kim, T. S., Rahn, H., and Farhi, L. E. (1966). Estimation of true venous and arterial P_{CO_2} by gas analysis of a single breath. *J. Appl. Physiol.* **21**, 1338–1344.

King, T. K. C., and Briscoe, (1967). Bohr integral isopleths in the study of blood gas exchange in the lung. *J. Appl. Physiol.* **22**, 659–674.

King, T. K. C., and Mazal, D. (1976). Alveolar–capillary CO_2 and O_2 gradients due to uneven hematocrits. *J. Appl. Physiol.* **40**, 673–678.

Kjerulf-Jensen, K., and Kruhøffer, P. (1954). The lung diffusion coefficient for carbon monoxide in patients with lung disorders as determined by $C^{14}O$. *Acta Med. Scand.* **150**, 395–406.

Kreuzer, F., and Van Lookeren Campagne, P. (1965). Resting pulmonary diffusing capacity for CO and O_2 at high altitude. *J. Appl. Physiol.* **20**, 519–524.

Kruhøffer, P. (1954). Studies on the lung diffusion coefficient for carbon monoxide in normal human subjects by means of $C^{14}O$. *Acta Physiol. Scand.* **32**, 106–123.

Larson, C. P., and Severinghaus, J. W. (1962). Postural variations in dead space and CO_2 gradients breathing air and O_2. *J. Appl. Physiol.* **17**, 417–420.

Laszlo, G., Clark, T. J. H., Pope, H., and Campbell, E. J. M. (1971). Differences between alveolar and arterial P_{CO_2} during rebreathing experiments in resting human subjects. *Respir. Physiol.* **12**, 36–52.

Lawson, W. H., Jr. (1970). Rebreathing measurements of pulmonary diffusing capacity for CO during exercise. *J. Appl. Physiol.* **29**, 896–900.

Lee, G. de J., and DuBois, A. B. (1955). Pulmonary capillary blood flow in man. *J. Clin. Invest.* **34**, 1380–1390.

Lenfant, C., and Okubo, T. (1968). Distribution function of pulmonary blood flow and ventilation–perfusion ratio in man. *J. Appl. Physiol.* **24**, 668–677.

Lewis, B. M., Lin, T. H., Noe, F. E., and Hayford-Welsing, E. J. (1959). The measurement of pulmonary diffusing capacity for carbon monoxide by a rebreathing method. *J. Clin. Invest.* **38**, 2073–2086.

Liese, W., Warwick, W. J., and Cumming, G. (1974). Water vapour pressure in expired air. *Respiration* **31**, 252–261.

Lin, K. H., and Cumming, G. (1973). A model of time-varying gas exchange in the human lung during a respiratory cycle at rest. *Respir. Physiol.* **17**, 93–112.

McEvoy, J. D. S., Jones, N. L., and Campbell, E. J. M. (1973). Alveolar-arterial P_{CO_2} difference during rebreathing in patients with chronic hypercapnia. *J. Appl. Physiol.* **35**, 542–545.

Matell, G. (1963). Time-courses of changes in ventilation and arterial gas tensions in man induced by moderate exercise. *Acta Physiol. Scand.* **58**, Suppl. 206, 1–53.

Mazzone, R. W., Durand, C. M., and West, J. B. (1978). Electron microscopy of lung rapidly frozen under controlled physiological conditions. *J. Appl. Physiol.* **45**, 325–333.

Mendoza, C., Peavy, H., Burns, B., and Gurtner, G. (1977). Saturation kinetics for steady-state pulmonary CO transfer. *J. Appl. Physiol.* **43**, 880–884.

Menkes, H. A., Sera, K., Rogers, R. M., Hyde, R. W., Forster, R. E., and DuBois, A. B. (1970). Pulsatile uptake of CO in the human lung. *J. Clin. Invest.* **49**, 335–345.

Meyer, M. (1979). Experimental evidence against role of facilitated transport of carbon monoxide in alveolar gas. *Pfluegers Arch.* **379**, R20.

Meyer, M., and Piiper, J. (1978). Pulmonary diffusing capacity for carbon monoxide and oxygen in man during heavy exercise. *Pfluegers Arch.* **373**, Suppl., p. 117.

Meyer, M., Worth, H., and Scheid, P. (1976). Gas-blood CO_2 equilibration in parabronchial lungs of birds. *J. Appl. Physiol.* **41**, 302–309.

Michaelson, E. D., Sackner, M. A., and Johnson, R. L., Jr. (1973). Vertical distribution of pulmonary diffusing capacity and capillary blood flow in man. *J. Clin. Invest.* **52**, 359–369.

Micheli, J. L., and Haab, P. (1970). Estimation de la capacité de diffusion pulmonaire pour l'oxygène chez l'homme au repos par la méthode du rebreathing hypoxique. *J. Physiol. (Paris)* **62**, Suppl. 1, 194–195.

Miller, J. N., and Camporesi, E. M. (1977). Rebreathing DL_{CO} with ^{13}CO. *Fed. Proc., Fed. Am. Soc. Exp. Biol.* **36**, 629.

Mittman, C., and Burrows, B. (1959). Uniformity of pulmonary diffusion: Effect of lung volume. *J. Appl. Physiol.* **14**, 496–498.

Miyamoto, Y., and Moll, W. (1971). Measurement of dimensions and pathway of red cells in rapidly frozen lungs in situ. *Respir. Physiol.* **12**, 141–156.

Mochizuki, M. (1966). Study on the oxygenation velocity of the human red cell. *Jpn. J. Physiol.* **16**, 635–648.

Mochizuki, M., Anso, T., Goto, H., Hamamoto, A., and Makiguchi, Y. (1958). The dependency of the diffusing capacity on the HbO_2 saturation of the capillary blood and on anemia. *Jpn. J. Physiol.* **8**, 225–233.

Moll, W. (1962). Die Oxygenation der Erythrocyten in der Lunge durch Diffusion, Reaktion und spezifischen Transport. *Pfluegers Arch.* **275**, 420–438.

Newth, C. J. L., Cotton, D. J., and Nadel, J. A. (1977). Pulmonary diffusing capacity measured at multiple intervals during a single exhalation in man. *J. Appl. Physiol.* **43**, 617–625.

Nye, R. E. (1970). Influence of the cyclical pattern of ventilatory flow on pulmonary gas exchange. *Respir. Physiol.* **10**, 321–337.

Ogilvie, C. M., Forster, R. E., Blakemore, W. S., and Morton, J. W. (1957). A standardized breath holding technique for the clinical measurement of the diffusing capacity of the lung for carbon monoxide. *J. Clin. Invest.* **36**, 1–17.

Pande, J. N., Lipscomb, D. J., Forse, G., Jones, T., and Hughes, J. M. B. (1975). Regional differences in carbon monoxide uptake in the lung. *INSERM* **51**, 169–174.

Piiper, J. (1961a). Unequal distribution of pulmonary diffusing capacity and the alveolar–arterial P_{O_2} differences: theory. *J. Appl. Physiol.* **16**, 493–498.

Piiper, J. (1961b). Variations of ventilation and diffusing capacity to perfusion determining the alveolar–arterial O_2 difference: theory. *J. Appl. Physiol.* **16**, 507–510.

Piiper, J. (1962a). Theoretische Untersuchung der alveolär-capillären O_2-Differenz bei verschiedenen Annahmen über die Lage des Diffusionswiderstandes. *Pfluegers Arch.* **275**, 173–192.

Piiper, J. (1962b). O_2-Austausch der isolierten Hundelunge im hypoxischen Bereich bei Veränderungen der Erythrozytenkonzentration und der Durchblutung. *Pfluegers Arch.* **275**, 193–214.

Piiper, J. (1965). Physiological equilibria of gas cavities in the body. *In* "Handbook of Physiology. Sect. 3: Respiration" (W. O. Fenn and H. Rahn, eds.), Vol. 2, pp. 1205–1217. Am. Physiol. Soc., Washington, D.C.

Piiper, J. (1969). Apparent increase of the O_2 diffusing capacity with increased O_2 uptake in inhomogeneous lungs: theory. *Respir. Physiol.* **6**, 209–218.

Piiper, J. (1979). Blood–gas equilibration of CO_2 in pulmonary gas exchange of mammals and birds. *Physiologist* **22**, 54–59.

Piiper, J. and Meyer, M. (1978). Pulmonary diffusing capacity for CO and O_2 measured simultaneously by a rebreathing technique. *Fed. Proc., Fed. Am. Soc. Exp. Biol.* **37**, 905.

Piiper, J., and Scheid, P. (1971). Respiration: Alveolar gas exchange. *Annu. Rev. Physiol.* **33**, 131–154.

Piiper, J., and Sikand, R. S. (1966). Determination of D_{CO} by the single breath method in inhomogeneous lungs: theory. *Respir. Physiol.* **1**, 75–87.

Piiper, J., Haab, P., and Rahn, H. (1961). Unequal distribution of pulmonary diffusing capacity in the anesthetized dog. *J. Appl. Physiol.* **16**, 499–506.

Piiper, J., Cerretelli, P., Rennie, D. W., and Di Prampero, P. E. (1971a). Estimation of the pulmonary diffusing capacity for O_2 by a rebreathing procedure. *Respir. Physiol.* **12**, 157–162.

Piiper, J., Dejours, P., Haab, P., and Rahn, H. (1971b). Concepts and basic quantities in gas exchange physiology. *Respir. Physiol.* **13**, 292–304.

Piiper, J., Gatz, R. N., and Crawford, E. C., Jr. (1976). Gas transport characteristics in an exclusively skin-breathing salamander, *Desmognathus fuscus (Plethodontidae). In* "Respiration of Amphibious Vertebrates" (G. M. Hughes, ed.), pp. 339–356. Academic Press, New York.

Plaas-Link, A., Mueller, J., Luttmann, A., Mückenhoff, K., and Loeschcke, H. H. (1977). Measurement of natural arterial CO_2 oscillations and production of artificial ones in cats. *Fed. Proc. Fed. Am. Soc. Exp. Biol.* **36**, 425.

Plesch, J. (1909). Hämodynamische Studien. *Z. Exp. Pathol. Ther.* **6**, 380–618.

Power, G. G., and Bradford, W. C. (1969). Measurement of pulmonary diffusing capacity during blood-to-gas exchange in humans. *J. Appl. Physiol.* **27**, 61–66.

Purves, M. J. (1966). Fluctuations of arterial oxygen tension which have the same period as respiration. *Respir. Physiol.* **1**, 281–296.

Rahn, H. (1949). A concept of mean alveolar air and the ventilation–blood flow relationships during pulmonary gas exchange. *Am. J. Physiol.* **158**, 21–30.

Rahn, H. (1954). The sampling of alveolar gas. *In* "Respiratory Physiology in Aviation" (W. B. Boothby, ed.), pp. 29–37. USAF Sch. Aviat. Med., Randolph Field, Texas.

Rapaport, E., Kuida, H., Haynes, F. W., and Dexter, L. (1956). Pulmonary red cell and plasma volumes and pulmonary hematocrit in the normal dog. *Am. J. Physiol.* **185**, 127–132.

Riley, R. L., and Cournand, A. (1949). "Ideal" alveolar air and the analysis of ventilation–perfusion relationships in the lungs. *J. Appl. Physiol.* **1**, 825–847.

Riley, R. L., and Cournand, A. (1951). Analysis of factors affecting partial pressures of oxygen and carbon dioxide in gas and blood of the lungs: theory. *J. Appl. Physiol.* **4**, 77–101.

Riley, R. L., and Permutt, S. (1973). Venous admixture component of the AaP_{O_2} gradient. *J. Appl. Physiol.* **35**, 430–431.

Riley, R. L., Shephard, R. H., Cohn, J. E., Carroll, D. G., and Armstrong, B. W. (1954). Maximal diffusing capacity of the lungs. *J. Appl. Physiol.* **6**, 573–587.

Robertson, H. T., and Hlastala, M. P. (1977). Elevated alveolar P_{CO_2} relative to predicted values during normal gas exchange. *J. Appl. Physiol.* **43**, 357–364.

Roughton, F. J. W., and Forster, R. E. (1957). Relative importance of diffusion and chemical reaction rates in determining rate of exchange of gases in the human lung, with special reference to true diffusing capacity of pulmonary membrane and volume of blood in the lung capillaries. *J. Appl. Physiol.* **11**, 291–302.

Sackner, M. A., Greeneltch, G., Heiman, M. S., Epstein, S., and Atkins, N. (1975). Diffusing capacity, membrane diffusing capacity, capillary blood volume, pulmonary tissue volume, and cardiac output measured by a rebreathing technique. *Am. Rev. Respir. Dis.* **111**, 157–165.

Scheid, P., and Piiper, J. (1970). Analysis of gas exchange in the avian lung: Theory and experiments in the domestic fowl. *Respir. Physiol.* **9**, 246–262.

Scheid, P., and Piiper, J. (1972). Cross-current gas exchange in avian lungs: Effects of reversed parabronchial air flow in ducks. *Respir. Physiol.* **16**, 304–312.

Scheid, P., and Piiper, J. (1976). Quantitative functional analysis of branchial gas transfer: Theory and application to *Scyliorhinus stellaris (Elasmobranchii)*. *In* "Respiration of Amphibious Vertebrates" (G. M. Hughes, ed.), pp. 17–38. Academic Press, New York.

Scheid, P., and J. Piiper (1980). Blood/gas equilibrium of carbon dioxide in lungs. A critical review. *Respir. Physiol.* **39**, 1–31.

Scheid, P., Slama, H., and Piiper, J. (1971). Electronic compensation of the effects of water vapor in respiratory mass spectrometry. *J. Appl. Physiol.* **30**, 258–260.

Scheid, P., Teichmann, J., Adaro, F., and Piiper, J. (1972). Gas–blood CO_2 equilibration in dog lungs during rebreathing. *J. Appl. Physiol.* **33**, 582–588.

Scheid, P., Adaro, F., Teichmann, J., and Piiper, J. (1973). Rebreathing and steady state pulmonary D_{O_2} in the dog and in inhomogeneous lung models. *Respir. Physiol.* **18**, 258–272.

Scheid, P., Meyer, M., and Piiper, J. (1979a). Arterial-expired P_{CO_2} differences in the dog during acute hypercapnia. *J. Appl. Physiol.* **47**, 1074–1079.

Scheid, P., Meyer, M., and Slama, H. (1979b). Use of a mass spectrometer to measure lung diffusing capacity for O_2 and CO by rebreathing stable isotopes at tracer levels. *Bull. Europ. Physiopath. Resp.* **15**, 11P–14P.

Schmidt, W., Thews, G., and Schnabel, K. H. (1972). Results of distribution analysis of ventilation, perfusion and O_2 diffusing capacity in the human lung. *Respiration* **29**, 1–16.

Shepard, R. H., Varnauskas, E., Martin, H. B., White, H. A., Permutt, S., Cotes, J. E., and Riley, R. L. (1958). Relationship between cardiac output and apparent diffusing capacity of the lung in normal men during treadmill exercise. *J. Appl. Physiol.* **13**, 205–210.

Sikand, R. S., and Piiper, J. (1966). Pulmonary diffusing capacity for CO in dogs by the single breath method. *Respir. Physiol.* **1**, 172–192.

Slama, H., and Scheid, P. (1975). Electronic feedback circuit for increasing signal-to-noise ratio in a mass spectrometer. *Pneumonologie* **151**, 247–249.

Sølvsteen, P. (1964). Measurement of lung diffusing capacity by means of $C^{14}O$ in a closed system. *J. Appl. Physiol.* **19**, 59–74.

Sølvsteen, P. (1965a). Lung diffusing capacity: Cyclically and continuously ventilated closed systems. *J. Appl. Physiol.* **20**, 92–98.

Sølvsteen, P. (1965b). Lung diffusing capacity: Rebreathing method, applicability in nonuniform ventilation. *J. Appl. Physiol.* **20**, 99–102.

Staub, N. C., Bishop, J. M., and Forster, R. E. (1962). Importance of diffusion and chemical reaction rates in O_2 uptake in the lung. *J. Appl. Physiol.* **17**, 21–27.

Suwa, K., and Bendixen, H. H. (1972). Pulmonary gas exchange in a tidally ventilated single alveolus model. *J. Appl. Physiol.* **32**, 834–841.

Sybert, A., Ayash, R., Mendoza, C., and Gurtner, G. (1978). Abolition of carrier mediated pulmonary CO transport by hyperoxia. *Fed. Proc., Fed. Am. Soc. Exp. Biol.* **37**, 906.

Teichmann, J., Adaro, F., Veisteinas, A., Cerretelli, P., and Piiper, J. (1974). Determination of pulmonary blood flow by rebreathing of soluble inert gases. *Respiration* **31**, 296–309.

Thews, G. (1963). Die theoretischen Grundlagen der Sauerstoffaufnahme in der Lunge. *Ergeb. Physiol., Biol. Chem. Exp. Pharmakol.* **53**, 42–107.

Thews, G. (1968). The theory of oxygen transport and its application to gaseous exchange in the lung. *In* "Oxygen Transport in Tissue" (D. W. Lübbers, U. C. Luft, G. Thews, and E. Witzleb, eds.), pp. 1–20. Thieme, Stuttgart.

Thews, G., and Vogel, H. R. (1968). Die Verteilungsanalyse von Ventilation, Perfusion und
    O₂-Diffusionskapazität in der Lunge durch Konzentrationswechsel dreier Inspira-
    tionsgase. I. Theorie. *Pfluegers Arch.* **303**, 195–205.
Thews, G., Schmidt, W., and Schnabel, K. H. (1971). Analysis of distribution inhomogene-
    ities of ventilation, perfusion and O₂ diffusing capacity in the human lung. *Respiration*
    28, 197–215.
Turino, G. M., Bergofsky, E. H., Goldring, R. M., and Fishman, A. P. (1963). Effect of ex-
    ercise on pulmonary diffusing capacity. *J. Appl. Physiol.* **18**, 447–456.
Ulmer, W. T., and Reichel, G. (1961). Physiologie und Pathologie des Gasaustausches in
    den Lungen, Untersuchungen zum alveolär/arteriellen Kohlensäuredruckgradienten.
    In "Bad Oeynhausener Gespräche" (H. Bartels and E. Witzleb, eds.), Vol. IV,
    pp. 53–65. Springer-Verlag, Berlin and New York.
Veicsteinas, A., Magnussen, H., Meyer, M., and Cerretelli, P. (1976). Pulmonary O₂ dif-
    fusing capacity at exercise by a modified rebreathing method. *Eur. J. Appl. Physiol.*
    35, 79–88.
Vogel, H. R., and Thews, G. (1968). Die Verteilungsanalyse von Ventilation, Perfusion und
    O₂-Diffusionskapazität in der Lunge durch Konzentrationswechsel dreier Inspira-
    tionsgase. II. Durchführung des Verfahrens. *Pfluegers Arch.* **303**, 206–217.
Vogel, H. R., Thews, G., Schulz, V., and von Mengden, H. J. (1968). Die Verteilungsana-
    lyse von Ventilation, Perfusion und O₂-Diffusionskapazität in der Lunge durch Kon-
    zentrationswechsel dreier Inspirationsgase. III. Untersuchung von Jugendlichen, äl-
    teren Personen und Schwangeren. *Pfluegers Arch.* **303**, 218–229.
Vreim, C. E., and Staub, N. C. (1973). Indirect and direct capillary blood volume in anesthe-
    tized open-thorax cats. *J. Appl. Physiol.* **34**, 452–459.
Wagner, P. D. (1977). Diffusion and chemical reaction in pulmonary gas exchange. *Physiol.
    Rev.* **57**, 257–312.
Wagner, P. D., and West, J. B. (1972). Effects of diffusion impairment on O₂ and CO₂ time
    courses in pulmonary capillaries. *J. Appl. Physiol.* **33**, 62–71.
Wagner, P. D., Mazzone, R. W., and West, J. B. (1971). Diffusing capacity and anatomic
    dead space for carbon monoxide (C¹⁸O). *J. Appl. Physiol.* **31**, 847–852.
Wagner, P. D., Laravuso, R. B., Goldzimmer, E., Naumann, P. F., and West, J. B. (1975).
    Distributions of ventilation–perfusion ratios in dogs with normal and abnormal lungs.
    J. Appl. Physiol. **38**, 1099–1109.
Warrell, D. A., Evans, J. W., Clarke, R. O., Kingaby, G. P., and West, J. B. (1972). Pattern
    of filling in the pulmonary capillary bed. *J. Appl. Physiol.* **32**, 346–356.
Weibel, E. R. (1963). "Morphometry of the Human Lung." Springer-Verlag, Berlin and
    New York.
Weibel, E. R. (1973). Morphological basis of alveolar–capillary gas exchange. *Physiol. Rev.*
    53, 419–495.
West, J. B. (1962). Regional differences in gas exchange in the lung of erect man. *J. Appl.
    Physiol.* **17**, 893–898.
West, J. B. (1965). Topographical distribution of blood flow in the lung. *In* "Handbook of
    Physiology. Sect. 3: Respiration" (W. O. Fenn and H. Rahn, eds.), Vol. 2, pp.
    1437–1451. Am. Physiol. Soc., Washington, D.C.
West, J. B. (1969). Ventilation–perfusion inequality and overall gas exchange in computer
    models of the lung. *Respir. Physiol.* **7**, 88–110.
West, J. B., and Dollery, C. T. (1960). Distribution of blood flow and ventilation–perfusion
    ratio in the lung, measured with radioactive CO₂. *J. Appl. Physiol.* **15**, 405–410.
West, J. B., Holland, R. A. B., Dollery, C. T., and Matthews, C. M. E. (1962). Interpreta-
    tion of radioactive gas clearance rates in the lung. *J. Appl. Physiol.* **17**, 14–20.

Whipp, B. J., and Wasserman, K. (1969). Alveolar–arterial gas tension differences during graded exercise. *J. Appl. Physiol.* **27,** 361–365.
Wolffberg, S. (1871). Über die Spannung der Blutgase in den Lugencapillaren. *Arch. Gesamte Physiol. Menschen Tiere* **4,** 465–492.
Yu, C. J., Lutherer, B., Guyatt, A. R., and Otis, A. B. (1973). Comparison of blood and alveolar gas composition during rebreathing in the dog lung. *Respir. Physiol.* **17,** 162–177.
Zander, R., and Schmid-Schönbein, H. (1973). Intracellular mechanisms of oxygen transport in flowing blood. *Respir. Physiol.* **19,** 279–289.

6

Kinetics of Pulmonary Gas Exchange

Robert A. Klocke

In a single day the lung must exchange over 300 liters of oxygen and a somewhat lesser quantity of carbon dioxide between the environment and blood just to maintain human life. These rates may increase severalfold for hours at a time, and during short bursts of activity may increase by an order of magnitude over resting values. Gas exchange dynamics are even more striking since blood remains in the gas exchange vessels for an average of less than 1 sec at rest (Piiper, 1969) and perhaps as little as one-half of that time during exercise (Johnson *et al.*, 1960). Therefore, diffusion of O_2 and CO_2 from the gas phase and chemical reactions in blood must take place with extreme rapidity.

Knowledge of the kinetic events occurring during these processes has increased substantially in the last 15 years, requiring reassessment of commonly held beliefs. Previously most attention was focused on oxygen uptake with CO_2 exchange assumed to be complete because of the high solubility of CO_2 in the alveolar–capillary membrane. Current thought is that O_2 exchange is completed early in capillary transit, but that CO_2 barely reaches equilibrium even under normal circumstances (Wagner, 1977). Under abnormal conditions, both gases do not reach exchange equilibrium in the lung, but oxygen is affected to a greater degree than carbon dioxide (Wagner and West, 1972). In spite of the demands placed on the system, most investigators feel that kinetic processes are not commonly the cause of significant blood gas abnormalities, although this conviction is not held universally (King and Briscoe, 1967).

Technical difficulties have confined most work to *in vitro* experiments. Data from these observations have been inserted into computer models and extrapolated to physiological circumstances to construct a representation of the kinetic events that take place *in vivo*. This approach has greatly advanced our understanding of pulmonary gas exchange since it allows investigation of the influence of interactions of different processes. These interactions often are not apparent from *in vitro* work in which only a single or a few variables can be manipulated at any one time. The danger of this approach is that unknown factors are not included in models and their absence may vitiate theoretical conclusions. Although kinetic work is being extended to isolated organs (Effros *et al.*, 1978; Crandall and O'Brasky, 1978; Klocke, 1978a) and even the intact animal (Hill *et al.*, 1977; Bidani and Crandall, 1978), further substantial progress is necessary to verify conclusions reached in modeling experiments.

The kinetics of gas exchange have been thoroughly and excellently reviewed in the previous decade (Forster, 1964; Roughton, 1964). Therefore this chapter focuses primarily on work that has advanced our knowledge since that time.

I. EXPERIMENTAL TECHNIQUES

The special techniques necessary to study kinetic events place constraints upon experimental conditions and presently preclude exact duplication of physiological circumstances. Review of these methods is helpful in understanding the limitations of the data present in the literature.

A. Steady State Methods

The rapid-reaction flow technique, first developed by Hartridge and Roughton (1923) to study reactions in blood, has also been used extensively in areas other than biology. The method is limited to the liquid medium; hence it is suitable for estimating reaction times in blood but cannot duplicate exchange between two phases across the alveolar–capillary membrane. Reactants are driven rapidly into a mixing chamber using motor-driven syringes or pressurized reservoirs, and uniformly mixed in less than 1 msec (Fig. 1). The reaction continues as fluid moves out of the mixing chamber and through the flow tube. Since flow is continuous, the elapsed reaction time remains constant at any given point along the flow tube. The reaction mixture is monitored at the end of the flow tube and the reaction time is linearly related to the length of the tube. Instruments with relatively slow response times can be used to monitor rapid reactions as long as constant flow is maintained during the period of measurement. The progression of a reaction with time is determined by multiple observations made with flow tubes of different lengths. Thus, rapid reactions involving O_2 (Craw et al., 1963) and CO_2 (Constantine et al., 1965) can be investigated even though the electrodes used have a response time much greater than the duration of the reaction. Large quantities of reactants are required to maintain high flows for relatively long periods of time, but less volume is required if the reaction can be monitored at several points along the flow tube during a single flow observation (Tosteson, 1959; Edwards and Staub, 1966). Reactions involving exchange across cell membranes, such as transmembrane ionic exchange,

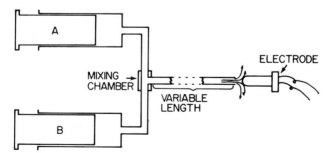

Fig. 1. Continuous-flow rapid-reaction apparatus. Reactants in syringes A and B are mixed in the chamber and continue to react as they are driven through the variable-length flow tube. Reactants are monitored at the end of the flow tube and the elapsed time is proportional to the tube length.

can be monitored by ultrafiltration of extracellular fluid with subsequent measurements made outside the reaction apparatus (Brahm, 1977).

Steady state transport can be utilized to determine chemical reaction rates providing that exchange is limited primarily by chemical rather than diffusional processes. Donaldson and Quinn (1974) studied facilitated diffusion of $^{14}CO_2$ through thin layers of aqueous bicarbonate solutions. The rate of conversion of CO_2 to bicarbonate limits the facilitation of diffusion and measurements of facilitated diffusion reflect carbonic anhydrase activity in the solution. Similarly, Klocke (1978a) was able to assess lung carbonic anhydrase activity by studying steady state CO_2 production in isolated rabbit lungs. In both studies the experimental conditions favored limitation of gas exchange principally by chemical reaction rates and not gaseous diffusion.

B. Unsteady State Methods

Gibson (1954) adapted the rapid-mixing principle to design the stopped-flow instrument, the most commonly used unsteady state technique. Reactants are driven by syringe into a mixing chamber, where the reaction is initiated, and proceed through an observation chamber into a third syringe (Fig. 2). Flow is suddenly arrested, leaving freshly mixed reactants in the observation chamber. As the reaction proceeds to com-

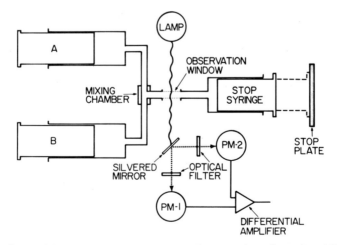

Fig. 2. Stopped-flow rapid-reaction apparatus. Reactants in syringes A and B are driven through the mixing chamber into the stop syringe. When the plunger of the stop syringe strikes the plate, flow stops and the reaction between the freshly mixed solutions is monitored in the observation chamber. A differential spectrophotometer is also illustrated.

pletion, a property of the mixture is monitored. Only rapidly responding instruments can be used to monitor the reaction, since response time must be considerably shorter than the duration of the reaction. In the past this has limited the stopped-flow method primarily to measurements of optical absorbance and electrical properties, but recently a rapidly responding pH electrode has been adapted to this apparatus (Crandall et al., 1971). A single run in the stopped-flow device provides a complete kinetic curve using only a few milliliters of reactants. Even cell suspensions can be studied using two wavelengths to cancel out light-scattering artifacts (Fig. 2).

In an effort to mimic physiological circumstances, some investigators have studied gas transport in a two-phase system. Luckner (1939) rapidly changed the CO_2 concentration in gas overlying a thin layer of blood and measured extracellular chloride concentration at the bottom of the layer. This approach enabled him to obtain an estimte of the speed of transmembrane $HCO_3^- - Cl^-$ exchange. Kreuzer and Yahr (1960) performed similar experiments, observing the rate of oxygen binding in thin layers of hemoglobin and blood by spectrophotometry. The major difficulty with this experimental approach has been that the layers are much thicker ($100-200$ μm) than the normal capillary diameter ($6-10$ μm). However, more recently studies have been conducted using very thin layers (Frech et al., 1968) or single cells (Sinha, 1969).

Investigations of the kinetics of gas exchange have been undertaken in intact animals using both plethysmography (Feisal et al., 1963). Instantaneous changes in lung volumes will reflect transport between the alveolar and capillary spaces, but experimental conditions must be manipulated so that only a single gas is exchanged.

C. Potential Artifacts

The in vitro measurements of chemical reactions are particularly prone to error. To prevent errors in estimating reaction time, turbulent flow must be maintained in both the stopped and continuous flow reaction apparatus. Even high flow rates do not always prevent the formation of stagnant layers (Rotman et al., 1970). Even with turbulent flow, eddies may exist, leading to diffusion gradients within the medium (Gad-el-Hak et al., 1977) and underestimation of the speed of a chemical reaction.

The presence of only a single phase in most experiments prevents duplication of physiological conditions. The lack of a gas phase and the relatively low solubility of respiratory gases in aqueous media result in wide fluctuations of gas tensions during the course of a reaction. In the measurements of oxygen uptake by red cells, experiments are performed with dilute erythrocyte suspensions and P_{O_2} may vary by 100–200 torr. As a result, measurements are often made under one set of conditions and extrapolated to events taking place under different circumstances. This problem is worrisome since our understanding of the actual kinetic mechanisms is incomplete and many observations are merely descriptive in nature.

Recently *in vitro* measurements of cellular reaction rates have come under attack from another direction. The erythrocyte is usually depicted as a biconcave disc of constant shape in which gases reach the interior primarily by diffusion. Convective intracellular mixing is ignored. Photographs of red cell suspensions indicate that the biconcave shape is maintained during flow under conditions similar to those encountered in most rapid reaction apparatus (Miyamoto and Moll, 1972). However, in rapidly frozen lungs erythrocytes appear to have a parachutelike configuration (Miyamoto and Moll, 1971). On the basis of *in vitro* work, Zander and Schmid-Schönbein (1973) concluded that the relative role of intracellular convection caused by distortion of the cell is greater than diffusive transport. Hence, an important factor present *in vivo* may be missing in experiments performed *in vitro*. There is no clear-cut answer to this question but confirmation of the currently accepted cellular reaction rates must be obtained under more physiological circumstances.

II. OXYGEN REACTIONS

Extensive studies have been conducted upon the reactions of hemoglobin and oxygen. The character and speed of these reactions are markedly influenced by the presence or absence of intact cells. The biology of the hemoglobin molecule is best studied in free solution, but the physiological consequences are reflected more clearly in cell suspensions.

A. Hemoglobin Solution

1. Kinetic Constants

In purely chemical terms, the equilibrium position of a system depends on both the reaction rate proceeding in one direction (k_f) and upon the rate in the reverse direction (k_b). The equilibrium constant is given by the ratio of the two kinetic constants ($K = k_f/k_b$). This straightforward kinetic approach is not strictly applicable in this case because the hemoglobin–oxygen relationship is sigmoid-shaped and cannot be described by a single constant. In the classic Adair hypothesis (Antonini and Brunori, 1971), four equilibrium constants, and hence eight kinetic constants are utilized to characterize the oxygen dissociation curve. Values for individual kinetic constants have been fitted to reaction data for hemoglobin in solution (Gibson, 1970), but this approach seems futile under present circumstances. Extraction of eight constants from kinetic data is prone to large errors due to the ill-conditioned nature of the problem. In addition, there is no certainty that the Adair hypothesis is correct, and the functional unit of hemoglobin may be a dimer rather than monomer (Antonini and Brunori, 1971). Accordingly, most workers describe hemoglobin reactions by a single association (k') and dissociation (k) constant

$$d([HbO_2])/dt = k'[Hb][O_2] - k[HbO_2] \qquad (1)$$

Although an entire reaction curve cannot be fitted with single values of k' and k, the fit is remarkably good and more elaborate calculations are not indicated considering the gaps in understanding of the basic mechanisms involved in hemoglobin–oxygen reactions (Bauer *et al.*, 1973).

2. Factors Influencing k', k

Since the equilibrium position of any reaction is dependent upon the ratio of forward and reverse kinetic constants, alteration of chemical equilibrium is effected through changes in one or both kinetic constants. Hence, any factor that influences the hemoglobin–oxygen equilibrium, usually characterized by the P_{50}, must influence the association and/or dissociation constants. Principal variables are hydrogen ion, temperature, and 2,3-diphosphoglyceric acid (2,3-DPG). Although CO_2 has a direct effect on the oxygen dissociation curve, the majority of its effect is exerted through its influence on pH (Roughton, 1964).

The kinetic bases of the major determinants of the position of the dissociation curve are shown in Fig. 3. Data in the panel on the left were obtained at 10°C, those on the right at 37°C. The lowest oxygen affinity, as measured by an increase in P_{50}, occurs at approximately pH 6.4 at both temperatures. As illustrated in the figure, the change in P_{50} with pH at both temperatures is the result of approximately equal changes in both k' and k. Likewise the increase in P_{50} mediated by 2,3-DPG (closed symbols) compared to phosphate-free media (open symbols) is the result of similar changes in both reaction constants. The effect of 2,3-DPG on all constants is greater at the lower temperature. In contrast to the equal changes in k' and k mediated through hydrogen ions and 2,3-DPG, temperature variation of the dissociation constant is greater than the association constant. Between 10 and 37°C, the latter increases approximately fivefold at pH 7.0, while the change in dissociation constant is greater than an order of

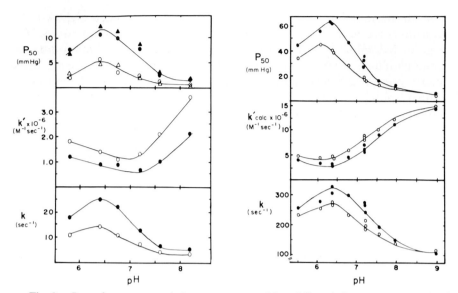

Fig. 3. P_{50} and oxygen association rate constant (k') and dissociation rate constant (k) of human hemoglobin solutions as a function of pH. Left-hand panel: temperature, 10°C, average hemoglobin concentration, 1.91×10^{-5} M. Right-hand panel: temperature, 37°C, average hemoglobin concentration, 5×10^{-3} M. Open symbols: dialyzed hemoglobin solution with no added 2,3-DPG. Filled symbols: 5×10^{-3} M 2,3-DPG added. Triangles: P_{50} calculated from k' and k. From Bauer *et al.*, 1973, reproduced by permission.)

magnitude. In obtaining the data in Fig. 3, Bauer *et al.* (1973) had to calculate k' from P_{50} and k at 37°C because of technical difficulties encountered in measurement of k'. They felt this procedure was acceptable since P_{50} calculated from k' and k (triangles) at 10°C agreed well with experimental data (circles). This illustrates that treating the oxygenation and deoxygenation reactions of hemoglobin as a single-step reaction provides a reasonable approximation of the true reaction, at least in the range of 50% saturation. However, this assumption becomes tenuous at the extremes of the dissociation curve.

In contrast to hemoglobin A, the oxygen affinity of fetal hemoglobin is less affected by 2,3-DPG. The apparent kinetic basis for this diminished 2,3-DPG effect is a failure of the organic phosphate to modify the dissociation rate constant (Salhany *et al.*, 1971). The influence of 2,3-DPG on the association constant has not been investigated but the lack of change in k is sufficient to explain the reduced effect of 2,3-DPG on the fetal hemoglobin P_{50}.

B. Erythrocyte Suspensions

Comparison of the rate of association–dissociation reactions of oxygen in hemoglobin solution and erythrocyte suspension indicates that the speed of the processes is 10–60 times slower in cell suspension (Roughton, 1964; Bauer *et al.*, 1973). As a result, the rate of oxygen exchange between the alveoli and pulmonary vessels not only is dependent upon diffusion across the alveolar–capillary membrane, but also is limited by the rate of oxygen uptake by red cells (Roughton and Forster, 1957). The marked discrepancy in the speed of oxygen reactions with hemoglobin in free solution and red cell suspensions has been attributed to a variety of factors.

1. Factors Influencing Reaction Rates

a. Erythrocyte Membrane. A highly structured lipid monolayer can offer considerably more resistance to diffusion of gases than a randomly organized film of the same thickness (Blank and Roughton, 1960). Since this alteration of the diffusion constant may be as great as several orders of magnitude, erythrocyte membrane permeability must be considered as a potential factor in slowing the rate of oxygen transfer. Nicolson and Roughton (1951) calculated the initial rate of oxygen uptake in a layer of hemoglobin unbounded by a membrane but of thickness equal to an erythrocyte. Comparing this rate with the value determined experimentally in erythrocyte suspensions, they concluded that the cell membrane was responsible for a portion of the difference in solution and suspension reaction rates. The relative importance of the membrane was expressed as λ, the ratio of permeability in the membrane to that in the cell interior. Forster (1964) refined these calculations using numerical techniques and applied them to a discoid-shaped packet of hemoglobin without a membrane (Fig. 4). On the basis of these calculations and agreement of the value of λ obtained under a variety of conditions, he concluded that the red cell membrane is a significant factor in oxygen transfer.

Conflicting experimental evidence concerning the importance of the cell membrane has been reported from two laboratories (Kreuzer and Yahr, 1960; Kutchai and Staub, 1969). The rate of steady state oxygen diffusion through layers of packed red cells is identical to that through concentrated hemoglobin solutions, implying that the membrane offers negligible resistance to diffusion. In addition, Kutchai (1975) has performed new calculations that do not support the concept of the cell membrane being an important factor. However, calculations of oxygen uptake by cells are critically dependent upon the values chosen for physical and

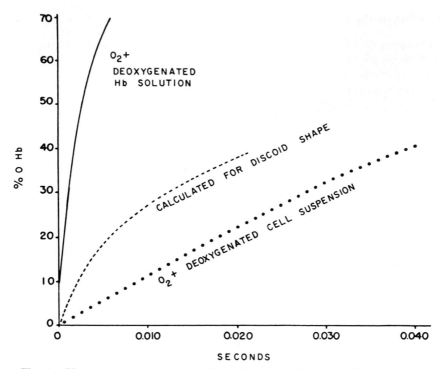

Fig. 4. Observed and calculated reactions of oxygen with hemoglobin in solution and cell suspension. Solid and dotted lines indicate experimental data. Dashed line represents calculated uptake by a discoid shape of hemoglobin unbounded by a cell membrane. The time lag between the calculated curve and experimental curve for the cell suspension is postulated to be due to the influence of the cell membrane on oxygen uptake. (From Forster, 1964, reproduced by permission.)

chemical constants. Although more recent work suggests a less prominent role of the erythrocyte membrane, the matter will not be completely resolved until actual measurements of membrane permeability to oxygen are achieved.

b. Hemoglobin Reactions. The previous discussions have alluded to the rapidity of the reactions of hemoglobin and oxygen in free solution. The majority of the experimental data have been obtained in dilute hemoglobin solution and heme–ligand equilibria have been thought to be concentration dependent (Forster and Andersson, 1970). If this is truly the case, then the reaction rates must also be concentration dependent. However, as noted in Fig. 3 the P_{50} at 37°C in fairly concentrated hemoglobin solution (1.0 mM) is identical to the normal P_{50} of blood. Therefore, it is likely that the reaction constants given in the figure are applicable to the physiologic situation. These kinetic constants are sufficiently large to rule out the possibility that the speed of chemical reaction is rate limiting in oxygen transfer.

   c. *Combined Reaction and Diffusion.* In the case of small molecules that do not bind to hemoglobin, as a first approximation the interior of the red cell can be treated as a single well-mixed compartment (Klocke *et al.*, 1972). Even though diffusion constants are reduced in the concentrated protein solution present inside the erythrocyte, the constants are still relatively large and diffusion distances are small, so that diffusional equilibrium is reached rapidly.

   The situation is different in the case of either large molecules (hemoglobin) or small molecules that bind to large molecules (oxygen). The diffusion coefficient of oxygen is only moderately reduced inside the red cell, i.e., one-third of its value in an infinitely dilute solution (Kreuzer, 1970). Hemoglobin, which has a diffusion coefficient substantially less than O_2 in dilute solution, is affected even more in concentrated protein solutions. At the hemoglobin concentration (33 gm%) present inside the red cell, the hemoglobin diffusion coefficient is only one-twelfth as great as that of oxygen (Kreuzer, 1970). Hence, hemoglobin is relatively immobile inside the red cell. Thus, as successive oxygen molecules enter the red cell and bind to hemoglobin, they must diffuse further into the cell interior prior to reacting with a reduced molecule (Fig. 5). In addition to the resulting increase in diffusion distance, transfer is slowed by a sharp drop in the oxygen tension profile inside the cell. As oxygen combines with hemoglobin, local P_{O_2}, which is proportional to the concentration of unbound O_2 molecules, decreases. Since diffusion occurs down a pressure gradient, O_2 movement deep within the cell is slowed until the P_{O_2} in the peripheral portion of the cell increases. Thus, the combined process of chemical reaction and diffusion is substantially slower than simple chemical reaction in a well-mixed solution. This process has been modeled in a variety of ways. The advancing front theory assumes instantaneous chemical equilibrium and limitation of O_2 transfer solely by diffusion (Nicolson and Roughton, 1951). More sophisticated numerical analyses include finite reaction rates but reach essentially the same conclusions (Forster, 1964).

   Our understanding of the events occurring inside the cell is further clouded by two additional complicating factors. First, hemoglobin molecules are not completely immobile, and may facilitate diffusion of oxygen into the cell interior by carrying oxygen as oxyhemoglobin. Although hemoglobin diffusion is far slower than O_2 diffusion, the concentration of heme pigment inside the red cell is large in comparison to the unbound O_2

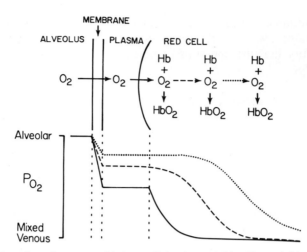

Fig. 5. Reaction of oxygen with intracellular hemoglobin. Hemoglobin molecules are relatively immobile and the distance oxygen must diffuse prior to reacting with a reduced molecule increases with time. Hypothetical P_{O_2} profiles in plasma and red cell are shown in the lower portion of the figure. Solid line represents initial profile; dashed and dotted lines represent profiles at progressively later points in time. Note the sharp drop in P_{O_2} inside the cell.

concentration. Hence, even though individual molecular movement is small, the total net movement may be substantial. Facilitated diffusion of oxygen in thin films of packed erythrocytes has been documented (Kutchai and Staub, 1969). However, experimental conditions were chosen to maximize facilitation and were quite different than those normally present inside a single red cell. Current data suggest that facilitated diffusion does not augment intracellular O_2 transfer by more than 10% (Kreuzer, 1970), but admittedly these estimates are quite speculative. The second unknown factor is the possible effect of convective mixing of cell contents because of deformation of erythrocytes during passage through capillaries (Miyamoto and Moll, 1972). The experiments of Zander and Schmid-Schönbein (1973) suggest that this may play an important role in cellular oxygen uptake or release in the intact organism. The only satisfactory approach to resolve this question is measurement of reaction rates *in vivo*, a task not yet achieved because of immense technical problems.

2. *Experimental Observations*

The same general approach used to characterize solution reaction rates is applied to cellular reactions. Association and dissociation rate constants are subscripted (k_c' and k_c) to indicate that they apply to erythrocyte suspensions. As noted previously, k' and k are not true kinetic constants because the assumption of a single-step reaction represents an oversimplification of the interactions between the different heme moieties and oxygen. The use of two constants permits a fairly good description of hemoglobin reactions in solution but is less satisfactory in cellular reactions. The simultaneous occurrence of chemical and diffusive processes cannot be described by a single constant. Accordingly, k'_c and k_c vary throughout a reaction and are dependent upon experimental conditions. These pseudoconstants provide a phenomenological description of the reactions and are usually derived from the observed rate of change in hemoglobin or oxyhemoglobin concentration at the start of a reaction. Representative values for k'_c and k_c are included in Table I under a variety of circumstances. A number of factors will influence actual values of these pseudoconstants.

TABLE I

Erythrocyte Rate Constants

Reference	$k'_c{}^a$ (mM^{-1}sec^{-1})	k_c (sec^{-1})	l'_c (mM^{-1}sec^{-1})	m'_c (sec^{-1})	Comments
Holland *et al.* (1977)	99 (3)[b]				
	136 (3)				O_2 saturation = 25%
	173 (3)				O_2 saturation = 49%
	347 (3)				O_2 saturation = 74%
	89 (2)				Fetal cells
Bauer *et al.*	76 (2)	13.5 (2)			Cells depleted of
(1973)	83 (2)	7.7 (2)			2,3-DPG
Rotman *et al.*	89 (8)	11.0 (8)			
(1974)	45 (6)	20.8 (6)			Cells containing hemoglobin S
Forster *et al.* (1957)	92 (3)		79 (3)		
Roughton *et al.*				8.4 (6)	P_{O_2} = 100 torr
(1957)				11.3 (6)	P_{O_2} = 319 torr
				12.8 (6)	P_{O_2} = 571 torr
Lawson (1971)	79 (3)	12.0 (3)	73 (3)		
	66 (4)	16.0 (4)	54 (3)		Cells containing hemoglobin S
				4.9 (8)	P_{O_2} = 75 torr
				7.8 (2)	P_{O_2} = 143 torr
				11.2 (5)	P_{O_2} = 357 torr

[a] Initial O_2 saturation = 0% unless otherwise noted.
[b] Number of subjects in parentheses.

a. Oxyhemoglobin Saturation. Most values of k'_c are obtained from experiments with an initial oxygen saturation of zero. However, k'_c is markedly dependent upon oxygen saturation, increasing five- to tenfold as saturation of an erythrocyte suspension increases from 0 to 100% (Staub *et al.*, 1961; Holland *et al.*, 1977). Hence, most measurements of k'_c cannot be applied directly to calculations of oxygen uptake under physiological circumstances. Another constant, Θ_{O_2}, has been defined to circumvent this problem. This is the quantity of oxygen taken up per minute by 1 ml of blood with a normal oxygen capacity (20 vol%) when exposed to a unit oxygen tension gradient between the cell surface and interior. Θ_{O_2} is related to k'_c by

$$\Theta_{O_2} = 0.00017 k'_c (100 - S_{O_2}) \tag{2}$$

where S_{O_2} is initial erythrocyte oxygen saturation (%) (Forster, 1964). k'_c increases with increasing oxygen saturation but the term $100 - S_{O_2}$ simultaneously decreases. Hence, Θ_{O_2} is relatively constant at approximately 1.5 ml/(ml · min · torr) from 0 to 80% saturation, and then decreases to zero as blood becomes fully saturated (Fig. 6). Initial estimates of Θ_{O_2}

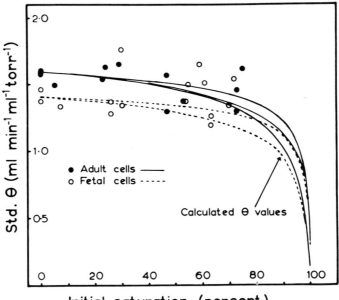

Fig. 6. The relationship between Θ_{O_2} and oxygen saturation at the start of the reaction in adult and fetal erythrocyte suspensions. Calculated values were obtained from theoretical consideration of combined chemical reaction and diffusion. Θ_{O_2} was adjusted to blood with oxygen capacity of 20 vol%. (From Holland *et al.*, 1977, reproduced by permission.)

were slightly higher (Staub *et al.*, 1961), but were subject to some technical artifacts (Rotman *et al.*, 1970; Lawson, 1966).

In contrast to k_c', the dissociation velocity constant is less affected by the initial oxygen saturation, changing less than 30% over the entire range of saturation (Lawson, 1966). Most of this observed variation is noted at low saturations. For practical purposes k_c can be assumed independent of oxygen saturation in the physiologic range.

b. Hemoglobin Type. Rotman *et al.* (1974) demonstrated that cells containing hemoglobin S have cellular association rate constants approximately one-half of normal (Table I). In contrast, k_c in sickle (SS) cells was twice normal. These differences do not appear to result from structural differences in the hemoglobin molecule since both have the same affinity (Rotman *et al.*, 1974) and have similar association rate constants with CO in dilute solution (Lawson, 1971). The changes in k_c' were confirmed by Harrington *et al.* (1977), although they did not observe any variations in k_c. This discrepancy may have been the result of different intracellular concentrations of 2,3-DPG since this organic phosphate markedly affects k_c (Bauer *et al.*, 1973). Harrington *et al.* (1977) also found no difference in k_c' of irreversibly sickled cells and ordinary SS cells, suggesting that hemoglobin concentration and alterations in the cell membrane are not responsible for the altered kinetics. These investigators caused sickling in sickle trait erythrocytes by changing extracellular osmolality and found that k_c' fell from a normal value to a level seen with SS cells. Addition of an antisickling agent returned k_c' in SS cells to normal. The authors concluded, based on these findings and the effect of temperature on k_c' in both types of cells, that the slower rate of oxygenation present in SS cells is the result of polymerization of deoxygenated hemoglobin S.

Cells containing predominantly fetal hemoglobin take up O_2 at a slightly slower rate than normal (Holland *et al.*, 1977). However, as saturation increases, this difference diminishes so that there probably is no difference in k_c' between fetal and adult cells under physiologic conditions. Deoxygenation rates have not been studied in fetal cells.

c. Other Factors. Even though 2,3-DPG has a pronounced effect on both association and dissociation reactions in hemoglobin solution, the effect of the organic phosphate is largely confined to k_c in cell suspensions (Bauer *et al.*, 1973). Most likely this difference is due to the predominant effect of simultaneous chemical reaction and diffusion in the association reaction. The actual chemical combination itself is great enough to have little influence on k_c' (Table I). The increase in k_c seen in cells containing

2,3-DPG probably is a function of both the organic phosphate per se and the lower intracellular pH produced by the presence of 2,3-DPG.

Both k'_c and k_c decrease as temperature is lowered, but the latter is affected to a greater degree (Lawson *et al.*, 1965; Lawson, 1966; Harrington *et al.*, 1977). Oxygen will be released more slowly in peripheral tissues such as the hand because tissue temperatures are less than 37°C. Although k_c may drop threefold under these circumstances, oxygen release probably is not impaired except under the most extreme conditions of anemia and exercise (Lawson and Forster, 1967).

III. CARBON MONOXIDE REACTIONS

Rate constants for the association and dissociation of carbon monoxide, l' and l, are analogous to the rate constants for oxygen in hemoglobin solution. Similarly, subscripted rate constants l'_c and l_c represent the CO reactions in cell suspensions. An additional set of constants m' and m'_c are also of interest. These constants describe the rate of replacement of bound oxygen by carbon monoxide in hemoglobin solution and cell suspensions, respectively. In fact, these constants are more important from a physiologic viewpoint since they are determinants of the carbon monoxide diffusing capacity.

A. Hemoglobin Solution

Despite the substantially greater affinity of CO for hemoglobin, surprisingly the association velocity constant l' is actually only one-tenth of the comparable oxygen association constant (k') (Antonini and Brunori, 1971). Carbon monoxide affinity is greater than O_2 affinity because carbon monoxide dissociation from hemoglobin is extremely slow; the dissociation constant is approximately three orders of magnitude less than the oxygen dissociation constant (Antonini and Brunori, 1971). These CO constants are influenced to a lesser degree by hydrogen ion than the O_2 constants.

The replacement of bound O_2 by CO has been viewed as a two-stage process (Roughton *et al.*, 1957). The reaction $HbO_2 \rightarrow Hb + O_2$ occurs first, followed by $CO + Hb \rightarrow HbCO$. If the ratio of gas concentrations in the reactant solution, $[CO]/[O_2]$, is less than 0.03, the first reaction is rapid and the combination of CO with hemoglobin becomes rate limiting. Unfortunately, it is not possible to achieve these conditions experimentally. In order to attain the true replacement constant m'_∞, the measured replacement constant m' must be corrected

$$m'_\infty = m'[1 + (r)l'_4/k'_4] \tag{3}$$

where r is the ratio of CO and O_2 concentrations and l'_4 and k'_4 are the rate constants for the combination of CO and O_2 with hemoglobin tetramer, which has already bound three ligand molecules (Roughton et al., 1957). The measured (m') and true (m'_∞) constants vary by a factor of approximately 25% under most experimental circumstances.

B. Erythrocyte Suspensions

The rate of CO uptake by cells (l'_c) is only slightly slower than the speed of O_2 combination (k'_c) (Forster et al., 1957) (Table I). The difference in rate constants between the two gases is substantially less in cell suspension than in hemoglobin solution because of the additional factor of diffusion of the ligand within the cell. The l'_c is reduced to 74% of normal in sickled cells (Lawson, 1971), but is unchanged in cells containing fetal hemoglobin (Holland, 1967). There are no data available on the rate of dissociation of CO (l_c) from cells completely saturated with carbon monoxide.

The rate of replacement of O_2 by CO in erythrocytes, m'_c, cannot be measured in vitro under conditions similar to those prevailing in the lung during measurement of the diffusing capacity. In vitro measurements of m' and m'_c are extrapolated to in vivo circumstances using a theoretical equation describing the intracellular events taking place during combined chemical reaction and diffusion (Roughton et al., 1957; Lawson, 1971). Although the correction is only 10–30%, the validity of this procedure has not been proven experimentally. m'_c is related to Θ_{CO}, the rate of uptake of carbon monoxide by blood (Roughton and Forster, 1957):

$$\Theta_{CO} = 46.2 \, m'_c [HbO_2]/P_{c_{O_2}} \tag{4}$$

θ_{CO} is a function of oxyhemoglobin concentration (ml/ml) and intracellular oxygen tension ($P_{c_{O_2}}$), and will vary with oxygen saturation. Θ_{CO} is relatively constant at approximately 1.0 ml/(ml · min · torr) from 0 to 75% oxyhemoglobin saturation, and then gradually decreases to zero at 100% saturation (Forster, 1964). Uncertainty of the true value of m'_c, and therefore Θ_{CO}, has physiologic implications. The latter is used to estimate the diffusing capacity of the pulmonary membrane (D_m) and pulmonary capillary blood volume (V_c) through the well-known relationship

$$\frac{1}{D_L} = \frac{1}{D_m} + \frac{1}{\Theta V_c} \tag{5}$$

where D_L is the pulmonary diffusing capacity. D_m is susceptible to error resulting from incorrect estimates of m'_c and Θ_{CO}. Unfortunately, at the present time m'_c cannot be measured without resorting to extrapolation procedures.

IV. CARBON DIOXIDE REACTIONS

Carbon dioxide is carried in the blood in three different forms— dissolved CO_2, bicarbonate ion, and hemoglobin carbamate compounds (Klocke, 1978b). The latter two species are not exchanged across the alveolar–capillary membrane and must be converted into free carbon dioxide prior to excretion in the lungs. These additional steps are potential rate limiting processes.

The complex nature of carbon dioxide exchange is indicated in Fig. 7. Bicarbonate reactions occur both in the red cell and plasma, but the former are quantitatively far more important. Carbamate compounds are formed by binding of CO_2 to free amino groups of proteins. Only hemoglobin carbamate compounds are shown in Fig. 7 since plasma carbamate compounds play no role in CO_2 excretion (Gros et al., 1976).

Less than 10% of the carbon dioxide in blood passing through the lung is excreted in the alveolar gas. Therefore, distinction must be made between the amount of carbon dioxide carried in each form in blood and the relative importance of each chemical species in CO_2 excretion. For

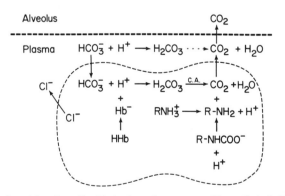

Fig. 7.   Reactions of carbon dioxide in the pulmonary capillary. C.A. indicates a reaction catalyzed by carbonic anhydrase. Dashed arrow indicates an uncatalyzed CO_2 reaction with a slow natural rate.

example, plasma carbamate concentration is approximately 0.6 mM, but the compound is unimportant in CO_2 exchange since there is no difference between arterial and venous concentrations. Conversely, the contribution of hemoglobin carbamate to CO_2 excretion is important since it has a relatively large ($a - \bar{v}$) difference. Carbon dioxide exchange must be viewed in the light of the concentration changes taking place as well as the actual speed of the individual processes.

A. Speed of CO_2 Movement

Carbon dioxide diffusion across membranes has been viewed as a rapid process because of the relatively high lipid solubility of the molecule. Direct measurements of CO_2 permeability are not technically feasible and only indirect estimates are available.

A CO_2 permeability coefficient of 0.58 cm/sec has been calculated (Forster, 1969) from measurements of red cell permeability to ammonia (Klocke et al., 1972) and the relative lipid solubilities and masses of the two molecules. This calculated permeability is several orders of magnitude larger than anion permeability, as would be expected of an uncharged, lipid-soluble molecule. Silverman et al. (1976) utilized measurements of the rate of depletion of isotopic oxygen-enriched CO_2 in erythrocyte suspensions to calculate CO_2 permeability of the red cell membrane. They obtained a value of 0.0075 cm/sec, approximately 1/100 of the previous estimate. If this estimate is accurate, CO_2 diffusion should be a major factor in gas exchange. However, the experimental approach was complex and required a number of assumptions. As acknowledged by the authors, resistance to diffusion of CO_2 in the cell interior as well as in the cell membrane could have been included in the derived permeability. The closest analog to direct measurement of red cell CO_2 permeability is observations of CO_2 diffusion through lipid bilayer membranes. Gutknecht et al. (1977) obtained a permeability of 0.35 cm/sec in this system, a value quite similar to that extrapolated from measured ammonia permeability (Forster, 1969). Gros and Moll (1971) found little difference in CO_2 diffusion between hemoglobin solution and erythrocyte suspension. From these data, they calculated a permeability of 3 cm/sec, far greater than other estimates. However, accuracy of this method is poor when membrane permeability is relatively large.

More direct experiments are required to reach a definite estimate of CO_2 permeability, but current knowledge suggests that diffusion across the red cell membrane is not a significant factor in limiting the speed of CO_2 exchange.

B. Carbamate Kinetics

Free amino groups on proteins can reversibly bind hydrogen ions where

$$R—NH_2 + H^+ \xrightleftharpoons{K_z} R—NH_3^+ \tag{6}$$

R represents the remainder of the protein moiety and K_z is the equilibrium constant of the reaction. Similarly, these amino groups can form carbamic acids with CO_2 that immediately dissociate into carbamate compounds and hydrogen ions since the pK of the overall reaction is much lower than

$$R—NH_2 + CO_2 \xrightleftharpoons{K_c} R—NHCOO^- + H^+ \tag{7}$$

body pH, where K_c is the equilibrium constant. The kinetics of the ionization reactions are essentially instantaneous, but binding of the uncharged CO_2 molecule occurs more slowly. Exchange of CO_2 transported as carbamate requires a finite period of time to reach completion. Carbon dioxide and hydrogen ion compete for the binding site on the free amino group ($R—NH_2$). As a result, carbamino binding is more prominent at higher pH. Carbon dioxide binding, as indicated in Eq. (7), releases hydrogen ions and lowers the concentration of free amino groups. The latter in turn shift the equilibrium of Eq. (6) to the left, increasing available amino groups and hydrogen ions. Binding of a single CO_2 molecule causes the release of an average of between one and two hydrogen ions via Eqs. (6) and (7). Obviously, carbamino transport is associated with significant effects on acid–base balance.

1. Plasma Protein Carbamate Formation

Gros *et al.* (1976) studied both the kinetic and equilibrium aspects of carbamate formation in protein solutions. Carbon dioxide binding is a first-order process with a half-time of less than 50 msec. Most investigators have assumed that CO_2 binding takes place only at the terminal α-amino groups of proteins (Roughton, 1964), but this study demonstrated significant binding to ϵ-amino groups of lysine residues. At pH 7.4 and P_{CO_2} 40 torr, 58% of the total CO_2 bound (0.56 mM) would be associated with α-amino groups and the remainder with ϵ-amino groups. As noted previously, a significant amount of CO_2 is bound to plasma proteins, but does not participate in CO_2 exchange. Differences in pH and P_{CO_2} between arterial and venous blood are never large enough to result in significant exchange via the plasma carbamate pathway. These compounds will be included, however, in measurements of total CO_2 content of blood, and thus may affect calculations based on such determinations.

2. Hemoglobin Carbamate Formation

Forster and colleagues (1968) have also studied binding of CO_2 to hemoglobin in solution. The rate of binding is rapid, reaching completion in 0.1 sec in both oxygenated and reduced hemoglobin solutions. Similar to carbamate binding to plasma proteins, hemoglobin–carbamate compounds would have little physiologic significance if CO_2 binding did not differ between the oxygenated and reduced states of the protein. Oxygenated hemoglobin binds significantly less CO_2 than the reduced heme molecule (Roughton, 1964). Hence, oxygenation of hemoglobin in the lung reduces carbamate affinity, causing the release of carbon dioxide. Rossi-Bernardi and Roughton (1967) estimated that this oxylabile mechanism accounted for more than one quarter of CO_2 excretion. However, these authors conducted their experiments in dialyzed hemoglobin solutions. Bauer (1970) demonstrated that 2,3-DPG sharply reduces the quantity of oxylabile carbon dioxide bound to hemoglobin because the organic phosphate also binds to amino groups involved in carbamino formation (Bunn and Briehl, 1970). These findings have been verified in intact cells (Bauer and Schröder, 1972; Klocke, 1973), and indicate that changes in arterial and venous carbamate concentrations normally account for only 11% of total CO_2 excretion (Bauer and Schröder, 1972).

The difference in carbamate formation between oxygenated and reduced hemoglobin presumably is the result of alterations in K_C and/or K_Z. Carbamic acids tend to be strong acids and dissociate completely at low pH. pK_c usually is in the range of 4.2 (Gros et al., 1976) and large changes would be required to have significant physiologic influence. It is more likely that changes in K_Z are related to the oxylabile effect. Exact definitions of these events is clouded by the fact that the functional amino groups do not behave uniformly. The N-terminal valines of β-chains are involved in 2,3-DPG binding, whereas those of the α-chains are not (Bunn and Briehl, 1970). Their relative importance in the carbamate pathway is unclear. The latter may be equally important (Kilmartin et al., 1973) or only one-third as important (Bauer et al., 1975) as β-chain groups in oxylabile carbamate transport. In view of the elegant studies of Gros et al. (1976), it seems likely that significant CO_2 binding to ϵ-amino groups also occurs with hemoglobin. However, there is no evidence that these groups are oxylabile so their contribution to CO_2 exchange would be effectively nil.

The binding of CO_2 to either reduced hemoglobin or oxyhemoglobin is relatively rapid (0.1–0.2 sec) (Forster et al., 1968) and proceeds at the same rate in solution or cell suspension (Kernohan and Roughton, 1968). However, when CO_2 binding in intact cells is altered by a change in hemo-

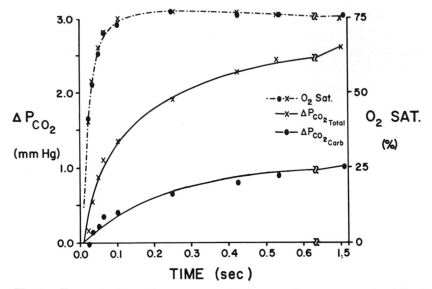

Fig. 8. Changes in P_{CO_2} and oxygen saturation in an erythrocyte suspension following mixture of an oxygenated buffer and reduced cell suspension. Both reactants had identical pH, P_{CO_2}, and $[HCO_3^-]$ at the start of the reaction. The dashed line represents change in oxygen saturation, and the solid lines changes in P_{CO_2}. Filled circles indicate that the reaction was performed with acetazolamide present and P_{CO_2} changes resulted from carbamate mobilization. $\times$'s represent reaction without carbonic anhydrase inhibition, and P_{CO_2} changes were due to combined carbamate and bicarbonate mobilization. (From Klocke, 1973, reproduced by permission.)

globin saturation, the rate is substantially slower (Klocke, 1973). This process follows an exponential course (Fig. 8) with a half-time of 0.120 sec, reaching completion in 0.5–0.6 sec after oxygenation. Thus, under normal circumstances carbamate exchange should reach completion in the pulmonary capillary, but the margin for error is less than would be expected from studies that do not involve a change in hemoglobin oxygenation.

C. Bicarbonate Reactions

1. Carbonic Anhydrase Catalysis

Reactions of carbonic acid (H_2CO_3), bicarbonate, and hydrogen ions are instantaneous, but the natural rate of the hydration–dehydration step between CO_2 and H_2CO_3 is slow. This is indicated by the dashed line between the two species in the plasma compartment in Fig. 7. Carbonic anhydrase in the cell interior catalyzes this reaction, permitting rapid interconversion of CO_2 and bicarbonate. Extrapolation of data obtained in hemoglobin solution indicates that physiologic concentrations of the enzyme increase the natural rate of the reaction by a factor of 13,000 (Kernohan et al., 1963; Donaldson and Quinn, 1974). This has been confirmed indirectly in the intact erythrocyte (Kernohan and Roughton, 1968; Klocke, 1973). Catalysis permits the rapid release of large amounts of CO_2 from bicarbonate stores and changes in bicarbonate concentration during pulmonary capillary transit are responsible for 80% of CO_2 excreted in the lung (Klocke, 1976; Swenson and Maren, 1978). The initial rate of CO_2 elimination in the pulmonary capillary is determined by the extent of the enzyme-mediated catalysis of the dehydration reaction (Klocke, 1973; Holland and Forster, 1975). A modest decrease in the extent of catalysis would slow the initial rate of CO_2 exchange in the capillary, but probably would not affect CO_2 excretion significantly since a sixfold excess of enzyme is available under conditions of maximal stress (Swenson and Maren, 1978). Inhibition of carbonic anhydrase activity does not impair survival but alters the relative contributions of the chemical pathways responsible for CO_2 exchange (Swenson and Maren, 1978). Changes in dissolved CO_2 increase to compensate for reduced bicarbonate mobilization. This leads to large swings in arterial and venous P_{CO_2}. Moderate exercise is possible with complete enzyme inhibition, but maximal exercise is limited.

2. Bicarbonate–Chloride Exchange

The conversion of large quantities of bicarbonate to CO_2 during pulmonary gas exchange rapidly depletes intracellular bicarbonate stores. If intracellular $[HCO_3^-]$ is not repleted after the initial surge of CO_2 excretion, the reduction will slow dehydration of carbonic acid by a mass action effect. Extracellular bicarbonate concentration remains unchanged during the initial stage of gas exchange due to the absence of carbonic anhydrase in plasma. As intracellular bicarbonate concentration decreases, an electrochemical gradient is established across the erythrocyte membrane and bicarbonate enters the cell (Klocke, 1976). Exchange of chloride ion in the opposite direction maintains electrical neutrality.

The exact mechanism of bicarbonate–chloride exchange is unclear. Traditionally, anion exchange has been viewed as passive diffusion of each ion down individual electrochemical gradients that are opposite in sign (Goldman, 1943). Linkage of the two fluxes by a common membrane potential requires simultaneous transport of anions in the opposite direction in order to maintain electrical neutrality. If the ions have differing permeabilities, more rapid transport of one causes a change in membrane potential, which slows movement of the more permeabile ion and increases the flux of the slower ion. This concept has been challenged following the demonstration that chloride self-exchange at $0°-10°C$ is highly temperature sensitive and exhibits apparent saturation kinetics. These findings are more consistent with a transport system than with simple diffusion (Sachs *et al.*, 1975). In addition, Rothstein and colleagues (1976) have isolated membrane proteins that appear to be involved in chloride transport, and have shown that anion exchange can be blocked by amino reagents that bind to these proteins.

These conflicting findings are compatible with the concept that anion exchange may be accomplished through more than one mechanism or may have several rate-limiting steps in a single process. Chow *et al.* (1976) have shown that the rate of bicarbonate–chloride exchange is quite temperature sensitive in the $0°-10°C$ range, but is less affected by thermal variation above $25°C$. They suggested that different processes may determine the rate of exchange in the two temperature ranges, possibly the result of thermally mediated changes in membrane properties. Brahm (1977) studied isotopic chloride self-exchange and found a qualitively similar thermal variation of flux. On the basis of these findings and observations of bromide self-exchange, he concluded that two separate steps in the same transport processes may limit flux. He postulated that the more temperature-dependent process is rate limiting below a critical turnover rate, and thereafter kinetics are limited by another less temperature-dependent step in the exchange process. Current evidence does not conclusively support either hypothesis. Nevertheless, exchange is mediated by two functionally different processes at varying temperatures and results at low temperature cannot be extrapolated to $37°C$.

Regardless of the correct mechanism, the speed of bicarbonate–chloride exchange under physiologic circumstances has been described and follows approximately first-order kinetics with a half-time of 0.1 sec (Chow *et al.*, 1976; Klocke, 1976). Thus, this ionic exchange by itself would not limit carbon dioxide excretion, but may become a limiting factor when acting in combination with other steps in the CO_2 exchange.

D. Carbon Dioxide Uptake by Erythrocytes

The processes involved in CO_2 exchange usually occur simultaneously rather than in serial fashion, even though one step may be predominant at a given point in time. The rate of carbon dioxide uptake by erythrocytes exposed to CO_2 dissolved in a buffer has been described under a variety of conditions (Constantine *et al.*, 1965; Holland and Forster, 1975). Although more analogous to CO_2 uptake in tissues than CO_2 excretion in the lung, these studies provide insight into both aspects of gas exchange. The initial uptake of CO_2 appears to be predominantly mediated through diffusion of CO_2 into the cell and hydration to carbonic acid with subsequent ionization to bicarbonate ion. At body temperature this rapid initial change accounts for approximately two-thirds of the total CO_2 uptake (Holland and Forster, 1975). Subsequently uptake of CO_2 slows and its rate appears to be mediated by the speed of transmembrane bicarbonate–chloride exchange. Finally, slow changes in P_{CO_2} occur over a period of seconds and apparently are the result of readjustment of hydrogen ion equilibrium across the cell membrane. Holland and Forster (1975) concluded that CO_2 uptake might not be complete in exercising muscle. Their work did not completely parallel the *in vivo* situation since significant carbamate formation did not occur in their experiments and simultaneous oxygen exchange was absent.

V. KINETICS OF O_2–CO_2 INTERACTIONS

In the previous sections, each respiratory gas and its exchange were viewed independently to simplify the concepts presented. However, oxygen and carbon dioxide are exchanged simultaneously. The two gases strongly interact in blood, and the exchange of each gas is linked to the other (Wyman, 1964). Carbon dioxide exchange is affected to a greater degree by oxygen exchange (Haldane effect) than the converse situation (Bohr effect) (Hill *et al.*, 1973). Figure 9 depicts the O_2 and CO_2 dissociation curves of blood and the reciprocal effects of the gases. Only the portions of the curves between the normal arterial and mixed venous points are shown in Fig. 9. Both curves are plotted on axes with identical scales to emphasize the different shapes and slopes. In the range shown, the CO_2 dissociation curve is steep and linear whereas the O_2 relationship is curvilinear with a more shallow slope.

The two curves in the left-hand panel of Fig. 9 demonstrate the effect of changes in P_{CO_2}, mediated principally through the resulting alteration in pH, on the arterial and venous curves. There is little lateral shift in the curve. Consequently, most of the $(a - \bar{v})$ difference in O_2 content is due to the decrease in oxygen pressure alone, indicated by $(\Delta O_2)_P$. The Bohr effect, the change in oxygen content produced by the shift in the O_2 dissociation curve, is labeled $(\Delta O_2)_{CO_2}$ and contributes little to the $(a - \bar{v})$ content difference.

The CO_2 dissociation curve in the right-hand panel of Fig. 9 presents a marked contrast. Oxygenation results in a significantly greater lateral shift than the Bohr effect. This shift is accentuated by the steep nature of the

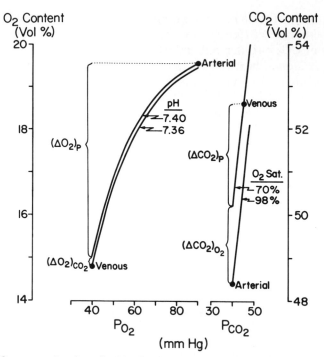

Fig. 9. Oxygen and carbon dioxide dissociation curves of blood. Oxygen curves on the left illustrate the displacement due to the Bohr effect. Carbon dioxide curves on right illustrate the displacement due to the Haldane effect. Changes in O_2 or CO_2 content produced by a change in gas tension are indicated by the subscript P. Changes in gas content resulting from a shift in the dissociation curve by changes in CO_2 or O_2 are indicated by the respective subscript.

CO_2 dissociation curve. As a result, the Haldane effect $(\Delta CO_2)_{O_2}$ is responsible for a change in CO_2 content approximately equal to that resulting from the $(a - \bar{v})$ difference in P_{CO_2}, $(\Delta CO_2)_P$. The Haldane effect is substantially more important in gas exchange than the Bohr effect. Hill *et al.* (1973) have calculated that 46% of CO_2 exchange in normal resting man is mediated through the Haldane effect, while the Bohr effect augments pulmonary O_2 uptake by only 2%.

Usually the Bohr effect has little influence on O_2 exchange. However, if alveolar P_{O_2} is reduced, a concomitant acidemia can markedly shift the O_2 dissociation curve to the right and thereby limit oxygen uptake. Normally plasma pH is maintained within narrow limits but may vary widely in disease.

Previous discussion has centered on the rate of gas exchange in response to alteration in tension. Gas exchange *in vivo* is not only determined by the rate of movement between the arterial and venous tensions on individual dissociation curves, but also upon the time required to shift the curves between the arterial and venous positions.

A. Rate of the Bohr Shift

The position of the O_2 dissociation curve can be altered by either fixed acid or carbon dioxide. The Bohr factor is slightly greater when mediated through changes in CO_2 because of carbamate formation (Hlastala and Woodson, 1975). Craw *et al.* (1963) and Forster and Steen (1968) produced step changes in P_{CO_2} in cell suspensions and measured the speed of the resultant decrease in oxygen saturation. The approach to equilibrium approximated a first-order process (Craw *et al.*, 1963) with a half-time of 0.120 sec at 37°C (Forster and Steen, 1968). In these experiments CO_2 had to diffuse into the cell, hydrate to carbonic acid, and dissociate into bicarbonate and hydrogen ions. The latter then produced a change in the O_2 affinity of hemoglobin and bound oxygen was released. The major limiting step in this chain appears to be the intracellular hydration of CO_2 under the influence of carbonic anhydrase. When the pH of the cell suspension was changed by addition of lactic acid, the process was much slower and the half-time rose to 0.350 sec (Forster and Steen, 1968). Even though lactic acid per se enters the red cell fairly rapidly (Klocke *et al.*, 1972), at physiologic pH it is completely ionized to lactate and hydrogen ions. The transmembrane hydrogen ion gradient is too small to foster rapid proton movement (Crandall *et al.*, 1971). Carbon dioxide formed from extracellular bicarbonate and the added hydrogen ions enters the cell and is converted back into H^+ and HCO_3^-. This process occurs slowly because of the absence of carbonic anhydrase in the extracellular fluid.

The Bohr shift mediated through addition of CO_2 appears to be sufficiently rapid to approach equilibrium during capillary transit. The increase in P_{CO_2} produces only a small enhancement of O_2 delivery. However, addition of large quantities of lactic acid, particularly in exercising muscle, has a potentially much greater influence on O_2 exchange. The slower shift of the curve produced by addition of fixed acid probably does not exert its full effect before blood leaves the exchange vessels. Obviously, the duration of capillary transit time is a critical factor. The fixed-acid Bohr effect certainly attains equilibrium by the time blood reaches the pulmonary vessels so that acid production in the peripheral tissues will influence subsequent oxygen loading in the lung.

Forster and Steen (1968) also studied the speed of the Bohr shift produced by a decrease in P_{CO_2}, analogous to the events occurring in the pulmonary capillary. As expected, the initial portion of this process was rapid and appeared to be governed predominantly by the catalyzed CO_2 reactions inside the cell. The later portions of the reactions proceeded more slowly because of extracellular CO_2 reactions. These reactions do not occur to the same extent *in vivo* since CO_2 enters the alveoli. The slower attainment of equilibrium in this case appears to be a consequence of the experimental conditions and does not reflect physiologic events. In the intact organism, most likely the Bohr reaction probably reaches equilibrium in the pulmonary capillary.

Nakamura and Staub (1964) hypothesized, based on their studies of the Bohr shift in cell suspensions, that the simultaneous occurrence of O_2 and CO_2 reactions increased the rate of the individual reactions. The cause of this apparent synergistic relationship was obscure. However, Forster and Steen (1968) have criticized the method used to calculate rate constants in this study. They modified the computations and concluded that the data of Nakamura and Staub (1964) did not support kinetic synergism.

B. Kinetics of the Haldane Effect

The Haldane effect is not the result of a single chemical event. As discussed previously, hemoglobin carbamate is oxylabile, i.e., the binding of CO_2 to terminal α-amino groups is much greater when hemoglobin is reduced. In addition, as hemoglobin is oxygenated, large numbers of hydrogen ions are released. These Bohr protons combine with bicarbonate to form CO_2. Thus, a portion of oxylabile carbon dioxide is generated from bicarbonate stores. The relative contributions of bicarbonate and carbamino compounds to the Haldane effect have been controversial (Roughton, 1964; Bauer, 1970).

The relative importance of oxylabile carbamate and bicarbonate, and the kinetics of the two pathways have been elucidated through simultaneous kinetic measurements of P_{O_2} and P_{CO_2} (Klocke, 1973). In these experiments a reduced erythrocyte suspension was rapidly mixed with an oxygenated bicarbonate buffer; both reactants had identical pH, P_{CO_2}, and bicarbonate concentrations. After oxygenation of hemoglobin, oxylabile carbamate and bicarbonate were mobilized and P_{CO_2} in the reactant mixture rose (Fig. 8). When the reaction was performed in the presence of acetazolamide, a potent carbonic anhydrase inhibitor, bicarbonate reactions were inhibited and initially only oxylabile carbamate was mobilized. These experiments provide quantitative data concerning the total Haldane effect and its component portions in human erythrocytes with normal 2,3-DPG concentration (Fig. 10). The Haldane effect, expressed as the quantity of CO_2 released per unit oxygen bound, is greatest at normal plasma pH, but decreases at lower pH. Although the total

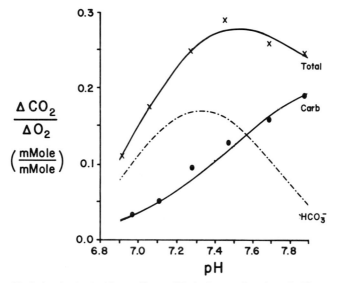

Fig. 10.   Variation in the Haldane effect $\Delta CO_2/\Delta O_2$ as a function of pH at mean P_{CO_2} of 42.5 torr. $\times$'s indicate total effect, closed circles carbamate portion, and dashed line bicarbonate contribution. (From Klocke, 1973, reproduced by permission.)

$\Delta CO_2/\Delta O_2$ is relatively constant at alkaline pH, the oxylabile carbamate component assumes greater relative importance for three reasons. First, more terminal α-amino groups exist in the uncharged form, which react with CO_2. Second, 2, 3-DPG binding to the terminal amino groups of beta chains is inversely proportional to pH (Garby and deVerdier, 1971), providing less competition for binding sites at higher pH. Finally, both bicarbonate and carbamate reactions consume hydrogen ions, and the number of Bohr protons available for bicarbonate transformation decreases as carbamate formation increases. Depending on the pH, 1.2 to 1.8 hydrogen ions are required for each CO_2 molecule released via the carbamate pathway (Klocke, 1973).

The two processes involved in the Haldane effect have different kinetics. The individual rate constants of each amino group involved in the carbamino pathway are not known, but the overall process follows an exponential course with a half-time of 0.120 sec (Klocke, 1973). As indicated in Fig. 8, oxylabile bicarbonate mobilization is a slower process. The initial portion of the reaction is limited by dehydration of CO_2. The degree of catalysis by carbonic anhydrase calculated from this portion of the reaction averaged 16,000. This is in good agreement with the value of 13,000 observed by Kernohan *et al.* (1963) in stopped-flow experiments. The transmembrane exchange of bicarbonate and chloride apparently limited the rate of reaction in latter stages. Both factors played a role in determining the speed of the intermediate portions.

The reactions shown in Fig. 8 reach equilibrium within most estimates of capillary transit time (Piiper, 1969). However, oxygenation was accomplished rapidly because a high oxygen tension was initially present in the reaction mixture. In addition, the oxygen did not have to cross the alveolar–capillary membrane prior to reacting with the red cell suspension. This is not the case *in vivo,* and the Haldane effect may not reach equilibrium before blood leaves the pulmonary capillary if oxygenation is delayed. In addition, partial oxygenation of blood, as occurs in maldistribution of ventilation and blood flow, will also decrease CO_2 excretion since the full potential of the Haldane effect will not be utilized.

VI. TIME COURSE OF PULMONARY O_2 AND CO_2 EXCHANGE

Unfortunately, current technology does not permit direct observation of the progress of gas exchange along the pulmonary capillary. Characteristics of the exchange process can be inferred indirectly, but present concepts of the events taking place in the capillary are based largely on mathematical models. These simulations are limited both by the theoretical framework chosen and the availability of experimentally determined rate constants. Constraints imposed by computing time have required additional compromises and any single model focuses on a restricted number of variables. For example, capillary length and transit time vary throughout the lung (Fung and Sobin, 1969); only a single study (Wagner and West, 1972) has addressed this problem. Diffusive movement of O_2 has been studied; the effect of a postulated oxygen carrier system (Mendoza *et al.,* 1977) has been ignored.

A. Constant Ventilation and Perfusion

Even though pulmonary blood flow is pulsatile (Lee and DuBois, 1955) and ventilation cyclic, computations are enormously simplifed by the assumptions that capillary volume, perfusion, and alveolar gas tensions are constant.

1. Oxygen Uptake

Computations of the time required for O_2 uptake are amazingly consistent despite a variety of different approaches and assumptions. Wagner (1977) has pointed out that O_2 transfer is optimized because Θ_{O_2} is large and the slope of the oxygen dissociation curve relatively steep during the

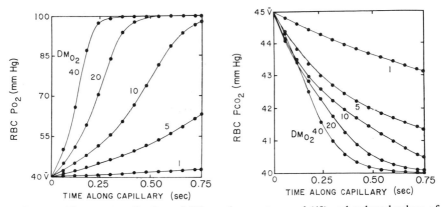

Fig. 11. Time courses for O_2 and CO_2 exchange at normal (40) and reduced values of $D_{m_{O_2}}$. $P_{A_{O_2}}$ and $P_{A_{CO_2}}$ fixed at 100 and 40 torr, respectively. (From Wagner and West, 1972, reproduced by permission.)

major portion of oxygen uptake. The effect of decreasing chemical reaction rates is greatest at high O_2 saturation when most of the uptake has already been completed.

All calculations indicate that O_2 uptake normally is complete within 0.2–0.3 sec (Fig. 11), well within capillary transit time even during exercise (Johnson *et al.*, 1960). Under boundary conditions simulating exposure to high altitude, oxygen exchange is not complete as blood leaves the capillary (Hlastala, 1973). A small alveolar–end-capillary P_{O_2} difference occurs as a consequence of the reduced alveolar P_{O_2}. Most authors have used Eq. (5), which includes the influence of chemical reaction rates, to compute the time course of capillary P_{O_2}. This equation serves quite well even though it treats oxygen reactions in plasma and the erythrocyte as a single parameter. In contrast to CO_2 excretion, interactions with other plasma and cellular processes is minimal in O_2 uptake (Hill *et al.*, 1973).

2. CO_2 Excretion

Kinetic models of CO_2 exchange are less consistent and results are diverse. Estimates for the time required to reach equilibrium between alveolar and capillary P_{CO_2} range from 0.2 sec to a duration greater than capillary transit time (Wagner, 1977). As a first step, models that do not allow for interactions of the respiratory gases and the finite rates of CO_2 reactions in blood can be ignored. As discussed previously, the Haldane effect accounts for approximately one-half of all CO_2 exchange (Hill *et al.*, 1973), and the associated kinetics lag considerably behind the oxygenation process (Klocke, 1973). Studies that take these factors into consideration are more uniform in their conclusions (Wagner, 1977).

Carbon dioxide reactions in blood are complex, but as a first approximation these can be viewed as a single exponential process (Wagner and West, 1972; Hlastala, 1973; Bidani *et al.*, 1978b). A value of Θ_{CO_2}, analogous to Θ_{O_2} and Θ_{CO}, is calculated from experimental observations of CO_2 exchange in erythrocyte suspensions. With this information carbon dioxide excretion can be computed from Eq. (5), viewing the exchange as two rate-limiting processes in series. Membrane-diffusing capacity for CO_2 is taken to be twentyfold greater than $D_{m_{O_2}}$ on the basis of the relative molecular weights and solubilities of the two gases. Despite the potential pitfalls resulting from the assumption of a single monoexponential reaction process, this approach has provided significant insight into gas exchange under a variety of circumstances.

However, the use of a lumped parameter, Θ_{CO_2}, rather than inclusion of the reactions of each individual chemical species (Fig. 7) can lead to misinterpretations. Equation (5) provides a reasonable assessment of the total quantity of CO_2 exchanged with time, but will not reflect the actual P_{CO_2} present. With this approach the calculated mass transfer of CO_2 is used to ascertain the quantity of CO_2 in all forms remaining in blood at each point in time. Then P_{CO_2} is computed from blood CO_2 content using subroutines for the dissociation curve obtained under *equilibrium* conditions (Wagner and West, 1972; Hlastala, 1973; Bidani *et al.*, 1978b). This provides a virtual P_{CO_2} or, as designated by Forster and Crandall (1975), an "equilibrated P_{CO_2}," i.e., the CO_2 tension that would exist if all chemical species were at equilibrium. Actual P_{CO_2} can only be obtained by considering the individual components of the CO_2 chain and their finite reaction rates (Hill *et al.*, 1973; Forster and Crandall, 1975; Bidani *et al.*, 1978a). This is underscored by comparing the time course of calculated P_{CO_2} under normal conditions in Figs. 11 and 12. The time course is markedly different, yet both studies reach similar conclusions concerning the rate of mass transfer of CO_2. P_{CO_2} in Fig. 12 is the actual P_{CO_2}; P_{CO_2} in Fig. 11 represents the total CO_2 content of blood. The latter approach is perfectly valid for calculating total exchange but should not be interpreted as evidence that diffusion through the pulmonary membrane is a limiting factor. A simple calculation underscores this point. The rate of change of blood P_{CO_2} during diffusion of CO_2 into alveolar gas is given by

$$\frac{-dP_b}{dt} = \frac{D_{m_{CO_2}}(P_b - P_A)}{\alpha V_c} \tag{8}$$

where α is the solubility of dissolved CO_2 in blood, V_c capillary blood volume, and P_b and P_A the respective P_{CO_2} in blood and alveolar gas. If P_A remains constant, Eq. (8) can be integrated to give a simple exponential function with the exponent equal to $-(D_{m_{CO_2}} t)/(\alpha V_c)$. If normal values for

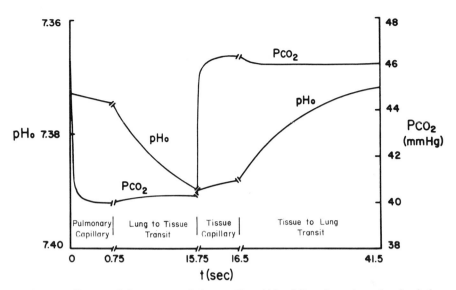

Fig. 12. Computed time course of plasma pH and blood P_{CO_2} throughout the circulation in normal man at rest, assuming no carbonic anhydrase activity available to the plasma. Note the broken time scale. (From Bidani *et al.*, 1978a, reproduced by permission.)

these variables (Bidani *et al.*, 1978a) are used, the half-time $t_{1/2}$ for CO_2 diffusion from blood into alveolar gas is 2.4 msec. It is important to note that α is the solubility of dissolved CO_2, not the slope of the CO_2 dissociation curve, which includes bicarbonate and carbamate compounds. Although there are potential problems in considering a single reaction in a series as an isolated event (Forster, 1964), it seems unlikely that a process with $t_{1/2}$ of 2.4 msec will be rate limiting when the $t_{1/2}$ of other processes in the series is 50 times greater.

Under normal circumstances the rates of chemical reactions and transmembrane ionic exchanges are the major determinants of the speed of CO_2 exchange. This conclusion could be challenged on the basis of findings in two studies (Wagner and West, 1972; Hlastala, 1973) in which variation of Θ_{CO_2} appeared to have little effect on exchange kinetics. Hlastala (1973) altered Θ_{CO_2} in his computations, but also included a separate reaction describing the rate of the Bohr shift. These two reactions were in series, and when Θ_{CO_2} was increased, the other was simultaneously decreased. Hence, overall reaction rates were varied little and no conclusion can be reached concerning their importance. In their study of the influence of $\dot{V}_A/\dot{Q}$ and D_m variations, Wagner and West (1972) found little change in end-capillary–alveolar P_{CO_2} differences when Θ_{CO_2} was varied by a factor of six. This is the result of two factors. First, if transfer for the most part is complete at the end of the capillary when $D_{m_{CO_2}}$ is normal or only moderately reduced, then the end-capillary–alveolar P_{CO_2} difference is a poor indicator of the speed of the overall process. The actual time course or half-time for equilibration would be better indicators. Second, their work was focused on the influence of reduction in D_m. In these abnormal circumstances diffusion of CO_2 across the pulmonary membrane can become a significant factor. When the exponent derived from Eq. (8) and the lowest $D_{m_{CO_2}}$ investigated in this study, are used, the calculated $t_{1/2}$ for diffusion of CO_2 from blood into the alveolus is 97 msec. This is identical to the time required for bicarbonate–chloride exchange (Klocke, 1976) and obviously must slow CO_2 excretion.

The relative importance of diffusion and chemical reaction can be illustrated by rearrangement of Eq. (5):

$$D_L = \frac{D_m(\Theta V_c)}{D_m + (\Theta V_c)} \qquad (9)$$

Taking the limit of Eq. (9) as D_m increases and Θ remains constant, Θ becomes the major determinant of the diffusing capacity. The converse occurs as Θ increases relative to D_m. Under normal circumstances $D_{m_{CO_2}}$ is 5 to 7 times the product of Θ_{CO_2} and V_c, and chemical processes rather than diffusion principally limit CO_2 exchange.

Despite rapid equilibration of P_{CO_2} across the pulmonary membrane, the total CO_2 content of blood decreases more slowly (Fig. 11) and exchange barely reaches completion as blood leaves the capillary (Wagner and West, 1972; Hill et al., 1973; Bidani et al., 1978a,b). Hlastala (1973) calculated that equilibrium is not attained in the capillary, but this conclusion has been challenged because a low value of Θ_{CO_2} was used (Wagner, 1977). It is apparent from these findings that CO_2 exchange will not be complete when capillary transit is reduced during exercise (Johnson et al., 1960) or when gas exchange is abnormal (Wagner and West, 1972). Even though equilibrium may not be reached, CO_2 excretion probably is not compromised in vivo under these circumstances. A slight increase in ventilation should lower alveolar P_{CO_2} sufficiently to promote an increased rate of exchange, which will compensate for failure to reach chemical equilibrium.

B. Varying Blood Flow and Ventilation

Hlastala (1972) incorporated pulsatile flow, cyclic ventilation, and interaction of O_2 and CO_2 exchange into a lung model. Cyclic ventilation caused a larger variation in end-capillary blood tensions than pulsatile flow, but had no effect on achievement of chemical and diffusional equilibrium during capillary transit. P_{CO_2} and P_{O_2} varied by 2.7 and 4.5 torr, respectively, throughout the ventilatory cycle under conditions of resting gas exchange. If lung tissue gas stores were not included in the model, fluctuations in P_{CO_2} increased by 26%. The tissue stores serve as a buffer, releasing CO_2 as alveolar tension falls in inspiration and absorbing the gas during expiration. Tissue stores had no effect on steady state exchange but merely dampened oscillations in P_{CO_2}. As expected, P_{O_2} was not influenced by tissue stores because of the lower solubility of O_2 in tissue water.

Incorporation of pulsatile blood flow into models to mimic actual pulmonary flow profiles (Lee and DuBois, 1955) has had surprisingly small effects (Wagner and West, 1972; Hlastala, 1972). Even with moderate diffusion and distribution abnormalities, gas transfer is reduced only a few percent below a constant flow model (Wagner and West, 1972). Calculated O_2 and CO_2 exchange was pulsatile (Hlastala, 1972), similar to that observed experimentally by body plethysmography (Bosman *et al.*, 1965). The dynamics of the pulmonary circulation during pulsatile flow are not completely clear. However, the work of Menkes *et al.* (1970) indicates that capillary blood volume also changes in a rhythmic fashion. Pulsatile flow does not increase linear velocity (and conversely decrease contact time) in direct proportion to the pulse profile. Bidani *et al.* (1978b) incorporated both pulsatile flow and volume into their model and found that speed of gas exchange improved compared to the situations in which either volume or velocity alone was allowed to vary with the pulse wave. In fact, the O_2 and CO_2 tension profiles along the capillary were almost identical to the hypothetical case of a constant flow–constant volume system. This work indicates that the latter model with its attendant simplicity is adequate to describe exchange kinetics.

C. Influence of Exchange Abnormalities

Wagner and West (1972) extensively studied the time course of O_2 and CO_2 exchange in the pulmonary capillary in the presence of abnormal diffusion and $\dot{V}_A/\dot{Q}$ distribution. Interestingly, CO_2 exchange is quite sensitive to these abnormalities. As the membrane diffusing capacity falls, failure to reach end-capillary equilibrium occurs with both gases (Fig. 11). CO_2 reaction rates were handled as a lumped parameter, and so P_{CO_2} in this case is more representative of total CO_2 content in blood rather than the actual CO_2 tension. The delay in CO_2 excretion appears to be the cumulative result of several factors. First, a severe decrease in D_m can become a factor in retarding CO_2 diffusion (*vide supra*). Second, as emphasized by the authors, the steep slope of the blood CO_2 dissociation curve is important since large quantities of CO_2 must be transferred with a relatively small capillary–alveolar pressure gradient. Carbon dioxide tension in mixed venous blood (46 torr) is only slightly greater than mean alveolar tension (40 torr). Finally, oxygen-linked CO_2 exchange occurring via the Haldane pathways cannot be accomplished until oxygenation occurs. A portion of CO_2 exchange lags behind O_2 transfer and is quite sensitive to delays in the speed of oxygenation.

The detailed studies of Wagner and West (1972) also provided quantitative estimates of the interaction between distribution and diffusion abnormalities. Figure 13 illustrates alveolar–end-capillary P_{O_2} differences under these circumstances. Low $\dot{V}_A/\dot{Q}$ values with normal D_m might produce a minimal difference. With moderate to severe alteration of the diffusive characteristics of the pulmonary membrane, end-capillary equilibrium is not achieved and the tension differences are greatest when $\dot{V}_A/\dot{Q}$ matching is normal. With extreme diffusion abnormalities, O_2 exchange is severely impaired in units with normal and elevated $\dot{V}_A/\dot{Q}$. The situation is slightly different in the case of CO_2. When D_m is reduced, total ex-

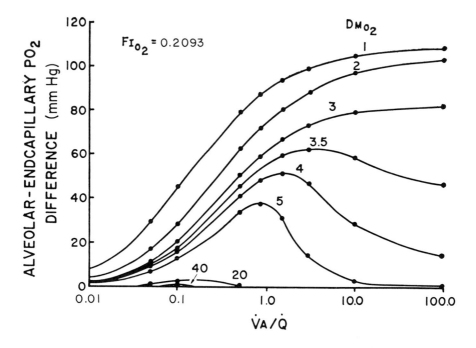

Fig. 13. Difference in P_{O_2} between alveolar gas and end-capillary blood with varying $\dot{V}_A/\dot{Q}$ relationships and $D_{m_{O_2}}$. (From Wagner and West, 1972, reproduced by permission.)

change is not as severely impaired with normal $\dot{V}_A/\dot{Q}$, but is as poor as O_2 exchange with high $\dot{V}_A/\dot{Q}$.

VII. SLOW pH AND P_{CO_2} CHANGES

Blood is not a homogeneous medium; chemical reactions and concentrations differ between plasma and cell compartments. Consequently, during gas exchange O_2 and CO_2 are not the only molecules that must cross the cell membrane before equilibrium is reached.

A. Theory of Disequilibrium

Rapid conversion of bicarbonate to CO_2 takes place during capillary transit inside the erythrocyte under the influence of carbonic anhydrase. Confinement of the enzyme to the red cell interior prompted Roughton (1935) to postulate many years ago that equilibrium between plasma and red cell pH would not be reached until long after blood has left the capillary. The large permeability of CO_2 (Forster, 1969) and the speed of trans-membrane bicarbonate–chloride exchange (Klocke, 1976) ensure that these two species are essentially in equilibrium between the plasma and cell interior as blood leaves the capillary. However, protons are required for the conversion of bicarbonate to CO_2 (Fig. 7), and intracellular hydrogen ion concentration becomes depleted in comparison to that outside the cell. Plasma pH apparently remains unchanged during capillary transit since the uncatalyzed dehydration of carbonic acid is quite slow. To achieve hydrogen ion equilibrium, substantial amounts of either H^+ or OH^- must be transported between the plasma and cell interior. Protons probably do not penetrate the cell membrane to a significant degree. Hydroxyl ion permeability is comparable to other anions, but the transmembrane concentration gradient is so small that significant movement does not occur (Crandall et al., 1971).

The disequilibrium is corrected after blood has left the capillary via the Jacobs–Stewart (1942) cycle. Plasma bicarbonate and CO_2 concentrations are reduced after CO_2 exchange in the capillary, but plasma $[H^+]$ remains unchanged. The product of $[HCO_3^-]$ and $[H^+]$ then is no longer in chemical equilibrium with $[CO_2]$ and the mass action effect causes the system to form CO_2 at the natural uncatalyzed rate. The CO_2 formed diffuses into the red cell, where it is rapidly hydrated back to a bicarbonate and a hydrogen ion. The bicarbonate ion disturbs the Donnan equilibrium, and this ion in turn exchanges for an extracellular chloride ion, leaving the hydrogen ion behind. Thus, the chloride shift that occurred during CO_2 exchange is reversed after blood has left the capillary. Each CO_2 molecule formed in the plasma that enters the cell in effect transfers a proton from plasma to cell interior. As a result, plasma pH rises as CO_2 carries protons into the cells. The slow dehydration of carbonic acid in the plasma limits the rate at which equilibrium is approached. As these readjustments take place, P_{CO_2} in postcapillary blood also rises slightly. These pH and P_{CO_2} changes have little direct effect on CO_2 exchange. E. D. Crandall (personal communication) has calculated that a twentyfold increase in CO_2 reaction rates in plasma would increase CO_2 excretion only 4%.

B. Evidence for Disequilibrium

Three different groups of investigators (Sirs, 1970; Hill *et al.*, 1973; Forster and Crandall, 1975) independently investigated the theoretical aspects of the disequilibrium originally proposed by Roughton (1935). All reached the same conclusion that pH and P_{CO_2} increase after blood leaves the pulmonary capillary. Similar postcapillary readjustments, but opposite in direction, occur following CO_2 exchange in the tissues. Bidani *et al.* (1978a) calculated that plasma pH is continually changing as blood circulates throughout the body (Fig. 12). They concluded that the slow uncatalyzed rate of hydration–dehydration reactions in plasma prevents attainment of true equilibrium at any time.

The first experimental evidence for this disequilibrium was presented by Forster and Crandall (1975). They reacted cell suspensions with CO_2 solutions in a stopped-flow apparatus and observed a slow readjustment of extracellular pH over a period of 10–15 sec. Addition of carbonic anhydrase to the extracellular fluid reduced the period of readjustment to less than 1 sec, confirming the rate-limiting nature of the slow extracellular CO_2 reactions.

Extension of these concepts into the intact organ and animal has resulted in provocative observations. Hemolysis in the experimental animal with subsequent spillage of carbonic anhydrase into the plasma frustrated initial efforts, but finally slow *in vivo* pH changes were demonstrated in two different laboratories (Hill *et al.*, 1977; Bidani and Crandall, 1978). In both reports blood was rapidly withdrawn from the carotid artery through a temperature-controlled pH cuvette. Following sudden arrest of flow, slow pH changes with half-times of 4–7 sec were observed. Addition of carbonic anhydrase to the circulation abolished the pH changes. The observed pH changes averaged 0.01 units, only one-third of the values predicted from theoretical considerations. Presumably a portion of the pH change had already occurred during the lag time (4–6 sec) between capillary exchange and pH measurement, but this could not explain the entire discrepancy.

C. Tissue Carbonic Anhydrase

A variety of tissues, the lung included, contain a significant quantity of carbonic anhydrase (Maren, 1967). Recent evidence from three independent sources (Effros et al., 1978; Crandall and O'Brasky, 1978; Klocke, 1978a) suggests that plasma may have access to pulmonary carbonic anhydrase, perhaps increasing the speed of plasma CO_2 reactions and decreasing slow pH and P_{CO_2} changes. These studies were all conducted in isolated lungs perfused with buffer free of erythrocytes.

Effros et al. (1978) observed the volume of distribution of radioactive CO_2 or bicarbonate following bolus injection into the circulation to the rabbit lung. Both had similar volumes of distribution, which included a portion of the interstitium and alveolar space. Addition of acetazolamide, a potent carbonic anhydrase inhibitor, sharply limited bicarbonate distribution to the vascular space but modified CO_2 distribution to a far less degree. The authors concluded that a portion of the tissue enzyme was localized to the pulmonary vascular endothelium and catalyzed conversion of HCO_3^- to CO_2.

Analogous to physiologic circumstances, Klocke (1978a) studied steady state CO_2 excretion in rabbit lungs during perfusion with bicarbonate buffer equilibrated with CO_2. When buffer reached gas exchange vessels, dissolved CO_2 left the perfusate, promoting production of more CO_2 from bicarbonate. The quantity of dissolved CO_2 in the expired ventilation was calculated from simultaneous measurements of acetylene excretion. The shaded areas in Fig. 14 indicate the quantities of excreted CO_2 that were generated from bicarbonate during capillary transit. In the presence of acetazolamide, a small amount of bicarbonate was mobilized because of the natural rate of the dehydration reaction. Without inhibition of carbonic anhydrase, CO_2 excretion was appreciably greater. Calculations indicated that the perfusate was exposed to sufficient enzyme to catalyze CO_2 reactions fivefold.

Crandall and O'Brasky (1978) used the stopped-flow pH technique to observe slow pH changes in buffer after perfusion through isolated rat lungs. Slow pH changes were not noted unless acetazolamide was added to the perfusate. pH measurements were made approximately 4 sec after perfusate left the pulmonary capillary, a sufficiently short period to observe pH changes if actually present.

These studies suggest that carbonic anhydrase may be associated with the vascular endothelium, akin to the association of angiotensin-

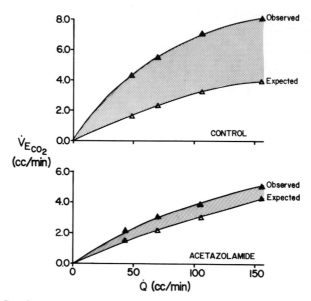

Fig. 14. Steady state carbon dioxide excretion in the isolated rabbit lung. Open symbols: expected excretion of dissolved CO_2 calculated from simultaneous acetylene excretion. Closed symbols: observed CO_2 excretion. Shaded areas: CO_2 produced from bicarbonate in the pulmonary capillary. Upper panel: no inhibition of carbonic anhydrase. Lower panel: 250 mg/liter acetazolamide added to perfusate. (From Klocke, 1978a, reproduced by permission.)

converting enzyme with the endothelium (Ryan *et al.*, 1972). Fain and Rosen (1973) have demonstrated that carbonic anhydrase is associated with the endothelium in reptiles, but the histochemical technique employed has been criticized (Muther, 1972). An alternative explanation of the experimental findings in the isolated lung preparations is that perfusate has access to enzyme present in the interstitium, either naturally or as a consequence of the experimental conditions. Data supporting either hypothesis are available in the intact animal. Feisal *et al.* (1963) observed that a bicarbonate bolus injected into the pulmonary artery of the dog has a volume of distribution greater than the vascular space. If the concept of catalysis of plasma CO_2 reactions in the lung is correct, slow pH and P_{CO_2} changes would be either reduced or absent entirely. Calculations from steady state CO_2 exchange (Klocke, 1978) and the *in vivo* slow pH observations (Hill *et al.*, 1977; Bidani and Crandall, 1978) support the concept of partial catalysis of these reactions. The remaining data (Effros *et al.*, 1978; Crandall and O'Brasky, 1978) suggest almost complete catalysis during pulmonary transit.

Skeletal muscle reputedly does not contain carbonic anhydrase (Maren,

1967), but studies of the volume of CO_2 distribution in the presence and absence of acetazolamide suggest that enzyme activity is present (Zborowska-Sluis et al., 1974). If the enzyme were located on the endothelium, it could effectively facilitate CO_2 movement but might be in small enough concentration not to be detected in assays of bulk tissue. Similar studies in cardiac muscle failed to supply any evidence of carbonic anhydrase activity (Zborowska-Sluis et al., 1975). Clearly further experimental evidence is needed to delineate the role of tissue carbonic anhydrase and the extent of slow pH and P_{CO_2} reactions throughout the body.

ACKNOWLEDGMENTS

The author appreciates the aid of Mrs. Anne Coe and Mrs. Marsha Barber in the preparation of this manuscript. This work was supported by grant HL-15194 from the National Heart, Lung and Blood Institute.

REFERENCES

Antonini, E., and Brunori, M. (1971). "Hemoglobin and Myoglobin in Their Reactions with Ligands," pp. 254–268, 383–398. Am. Elsevier, New York.

Bauer, C. (1970). Reduction of the carbon dioxide affinity of human haemoglobin solutions by 2,3-diphosphoglycerate. Respir. Physiol. 10, 10–19.

Bauer, C., and Schröder, E. (1972). Carbamino compounds of haemoglobin in human adult and foetal blood. J. Physiol. (London) 227, 457–471.

Bauer, C., Klocke, R. A., Kamp, D., and Forster, R. E. (1973). Effect of 2,3-diphosphoglycerate and H^+ on the reaction of O_2 and hemoglobin. Am. J. Physiol. 224, 838–847.

Bauer, C., Baumann, R., Engels, U., and Pacyna, B. (1975). The carbon dioxide affinity of various human hemoglobins. J. Biol. Chem. 250, 2173–2176.

Bidani, A., and Crandall, E. D. (1978). Slow postcapillary pH changes in blood in anesthetized animals. J. Appl. Physiol.: Respir. Environ. Exercise Physiol. 45, 674–680.

Bidani, A., Crandall, E. D., and Forster, R. E. (1978a). Analysis of postcapillary pH changes in blood in vivo after gas exchange. J. Appl. Physiol.: Respir. Environ. Exercise Physiol. 44, 770–781.

Bidani, A., Flumerfelt, R. W., and Crandall, E. D. (1978b). Analysis of the effects of pulsatile capillary blood flow and volume on gas exchange. Respir. Physiol. 35, 27–42.

Blank, M., and Roughton, F. J. W. (1960). The permeability of monolayers to carbon dioxide, Trans. Faraday Soc. 56, 1832–1841.

Bosman, A. R., Lee, G. deJ., and Marshall, R. (1965). The effect of pulsatile capillary blood flow upon gas exchange within the lungs of man. Clin. Sci. 28, 295–309.

Brahm, J. (1977). Temperature-dependent changes of chloride transport kinetics in human red cells. J. Gen. Physiol. 70, 283–306.

Bunn, H. F., and Briehl, R. W. (1970). The interaction of 2,3-diphosphoglycerate with various human hemoglobins. J. Clin. Invest. 49, 1088–1095.

Chow, E. I.-H., Crandall, E. D., and Forster, R. E. (1976). Kinetics of bicarbonate–

chloride exchange across the human red blood cell membrane. *J. Gen. Physiol.* **68,** 633–652.

Constantine, H. P., Craw, M. R., and Forster, R. E. (1965). Rate of the reaction of carbon dioxide with human red blood cells. *Am. J. Physiol.* **208,** 801–811.

Crandall, E. D., and O'Brasky, J. E. (1978). Direct evidence for participation of rat lung carbonic anhydrase in CO_2 reactions. *J. Clin. Invest.* **62,** 618–622.

Crandall, E. D., Klocke, R. A., and Forster, R. E. (1971). Hydroxyl ion movements across the human erythrocyte membrane. *J. Gen. Physiol.* **57,** 664–683.

Craw, M. R., Constantine, H. P., Morello, J. A., and Forster, R. E. (1963). Rate of the Bohr shift in human red cell suspensions. *J. Appl. Physiol.* **18,** 317–324.

Donaldson, T. L., and Quinn, J. A. (1974). Kinetic constants determined from membrane transport measurements: Carbonic anhydrase activity at high concentrations. *Proc. Natl. Acad. Sci. U.S.A.* **71,** 4995–4999.

Edwards, M. J., and Staub, N. C. (1966). Kinetics of O_2 uptake by erythrocytes as a function of cell age. *J. Appl. Physiol.* **21,** 173–176.

Effros, R. M., Chang, R. S. Y., and Silverman, P. (1978). Acceleration of plasma bicarbonate conversion to carbon dioxide by pulmonary carbonic anhydrase. *Science* **199,** 427–429.

Fain, W., and Rosen, S. (1973). Carbonic anhydrase activity in amphibian and reptilian lung: A histochemical and biochemical analysis. *Histochem. J.* **5,** 519–528.

Feisal, K. A., Sackner, M. A., and DuBois, A. B. (1963). Comparison between the time available and the time required for CO_2 equilibration in the lung. *J. Clin. Invest.* **42,** 24–28.

Forster, R. E. (1964). Rate of gas uptake by red cells. *In* "Handbook of Physiology. Sect. 3: Respiration" (W. O. Fenn and H. Rahn, eds.), Vol. 1, pp. 827–837. Am. Physiol. Soc., Washington, D.C.

Forster, R. E. (1969). The rate of CO_2 equilibration between red cells and plasma. *CO_2: Chem., Biochem., Physiol. Aspects, Symp. Haverford Coll., Haverford, Pa., 1968* **NASA SP-188,** pp. 275–286.

Forster, R. E., and Andersson, K. K. (1970). Effect of dilution and 2,3-diphosphoglycerate on the oxygen dissociation curve of human hemoglobin. *Fed. Proc., Fed. Am. Soc. Exp. Biol.* **29,** 852. (Abstr.)

Forster, R. E., and Crandall, E. D. (1975). Time course of exchange between red cells and extracellular fluid during CO_2 uptake. *J. Appl. Physiol.* **38,** 710–718.

Forster, R. E., and Steen, J. B. (1968). Rate limiting processes in the Bohr shift in human red cells. *J. Physiol. (London)* **196,** 541–562.

Forster, R. E., Roughton, F. J. W., Kreuzer, F., and Briscoe, W. A. (1957). Photocolorimetric determination of rate of uptake of CO and O_2 by reduced human red cell suspensions at 37°C. *J. Appl. Physiol.* **11,** 260–268.

Forster, R. E., Constantine, H. P., Craw, M. R., Rotman, H. H., and Klocke, R. A. (1968). Reaction of CO_2 with human hemoglobin solution. *J. Biol. Chem.* **243,** 3317–3326.

Frech, W.-E., Schultehinrichs, D., Vogel, H. R., and Thews, G. (1968). Modelluntersuchungen zum Austausch der Atemgase. I. Die O_2-Aufnahmezeiten des Erythrocyten unter den Bedingungen des Lungen-Capillarblutes. *Pfluegers Arch.* **301,** 292–301.

Fung, Y. C., and Sobin, S. S. (1969). Theory of sheet flow in lung alveoli. *J. Appl. Physiol.* **26,** 472–488.

Gad-el-Hak, M., Morton, J. B., and Kutchai, H. (1977). Turbulent flow of red cells in dilute suspensions. Effect on kinetics of O_2 uptake. *Biophys. J.* **18,** 289–300.

Garby, L., and deVerdier, C.-H. (1971). Affinity of human hemoglobin A to 2,3-diphosphoglycerate. Effect of hemoglobin concentration and pH. *Scand. J. Clin. Lab. Invest.* **27**, 345–350.

Gibson, Q. H. (1954). Stopped-flow apparatus for the study of rapid reactions. *Discuss. Faraday Soc.* **17**, 137–139.

Gibson, Q. H. (1970). The reaction of oxygen with hemoglobin and the kinetic basis of the effect of salt on binding of oxygen. *J. Biol. Chem.* **245**, 3285–3288.

Goldman, D. E. (1943). Potential, impedence, and rectification in membranes. *J. Gen. Physiol.* **27**, 37–60.

Gros, G., and Moll, W. (1971). The diffusion of carbon dioxide in erythrocytes and hemoglobin solutions. *Pfluegers Arch. Eur. J. Physiol.* **324**, 249–266.

Gros, G., Forster, R. E., and Lin, L. (1976). The carbamate reaction of glycylglycine, plasma, and tissue extracts evaluated by a pH stopped flow apparatus. *J. Biol. Chem.* **251**, 4398–4407.

Gutknecht, J., Bisson, M. A., and Tosteson, F. C. (1977). Diffusion of carbon dioxide through lipid bilayer membranes. *J. Gen. Physiol.* **69**, 779–794.

Harrington, J. P., Elbaum, D., Bookchin, R. M., Wittenberg, J. B., and Nagel, R. L. (1977). Ligand kinetics of hemoglobin S containing erythrocytes. *Proc. Natl. Acad. Sci. U.S.A.* **74**, 203–206.

Hartridge, H., and Roughton, F. J. W. (1923). A method of measuring the velocity of very rapid chemical reactions. *Proc. R. Soc. London, Ser. A* **104**, 395–415.

Hill, E. P., Power, G. G., and Longo, L. D. (1973). Mathematical simulation of pulmonary O_2 and CO_2 exchange. *Am. J. Physiol.* **224**, 904–917.

Hill, E. P., Power, G. G., and Gilbert, R. D. (1977). Rate of pH changes in blood plasma in vitro and in vivo. *J. Appl. Physiol.: Respir. Environ. Exercise Physiol.* **42**, 928–934.

Hlastala, M. P. (1972). A model of fluctuating alveolar gas exchange during the respiratory cycle. *Respir. Physiol.* **15**, 214–232.

Hlastala, M. P. (1973). Significance of the Bohr and Haldane effects in the pulmonary capillary. *Respir. Physiol.* **17**, 81–92.

Hlastala, M. P., and Woodson, R. D. (1975). Saturation dependency of the Bohr effect: Interactions among H^+, CO_2, and DPG. *J. Appl. Physiol.* **38**, 1126–1131.

Holland, R. A. B. (1967). Kinetics of combination of O_2 and CO with human hemoglobin F in cells and in solution. *Respir. Physiol.* **3**, 307–317.

Holland, R. A. B., and Forster, R. E. (1975). Effect of temperature on rate of CO_2 uptake by human red cell suspensions. *Am. J. Physiol.* **228**, 1589–1596.

Holland, R. A. B., van Hezewijk, W., and Zubzanda, J. (1977). Velocity of oxygen uptake by partly saturated adult and fetal human red cells. *Respir. Physiol.* **29**, 303–314.

Jacobs, M. H., and Stewart, D. R. (1942). The role of carbonic anhydrase in certain ionic exchanges involving the erythrocyte. *J. Gen. Physiol.* **25**, 539–552.

Johnson, R. L., Jr., Spicer, W. S., Bishop, J. M., and Forster, R. E. (1960). Pulmonary capillary blood volume, flow and diffusing capacity during exercise. *J. Appl. Physiol.* **15**, 893–902.

Kernohan, J. C., and Roughton, F. J. W. (1968). Thermal studies of the rates of the reactions of carbon dioxide in concentrated haemoglobin solutions and in red blood cells. A. The reactions catalysed by carbonic anhydrase. B. The carbamino reactions of oxygenated and deoxygenated haemoglobin. *J. Physiol. (London)* **197**, 345–361.

Kernohan, J. C., Forrest, W. W., and Roughton, F. J. W. (1963). The activity of concentrated solutions of carbonic anhydrase. *Biochim. Biophys. Acta* **67**, 31–41.

Kilmartin, J. V., Fogg, J., Luzzana, M., and Rossi-Bernardi, L. (1973). Role of the α-amino groups of the α and β chains of human hemoglobin in oxygen-linked binding of carbon dioxide. *J. Biol. Chem.* **248,** 7039–7043.

King, T. K. C., and Briscoe, W. A. (1967). Blood gas exchange in emphysema: An example illustrating method of calculation. *J. Appl. Physiol.* **23,** 672–682.

Klocke, R. A. (1973). Mechanism and kinetics of the Haldane effect in human erythrocytes. *J. Appl. Physiol.* **35,** 673–681.

Klocke, R. A. (1976). Rate of bicarbonate–chloride exchange in human red cells at 37°C. *J. Appl. Physiol.* **40,** 707–714.

Klocke, R. A. (1978a). Catalysis of CO_2 reactions by lung carbonic anhydrase. *J. Appl. Physiol.: Respir. Environ. Exercise Physiol.* **44,** 882–888.

Klocke, R. A. (1978b). Carbon dioxide transport. *In* "Extrapulmonary Manifestations of Respiratory Disease" (E. D. Robin, ed.), pp. 315–343. Dekker, New York.

Klocke, R. A., Andersson, K. K., Rotman, H. H., and Forster, R. E. (1972). Permeability of human erythrocytes to ammonia and weak acids. *Am. J. Physiol.* **222,** 1004–1013.

Kreuzer, F. (1970). Facilitated diffusion of oxygen and its possible significance; a review. *Respir. Physiol.* **9,** 1–30.

Kreuzer, F., and Yahr, W. Z. (1960). Influence of red cell membrane on diffusion of oxygen. *J. Appl. Physiol.* **15,** 1117–1122.

Kutchai, H. (1975). Role of the red cell membrane in oxygen uptake. *Respir. Physiol.* **23,** 121–132.

Kutchai, H., and Staub, N. C. (1969). Steady-state, hemoglobin-facilitated O_2 transport in human erythrocytes. *J. Gen. Physiol.* **53,** 576–589.

Lawson, W. H., Jr. (1966). Interrelation of pH, temperature, and oxygen on deoxygenation rate of red cells. *J. Appl. Physiol.* **21,** 905–914.

Lawson, W. H., Jr. (1971). Effect of anemia, species, and temperature on CO kinetics with red blood cells, *J. Appl. Physiol.* **31,** 447–457.

Lawson, W. H., Jr., and Forster, R. E. (1967). Oxygen tension gradients in peripheral capillary blood. *J. Appl. Physiol.* **22,** 907–973.

Lawson, W. H., Jr., Holland, R. A. B., and Forster, R. E. (1965). Effect of temperature on deoxygenation rate of human red cells. *J. Appl. Physiol.* **20,** 912–918.

Lee, G. deJ., and DuBois, A. B. (1955). Pulmonary capillary blood flow in man. *J. Clin. Invest.* **34,** 1380–1390.

Luckner, H. (1939). Über die Geschwindigkeit des Austauches der Atemgase im Beut. *Pfluegers Arch. Gesamte Physiol. Menschen Tiere* **241,** 753–778.

Maren, T. H. (1967). Carbonic anhydrase: Chemistry, physiology, and inhibition. *Physiol. Rev.* **47,** 595–781.

Mendoza, C., Peavy, H., Burns, B., and Gurtner, G. (1977). Saturation kinetics for steady-state pulmonary CO transfer. *J. Appl. Physiol.: Respir. Environ. Exercise Physiol.* **43,** 880–884.

Menkes, H. A., Sera, K., Rogers, R. M., Hyde, R. W., Forster, R. E., and DuBois, A. B. (1970). Pulsatile uptake of CO in the human lung. *J. Clin. Invest.* **49,** 335–345.

Miyamoto, Y., and Moll, W. (1971). Measurements of dimensions and pathway of red cells in rapidly frozen lungs *in situ. Respir. Physiol.* **12,** 141–156.

Miyamoto, Y., and Moll, W. (1972). The diameter of red blood cells when flowing through a rapid reaction apparatus. *Respir. Physiol.* **16,** 259–266.

Muther, T. (1972). A critical evaluation of the histochemical methods for carbonic anhydrase. *J. Histochem. Cytochem.* **20,** 319–330.

Nakamura, T., and Staub, N. C. (1964). Synergism in the kinetic reactions of O_2 and CO_2 with human red blood cells. *J. Physiol. (London)* **173,** 161–177.

Nicolson, P., and Roughton, F. J. W. (1951). A theoretical study of the influence of diffusion and chemical reaction velocity on the rate of exchange of carbon monoxide and oxygen between the red blood corpuscle and the surrounding fluid. *Proc. R. Soc. London, Ser. B* **138**, 241–264.

Piiper, J. (1969). Rates of chloride–bicarbonate exchange between red cells and plasma. *CO_2: Chem., Biochem., Physiol. Aspects, Symp. Haverford Coll., Haverford, Pa., 1968* **NASA SP-188**, pp. 267–273.

Rossi-Bernardi, L., and Roughton, F. J. W. (1967). The specific influence of carbon dioxide and carbamate compounds on the buffer power and Bohr effects in human haemoglobin solutions. *J. Physiol. (London)* **189**, 1–29.

Rothstein, A., Cabantchik, Z. I., and Knauf, P. (1976). Mechanism of anion transport in red blood cells: Role of membrane proteins. *Fed. Proc., Fed. Am. Soc. Exp. Biol.* **35**, 3–10.

Rotman, H. H., Klocke, R. A., and Forster, R. E. (1970). Artifact due to the stagnant layer on electrode surface in a continuous-flow reaction apparatus. *Physiologist* **13**, 297.

Rotman, H. H., Klocke, R. A., Andersson, K. K., D'Alecy, L., and Forster, R. E. (1974). Kinetics of oxygenation and deoxygenation of erythrocytes containing hemoglobin S. *Respir. Physiol.* **21**, 9–17.

Roughton, F. J. W. (1935). Recent work on carbon dioxide transport by the blood. *Physiol. Rev.* **15**, 241–296.

Roughton, F. J. W. (1964). Transport of oxygen and carbon dioxide. *In* "Handbook of Physiology. Sect. 3: Respiration" (W. O. Fenn and H. Rahn, eds.), Vol. 1, pp. 767–825. Am. Physiol. Soc., Washington, D.C.

Roughton, F. J. W.., and Forster, R. E. (1957). Relative importance of diffusion and chemical reaction rates in determining rate of exchange of gases in the human lung, with special reference to true diffusing capacity of pulmonary membrane and volume of blood in lung capillaries. *J. Appl. Physiol.* **11**, 290–302.

Roughton, F. J. W., Forster, R. E., and Cander, L. (1957). Rate at which carbon monoxide replaces oxygen from combination with human hemoglobin in solution and in the red cell. *J. Appl. Physiol.* **11**, 269–276.

Ryan, J. W., Smith, U., and Niemeyer, R. S. (1972). Angiotensin I: Metabolism by plasma membrane of lung. *Science* **176**, 64–66.

Sachs, J. R., Knauf, P. A., and Dunham, P. B. (1975). Transport through red cell membranes. *In* "The Red Blood Cell" (D. M. Surgenor, ed.), pp. 613–703. Academic Press, New York.

Salhany, J. M., Mizukami, H., and Eliot, R. S. (1971). The deoxygenation kinetic properties of human fetal hemoglobin: Effect of 2,3-diphosphoglycerate. *Biochem. Biophys. Res. Commun.* **45**, 1350–1356.

Silverman, D. N., Tu, C., and Wynns, G. C. (1976). Depletion of ^{18}O from $C^{18}O_2$ in erythrocyte suspensions. *J. Biol. Chem.* **251**, 4428–4435.

Sinha, A. K. (1969). O_2 uptake and release by red cells through capillary wall and plasma layer. Ph.D. Thesis, Univ. of California, San Francisco. (Xerox Univ. Microfilms, Ann Arbor, Michigan.)

Sirs, J. A. (1970). The interaction of carbon dioxide with the rate of the exchange of oxygen by red blood cells. *In* "Blood Oxygenation" (D. Hershey, ed.), pp. 116–136. Plenum, New York.

Staub, N. C., Bishop, J. M., and Forster, R. E. (1961). Velocity of O_2 uptake by human red blood cells. *J. Appl. Physiol.* **16**, 511–516.

Swenson, E. R., and Maren, T. H. (1978). A quantitative analysis of CO_2 transport at rest and during maximal exercise. *Respir. Physiol.* **35**, 129–159.

Tosteson, D. C. (1959). Halide transport in red blood cells. *Acta Physiol. Scand.* **46,** 19–41.

Wagner, P. D. (1977). Diffusion and chemical reaction in pulmonary gas exchange. *Physiol. Rev.* **57,** 257–312.

Wagner, P. D., and West, J. B. (1972). Effects of diffusion impairment on O_2 and CO_2 time courses in pulmonary capillaries. *J. Appl. Physiol.* **33,** 62–71.

Wyman, J., Jr. (1964). Linked functions and reciprocal effects in hemoglobin: a second look. *Adv. Protein Chem.* **19,** 223–286.

Zander, R., and Schmid-Schönbein, H. (1973). Extracellular mechanisms of oxygen transport in flowing blood. *Respir. Physiol.* **19,** 279–289.

Zborowska-Sluis, D. T., L'Abbate, A., and Klassen, G. A. (1974). Evidence of carbonic anhydrase activity in skeletal muscle: A role for facilitative carbon dioxide transport. *Respir. Physiol.* **21,** 341–350.

Zborowska-Sluis, D. T., L'Abbate, A., Mildenberger, R. R., and Klassen, G. A. (1975). The effect of acetazolamide on myocardial carbon dioxide space. *Respir. Physiol.* **23,** 311–316.

7

Ventilation–Perfusion Relationships

Peter D. Wagner and John B. West

I. INTRODUCTION

It would be natural to suppose that if a lung were supplied with adequate amounts of fresh gas and mixed venous blood, and if complete equilibration occurred between alveolar gas and pulmonary capillary blood in every lung unit, then normal pulmonary gas exchange would be assured. As is well known, however, this is not the case. Unless the proportion of the total ventilation and blood flow going to each gas-exchanging unit is the same, overall gas exchange becomes inefficient and, other things being equal, the arterial P_{O_2} falls and the P_{CO_2} rises.

A full understanding of how mismatching of ventilation and blood flow

PULMONARY GAS EXCHANGE, VOL. I

within the lung affects gas exchange remains one of the most challenging problems in the whole area of pulmonary gas exchange. Two factors greatly increase the complexity of this problem. First, the way in which the P_{O_2}, P_{CO_2}, and P_{N_2} in any lung unit change as the ventilation–perfusion ratio is altered depends on the shapes and positions of the oxygen and carbon dioxide dissociation curves. These are not only non-linear but also interdependent. As a consequence, closed-form solutions are not possible, and indeed until recently, only graphical solutions were possible. Second, any realistic approach must consider the gas exchange behavior of a series of lung units with some type of distribution of ventilation–perfusion ratios. The resultant complexity necessitates numerical analysis, and indeed the introduction of digital computing has revolutionized this area of research (see this volume, Chapter 8).

It is worth noting that pulmonary physiology seems to be well ahead of other areas of physiology in this regard. There is every reason to believe that functional inhomogeneity within other organs impairs their overall function. For example, in peripheral tissues such as skeletal muscle, inequalities in the ratio of blood flow to oxygen uptake must reduce the efficiency of oxygen transfer. In the kidney, inequalities in the ratio of glomerular filtration rate to plasma flow among different nephrons presumably affect renal function. However, relatively little interest has been directed toward the consequences of these types of functional inhomogeneity. By contrast, the sequelae of ventilation–perfusion inequality in the lung demand attention because this is the commonest mechanism of arterial hypoxemia and hypercarbia.

In this chapter we first review ways of analyzing ventilation–perfusion inequality based on the measurement of partial pressures of the three naturally occurring respiratory gases: oxygen, carbon dioxide, and nitrogen, as they exist under steady state conditions. This is the simplest approach, was historically the first, and is still employed extensively in the clinical setting. Next we turn to methods based on simple interventions such as the wash-out of nitrogen from the lung. Both compartmental and continuous distributions of ventilation–perfusion ratios have been obtained in this way. Finally, analyses based on the infusion of multiple infused inert gases are examined. Here we exploit the gas exchange behavior of specially chosen gases rather than rely on the respiratory gases that happen to be present. This is the most complex but the most informative approach available to date. The emphasis of the chapter is on general principles of gas exchange in the presence of ventilation–perfusion inequality rather than the patterns that occur in particular physiological conditions or specific disease states. Studies on both normal and abnormal lungs are included.

II. ANALYSIS USING P_{O_2}, P_{CO_2}, AND P_{N_2}

Since ventilation–perfusion inequality usually causes profound changes in the partial pressures of P_{O_2}, P_{CO_2}, and P_{N_2} in arterial blood and expired gas, these constitute the simplest way of assessing the inequality. However, although this approach has advantages, there are also drawbacks. The main advantage is that the gases are always available and that the measurements can be made relatively easily. A serious disadvantage is that the amount of resulting information is severely limited. The number of available measurements is small and, furthermore, the common respiratory gases do not have properties that are anywhere near ideal for this purpose. Nevertheless, for clinical purposes, this approach as originally formulated over 30 years ago by Riley and Cournand (1949) is still extensively used.

A. Oxygen–Carbon Dioxide Diagram

The oxygen–carbon dioxide diagram is the key to understanding how mismatching of ventilation and blood flow affect the arterial P_{O_2}, P_{CO_2}, and P_{N_2}, and how measurements of these gases can throw light on the type of ventilation–perfusion inequality that must exist. Some discussion of the O_2–CO_2 diagram can be found in Chapters 2 and 3 of this volume, where its historical background is considered, and a full description was given by Rahn and Fenn (1955). Figure 1 shows an O_2–CO_2 diagram with the points representing the compositions of inspired gas (I) and mixed

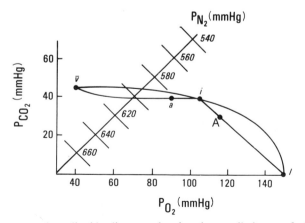

Fig. 1. Oxygen–carbon dioxide diagram showing the ventilation–perfusion ratio line joining the mixed venous ($\bar{v}$) to the inspired gas (I) point. Ideal (i), arterial (a), and alveolar (A) points are also shown. Lines of equal P_{N_2} have a slope of -1.

venous blood ($\bar{v}$). The curved line joining these indicates the alveolar gas composition of lung units having increasing ventilation–perfusion ratios from zero at point $\bar{v}$ to infinity at point I. No other alveolar gas composition in homogeneous lung units can exist in this lung. If we assume equilibration between alveolar gas and end-capillary blood in every lung unit, the line (called the ventilation–perfusion ratio line) also denotes the partial pressures of end-capillary blood.

The diagram also shows typical examples of the composition of mixed alveolar gas (A) and mixed arterial blood (a). These points lie on the gas and blood R lines corresponding to the respiratory exchange ratio of the whole lung. In a lung with no ventilation–perfusion inequality, the points would be superimposed at point i, known as the ideal point. With increasing ventilation–perfusion inequality they diverge further and further away. The corresponding alveolar–arterial P_{O_2} and P_{CO_2} differences can be read off the diagram.

Figure 1 also shows how the isopleths (lines of equal partial pressure) for nitrogen cut across the diagram at an angle of 45°. Inspection will show that as the ventilation–perfusion ratio is increased from zero to somewhat above normal (that is, beyond point i), the P_{N_2} decreases. With further rise in the ventilation–perfusion ratio the P_{N_2} increases again. Also note that while the P_{N_2} of mixed arterial blood rises steadily as the degree of ventilation–perfusion inequality is increased, the change in P_{N_2} of mixed alveolar gas is much less and will depend critically on the slope of the gas R line. Indeed when the gas R is 1.0, the alveolar P_{N_2} is constant irrespective of the degree of ventilation–perfusion inequality present in the lung.

It is clear that the partial pressure differences for all three gases— oxygen, carbon dioxide, and nitrogen—contain information about the *amount* of ventilation–perfusion inequality. Moreover, these differences give some information about the *type* of inequality present. For example, a lung with large amounts of blood flow to regions with low ventilation–perfusion ratios will substantially reduce the arterial P_{O_2} and also raise the arterial P_{N_2}. By contrast, the presence of areas of high ventilation–perfusion ratios will have much less influence on the mixed alveolar P_{O_2} and almost none on the P_{N_2}. Although the information value of these respiratory gases is limited, they have been extensively studied because no further interventions are necessary to get the information.

B. Riley Method

In this method (Riley and Cournand, 1949) the P_{O_2} and P_{CO_2} of arterial blood and mixed expired gas are used to construct a three-compartment model of the lung, as shown in Fig. 2. One compartment (physiologic

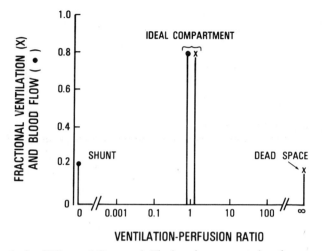

Fig. 2. Analysis of Riley and Cournand. The lung is represented as three compartments. One is perfused but not ventilated (physiologic shunt). Another is ventilated but not perfused (physiologic deadspace). The third (ideal) receives the remainder of the ventilation and blood flow.

shunt) is considered to be perfused but unventilated (point $\bar{v}$ on Fig. 1), another (physiologic dead space) ventilated but unperfused (point 1 on Fig. 1), and the third compartment (ideal) contains the remainder of the ventilation and blood flow (point i on Fig. 1).

In practice, the gas composition of the ideal compartment is first determined using the alveolar gas equation and taking the arterial P_{CO_2} to represent the ideal value. This is a reasonable approximation in most instances because the blood R line is so nearly horizontal (Fig. 1). Once this has been done, the blood flow to the shunt compartment is calculated from the familiar shunt equation, while the ventilation to the physiologic dead space is derived from the Bohr dead space equation. Details can be found in Chapter 3 of this volume, which also describes the historical development of this approach.

C. Alveolar–Arterial P_{N_2} Differences

As shown in Fig. 1, lung units with different ventilation–perfusion ratios generally have a different P_{N_2} (Canfield and Rahn, 1957). Therefore, in a lung with ventilation–perfusion inequality, the mixed alveolar P_{N_2} is a ventilation-weighted average

$$P_{E_{N_2}} = \frac{\Sigma P_{A_{N_2}} \dot{V}_A}{\Sigma \dot{V}_A}$$

while the arterial P_{N_2} is a blood-flow-weighted average

$$P_{a_{N_2}} = \frac{\Sigma P_{A_{N_2}} \dot{Q}}{\Sigma \dot{Q}}$$

The result is an alveolar–arterial difference for P_{N_2}, the arterial value being higher because poorly ventilated well-perfused units have a high P_{N_2} (Fig. 1).

A valuable feature of the alveolar–arterial P_{N_2} difference is that it is unaffected by direct shunts through unventilated lung because the P_{N_2} of arterial and mixed venous blood are the same. This property can therefore be used to distinguish between such shunts and blood flow through finitely but very poorly ventilated units. For example, by comparing the alveolar–arterial differences for P_{O_2} and P_{N_2}, Corbet and co-workers (1974) concluded that the hypoxemia of infants with hyaline membrane disease was caused almost exclusively by blood flow to unventilated regions. By contrast, in a group of patients with cystis fibrosis, the mechanism was blood flow through units with low but finite ventilation–perfusion ratios (Corbet et al., 1975).

Another theoretically useful property of the alveolar–arterial P_{N_2} difference is that it is unaffected by diffusion impairment within the lung, which can raise the P_{O_2} difference. This is because nitrogen and all the other inert gases (those which obey Henry's law) equilibrate very rapidly between alveolar gas and pulmonary capillary blood (Wagner, 1977b).

It should be emphasized that the measurement of the P_{N_2} in blood is technically a very arduous procedure. The analysis is generally done by gas chromatography (Lenfant and Aucutt, 1966) but the value is very sensitive to the temperature of the pulmonary blood, and nitrogen contamination from air leaks is difficult to avoid. Because of these difficulties, relatively little practical use has been made of the alveolar–arterial P_{N_2} difference.

D. Triple Gradient

A few investigators have combined measurements of the alveolar and arterial differences for P_{O_2}, P_{CO_2}, and P_{N_2} (the so-called triple gradient) to derive information about the pattern of ventilation–perfusion inequality in the lung. For example Lenfant (1963) studied a series of normal subjects at various inspired oxygen concentrations and by comparing the behavior of the three alveolar–arterial differences he concluded that the lungs had a significant number of units with very low and indeterminable ventilation–perfusion ratios. In a further study (Lenfant, 1964) made under hyperberic conditions (2.6 atm) the data were reported to be consistent with a bimodal distribution of ventilation–perfusion ratios composed of a large group of well-ventilated units and another small group having a very low but finite ventilation–perfusion ratio.

The most sophisticated analysis of the distribution compatible with measured P_{O_2}, P_{CO_2}, and P_{N_2} data was presented by Markello and colleagues (1973). These investigators used techniques of numerical analysis to find three compartment models that would fit the lungs of patients following induction with halothane anesthesia. The compartments consisted of one with a high ventilation–perfusion ratio, one with a low ratio, and a direct left-to-right shunt. No consistent pattern was found; in some patients a shunt was the predominant cause of impaired gas exchange, while in others ventilation–perfusion inequality was marked. The method was also used to investigate pulmonary gas exchange of patients in the intensive care setting (Markello et al., 1972).

III. ANALYSIS FOLLOWING GAS WASHOUT

Up to this point we have been considering analyses of ventilation–perfusion relationships based solely on the steady state partial pressures of the naturally occurring respiratory gases—oxygen, carbon dioxide, and nitrogen. When these data are combined with measurements of the wash-out of nitrogen during oxygen breathing (or wash-in or wash-out of other insoluble inert gases) additional information about the ventilation–perfusion inequality can be obtained.

A. Compartmental Analysis

Briscoe and colleagues (Briscoe, 1959; Briscoe et al., 1960; King and Briscoe, 1967; King et al., 1973) have been the most consistent proponents of this type of analysis over a period of many years. Chapter 8 in Volume II of this treatise is devoted mainly to this subject; a summary is included here to show how the method relates to other ways of measuring ventilation–perfusion inequality.

When an almost insoluble gas such as helium or nitrogen is washed out from the lungs, the pattern of end-tidal or mixed expired gas concentrations can be treated as if the lung consisted of two populations of lung units, one well ventilated and the other poorly ventilated. If these data are combined with measurements of arterial oxygen saturation (Briscoe, 1959) the resultant two-compartment model gives the ventilation, blood flow, and lung volume of each population of lung units consistent with all the data. For example, it has been shown that an emphysematous lung may behave as if nine-tenths of the total ventilation and one-half of the total blood flow go to one-quarter of the volume of the lung (the fast space), whereas the other three-quarters of the volume receive only one-tenth of the ventilation and the other half of the blood flow (the slow space).

An extension of this method of analysis allows the diffusion properties of each compartment to be estimated. This is done using the notion of "Bohr integral isopleths," which give the rate of rise of P_{O_2} along the pulmonary capillary for different values of diffusing capacity per unit blood flow. As an example of the application of this method, Arndt *et al.* (1970) reported that in 10 patients with interstitial lung disease the lung units in the fast space had an alveolar–end-capillary P_{O_2} difference of 10 mm Hg, and the value of this difference in the slow space was 56 mm Hg. The conclusion was that even at rest a substantial amount of the arterial hypoxemia of these patients was attributable to diffusion impairment. It might be noted that this conclusion is at variance with that of Wagner *et al.* (1976), who found that all the hypoxemia in a group of patients with interstitial lung disease was caused by ventilation–perfusion inequality at rest, although a component was caused by diffusion impairment on exercise.

B. Continuous Distributions

Although compartmental analysis is a convenient and simple way of looking at the relations between pulmonary ventilation, blood flow and gas exchange, it has been recognized for many years that the real lung must consist of some kind of distribution of ventilation–perfusion ratios. Rahn (1949) has the distinction of being the first to suggest that a logarithmic normal distribution might be present and he assumed this for some theoretical studies, later extended by Fàrhi and Rahn (1955). Other investigators have examined data on gas exchange in the light of the predicted behavior of distributions of ventilation–perfusion ratios. For example, as mentioned earlier, Lenfant (1964) measured the alveolar–arterial difference for P_{O_2}, P_{CO_2}, and P_{N_2} in subjects breathing 75% oxygen at sea level and again at an increased pressure of 2.6 atm and compared the results with those expected from bimodal distributions of ventilation–perfusion ratios. However, the first experiment designed specifically to recover distributions was that by Lenfant and Okubo (1968).

These investigators measured the arterial P_{O_2} and P_{CO_2} while the subjects breathed 100% oxygen and thus washed the nitrogen out of their lungs over a period of approximately 10 min. The time course of the calculated arterial oxygen content was then analyzed using Laplace transform techniques. A serious mathematical difficulty was posed by the nonlinearity of the oxygen dissociation curve but this was overcome by using an empirical exponential fit for the time course of oxygen bound to hemoglobin.

Figure 3 shows some of their results; subjects 1–5 were normal, whereas subjects 6–10 had chronic obstructive lung disease. The plots show both blood flow and lung volume plotted against ventilation–perfusion ratio, the latter on a log scale from 0.1 to 10. Note that the

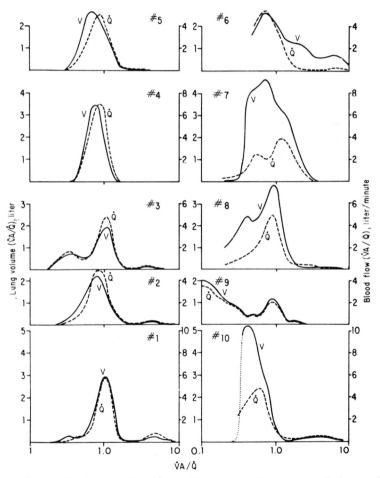

Fig. 3. Distributions of blood flow (Q) and lung volume (V) against ventilation–perfusion ratio reported by Lenfant and Okubo (1968). Note that the normal subjects (1–5) had relatively narrow distributions, whereas the patients with chronic obstructive lung disease (6–10) had broader and sometimes bizarre distributions. (From Lenfant and Okubo, 1969, reproduced by permission.)

normal patients (subjects 1–4) showed relatively narrow distributions although subject 3 had a well-defined shoulder on the low $\dot{V}_A/\dot{Q}$ side of the distribution. In the patients with lung disease (subjects 5–10) the distributions were generally much broader and some bizarre patterns were seen (for example, patient 9). It is worth noting here that the range of ventilation–perfusion ratios shown in Fig. 3 is considerably less than that studied by the multiple inert gas elimination technique (see below).

C. Limitations of These Methods

The gas wash-out methods to study ventilation–perfusion relationships are examples of the use of forcing functions to elucidate the gas exchange behavior of the lung. We can imagine the lung as a black box that, when perturbed by a known disturbing factor, responds in a way which depends on its ventilation–perfusion ratio distribution. A basic assumption of such a method is that the forcing function itself does not alter the distribution. However, there is every reason to believe that increasing the inspired P_{O_2} will alter the distribution of ventilation–perfusion ratios in some circumstances as pointed out by Lenfant (1965). For example, there may be hypoxic vasoconstriction in some regions, which will be relieved when the local alveolar P_{O_2} is increased. Again direct measurements of distributions of ventilation–perfusion ratios in patients with blood flow to very poorly ventilated regions have shown that the ventilation to these units may be abolished during high oxygen breathing (Dantzker et al., 1975). Clearly a technique that alters the distribution in an unpredictable way cannot reliably be used to measure the distribution.

Another objection to the method of Lenfant and Okubo (1968) was raised by Peslin et al. (1971). They pointed out that the Post–Widder equation, which was used by Lenfant and Okubo to obtain an approximate inversion of the Laplace integral, gave results that were highly sensitive to experimental error. Indeed, they argued that with the usual experimental accuracy, the data carried little information about the shape of the distribution function. This is an important question about any underdetermined system and it has been extensively investigated for the multiple inert gas elimination method (see later).

A further reservation applies to the compartmental analysis of Briscoe and colleagues. As indicated above, the first step is to divide the lung into fast and slowly ventilatory spaces by means of a gas wash-out. The blood flow is then apportioned to these compartments on the assumption that the blood flow within each compartment is uniform. In a final step the diffusion properties of each compartment are computed, again assuming that each compartment is homogeneous with respect to diffusion.

However, these are weak assumptions. There is no reason why the blood flow and diffusion properties of a lung unit should always be matched to its ventilation. It is possible that a lung might have some poorly perfused units that are well ventilated as well as others which are poorly ventilated. The same applies to the diffusion characteristics of the units. It therefore seems unwarranted (as the authors claim) to argue that because the hypoxemia of a given patient with interstitial lung disease is more severe than can be accounted for by the ventilation–perfusion inequality of a two-compartment model, an additional cause of hypoxemia may be present (Arndt et al., 1970). An alternative view is that the model with its limited number of compartments and severe assumptions is inadequate.

IV. USE OF FOREIGN (INERT) GASES

A. Introduction

Although the naturally occurring respiratory gases—oxygen, carbon dioxide, and nitrogen—are always affected by ventilation–perfusion inequality, there is no intrinsic reason why these should be the preferred gases for determining the distribution of ventilation–perfusion ratios. Indeed, they have obvious limitations. First, with only three gases available, the amount of information is severely limited. Second, it can be shown that the gas exchange behavior of a gas in the presence of ventilation–perfusion inequality is dominated by the slope of its dissociation curve in blood, that is, its physiologic "solubility" (West, 1969–1970). Although carbon dioxide has a steeper slope than oxygen in most physiological circumstances, the range of solubilities provided by these gases is very small. The solubility of nitrogen is irrelevant because the behavior of this gas is essentially determined by the other two.

For these reasons the pattern of uptake or elimination of a series of foreign gases by the lung potentially contains far more information about any ventilation–perfusion inequality that may be present than any possible measurements of oxygen, carbon dioxide, and nitrogen. Moreover, these gases have the following advantages. First, since they generally obey Henry's law of solubility, the complicating effects of a nonlinear dissociation curve on gas exchange are avoided. (Traditionally these gases have been called "inert" by physiologists because they do not combine with hemoglobin. The term is a poor one because several of the gases are anesthetic in high concentrations and therefore are not always physiologically inert. However, we shall follow this usage.) A second advantage is that an enormous range of solubilities is available, for example, a factor of approximately 10^5 between the solubilities of acetone and sulfur hexafluoride in blood.

The first measurements of inert gas exchange to derive information about ventilation–perfusion inequality were made by Yokoyama and Farhi (1967). They allowed anesthetized dogs to breathe a mixture of methane, ethane, and nitrous oxide with oxygen for 20 min and then followed the wash-out of these gases in expired gas, and arterial and mixed venous blood. They interpreted the data in terms of a two-compartment model based on simple mixing equations, which took account of the mass conservation that must be present (Farhi and Yokoyama, 1967). They found that the lungs behaved as if there was one compartment with a nearly normal ventilation–perfusion ratio and another with a low ratio of less than 0.1, which received 10–29% of the total bloodflow.

However, the potential of inert gases for elucidating the pattern of ventilation–perfusion inequality goes far beyond deriving a two-compartment model. The remainder of this chapter is devoted to a method based on multiple inert gas elimination, which has now been used extensively for obtaining basic physiologic information and also for studying various types of lung disease. We review both the theoretical and experimental aspects of the method, indicating the quality and quantity of information that can be potentially obtained, and the information that has, in fact, been gathered recently in the study of patients with asthma on the one hand, and patients undergoing general anesthesia on the other.

B. Principles of Inert Gas Elimination

The inert gas elimination method rests on the mass balance principle, which relates alveolar pressures of inert gases in the lung to the solubility of the gas and the ventilation–perfusion ratio of the area of lung under consideration. This expression has been derived and described many times in the past (Kety, 1951; Farhi, 1967) and has been further treated in Chapter 8 of this volume and Chapter 1 of Volume II. Specifically, in a small area of lung of homogeneous alveolar partial pressure, the relationship between alveolar (P_A) and end-capillary ($P_{c'}$) and mixed venous $P_{\bar{v}}$ partial pressures of an inert gas and the blood gas partition coefficient (λ) and ventilation–perfusion ratio ($\dot{V}_A/\dot{Q}$) is given by

$$\frac{P_{c'}}{P_{\bar{v}}} = \frac{P_A}{P_{\bar{v}}} = \frac{\lambda}{\lambda + \dot{V}_A/\dot{Q}} \tag{1}$$

Because much of the material to follow centers on the interpretation of results obtained with the inert gas elimination technique, it is important to state the specific assumptions that go into this relationship. These assumptions can be listed as follows:

1. Each homogeneous lung unit is in a steady state of gas exchange such that the net rate of transfer of gas from capillary blood to alveolar gas exactly equals the net rate of elimination through expiration. Thus, the amount of inert gas stored in the lung (in blood, lung tissue, and alveolar gas) is constant.

2. Both ventilation and blood flow are taken to be continuous processes. Thus, the tidal nature of ventilation and the pulsatile nature of perfusion are specifically not taken into account.

3. The lung is treated as a collection of separate "lung units," each of which is homogeneous. Each unit receives ventilation and blood flow, and the ratio of ventilation to blood flow in the various lung units (that make up the entire lung) varies from unit to unit.

4. Diffusion equilibration is assumed to be complete. This assumption applies both to diffusion between capillary blood and alveolar gas, resulting in the assumption that alveolar and end-capillary partial pressures of inert gas are the same, and to diffusion within the gas phase, resulting in the assumption of uniform partial pressure everywhere within the lung unit. This also implies that gases of different molecular weight do not behave differently other than through differences in their solubility.

5. All such lung units receive blood of the same hematocrit.

6. All lung units within the lung are arranged in parallel with one another so that they each receive inspired gas that traverses only their own conducting airway dead space. Thus, there is no transfer of gas either during inspiration or expiration between physically adjacent lung units.

These assumptions are precisely the ones that are made in all steady state gas exchange techniques in which attempts are made to quantitate the amount of ventilation–blood flow mismatching and shunt. It is generally held that if a patient or experimental animal is in a steady state as evidenced by constant tidal volume and frequency of respiration, constancy of heart rate and blood pressure, and constancy of end-tidal P_{O_2} and P_{CO_2} partial pressures, all of these assumptions are entirely reasonable. In other words, real data obtained under such conditions can be closely fitted by models that are based on the above assumptions. Further comments on the appropriateness of these assumptions are made below in reviewing the information content of the inert gas elimination method.

Given single lung units exchanging inert gas under the above assumptions, the behavior of a lung that is made up of many lung units of different ventilation–perfusion ratio can be studied mathematically in a straightforward manner by employing traditional mixing equations. Once again, these equations are statements of mass balance. The total amount of gas delivered from each unit is a product of the concentration of the gas and the ventilation of the unit (expired gas) or the blood flow of the unit (arterial blood). The sum of these quantities over all such units must be equivalent to the total amounts transported respectively in mixed expired gas and mixed arterial blood. This in turn is equal to the corresponding concentration of the gas multiplied by total ventilation ($\dot{V}_E$) and total blood flow ($\dot{Q}_T$). These concepts lead to the following equations for mixed expired gas [Eq. (2)] and mixed arterial blood [Eq. (3)]:

$$P_E \dot{V}_E = \sum_{j=1}^{j=N} P_{A_j} \dot{V}_{A_j} \tag{2}$$

$$P_a \dot{Q}_T = \sum_{j=1}^{j=N} P_{c_j'} \dot{Q}_j \tag{3}$$

In these equations the left-hand side reflects measurable quantities that form the experimental data base for the ensuing calculations. The right-hand side, consisting of the sum of many (N) terms, contains both the calculated alveolar gas and end-capillary partial pressures [Eq. (1)], multiplying the unknown ventilations ($\dot{V}_{A_j}$) [Eq. (2)] and perfusions ($\dot{Q}_i$) [Eq. (3)] of the various lung units. Equations (2) and (3) embody two different relationships. The first is that between expired (or mixed arterial) partial pressures and blood gas partial coefficient (excretion–solubility or retention–solubility curves). The second is the distribution of ventilation and blood flow. By distribution of ventilation we mean the plot, lung unit by lung unit, of ventilation on the ordinate against ventilation–perfusion ratio on the abscissa. By distribution of blood flow we mean the plot, lung unit by lung unit, of blood flow on the ordinate against ventilation–perfusion ratio on the abscissa. Equations (2) and (3) tie these two relationships to each other.

It can be seen intuitively then that measured retention and excretion–solubility curves are a reflection of the distributions of ventilation and blood flow with respect to $\dot{V}_A/\dot{Q}$. The multiple inert gas elimination technique exploits these principles by extracting information about the distribution of ventilation and blood flow from the retention solubility curves in a manner described in detail in Chapter 8 of this volume.

It is important to realize both the advantages and the limitations of the inert gas approach, and the results to follow that pertain to disease states have been interpreted in the light of these limitations, as discussed more fully in Chapter 8 of this volume.

Currently used computer algorithms for performing the fitting procedures for obtaining least-squares estimates of the distribution with enforced smoothing are available in the central depository, as indicated in Chapter 8 of this volume.

C. Information Content of the Multiple Inert Gas Elimination Method

The primary objective of the inert gas elimination technique is to estimate the qualitative and quantitative features of the distribution of ventilation–perfusion ratios in various normal and diseased states. Thus, when the technique is used in a particular setting, a smooth distribution is obtained and the appropriate interpretation is made. This section discusses the various forms of information that can be obtained from application of the inert gas technique. Much more can be learned about gas exchange in the lung than just a description of the $\dot{V}_A/\dot{Q}$ distribution. This is now illustrated.

1. The Residual Sum of Squares: Fitting the Model

In any mathematical approach in which data are fitted by some model by using a least-squares criterion, the residual sum of squares between the closest fit by the model and the data themselves can provide useful information about the acceptability of the model. For example, if the model is accurate and there is no experimental error in the measurement, the residual sum of squares would be zero. Thus, in the absence of experimental error, a nonzero sum of squares would indicate that some feature of the model is unacceptable. Which aspect could be determined by appropriate modifications of the components of the model in a systematic fashion, until a zero sum of squares could be obtained. Even then, it would be dangerous to claim that the particular model is the only one compatible with the data. Historically, however, most workers have been content to find even one model that can fit data (Riley and Cournand, 1951; Briscoe et al., 1960; Yokoyama and Farhi, 1967).

In the experimental setting, even when the model is accurate, the residual sum of squares will never be zero (that is, the fit to the data will not be perfect) except by chance, and then only under two circumstances. The first is if each of the measured data points in the specific case contains no error (even though this rarely, if ever, occurs). The second is when the errors are of appropriate magnitude and direction such that the data still lie within the province of the model. To illustrate these concepts, consider the calculation of venous admixture given a measured value of arterial oxygen saturation. If the true oxygen saturation were 95% and the measured value were reported as 95%, the calculated venous admixture would be correct. If, however, the measured arterial oxygen saturation were reported as 94% rather than the correct value of 95%, the model (venous admixture) would still yield a physiologically reasonable answer, but the value obtained would be in error. In this setting, whether the arterial oxygen saturation is correct or in error, an exact (and reasonable) model can be found that fits the data. If, however, the measured arterial oxygen saturation were reported as 103%, the calculated venous admixture would be negative and physiologically meaningless because oxygen saturation cannot exceed 100%. The smallest venous admixture that could be reported from a measured oxygen saturation of 103% would therefore be zero, and there would be a difference between the measured data (103%) and the nearest fit to the data (100% saturation).

These concepts can be applied to the multiple inert gas technique in exactly the same manner. If the inert gas data are error free and the model is correct, a sum of squares of zero will result when the least-squares analysis is performed (Chapter 8, this volume). If the inert gas data contain error, but still lie within the bounds of the model, it may be possible to fit the data and still have a residual sum of squares of zero.

Although in the above example a reported arterial oxygen saturation of 103% would be most unusual, the corresponding result when using the inert gas technique is by no means unusual—in fact, it is the rule. In other words, it is quite likely that in gathering inert gas elimination data in the presence of experimental error, the sum of squares will not be zero even if this model is correct. The reason lies in Eqs. (2) and (3), which decree a very tight relationship between the retention values for gases of different solubility. This has been described previously (Wagner *et al.*, 1974c).

This lengthy introduction is necessary to illustrate the potential complexity of interpreting a sum of squares in a least-fitting process. If the sum of squares is nonzero, as is the rule in most analyses of real data, two independent factors may contribute. The first is experimental error, and the second is inaccuracy in the model. The differentiation between these two causes for failure to fit the model will now be discussed because of its importance in the interpretation of real data.

The basis for understanding the cause of a nonzero sum of squares is in the knowledge of the coefficient of variation in the inert gas elimination data. If the coefficient of variation of retention and excretion is known, then the range of sum of squares to be expected from such a degree of random error can be determined either numerically (by generating such data repeatedly and attempting to fit them with the least-squares procedure) or more directly by consulting appropriate statistical tables. In our approach to the inert gas elimination technique (Evans and Wagner, 1977), we use the coefficient of variation for the measurement of retention of each gas to weight Eqs. (2) and (3) for each gas. In other words, these equations are multiplied throughout by a weighting factor that makes the weighted retention values have unit variance. If we use six gases, we have that many degrees of freedom and can examine the χ^2 table for that number. When this is done, it is seen that the normalized sum of squares (that expected when fitting six independent data points whose variance is each 1.0) would exceed 5.348 50% of the time. The sum of squares would exceed 10.645 only 10% of the time and 16.812 only 1% of the time on the basis of random error.

Thus, it is seen that knowledge of the error of the method together with the appropriate calculation allows an interpretation of the residual sum of squares that gives information on how well the model fits the data. In our experience, a residual sum of squares greater than 20 is exceedingly rare, and usual values are in the range of 2–10. In this way, taking account of experimental error in real inert gas data (obtained from both human and animal studies involving both normal and diseased lungs) reveals compatibility with the steady state model referred to above [Eq. (1)–(3)]. Specifically, this compatibility implies that none of the assumptions used are sufficiently unreasonable that they prevent an adequate analysis of the data.

We have recently used such an analysis in the study of mechanisms of gas exchange in different experimental animals (Powell and Wagner, 1979). All of our previous work had been done in mammalian lungs and is based on Eq. (1), which describes gas exchange in a mammalian alveolar lung unit. However, it has long been suspected that the appropriate model for gas exchange in most bird lungs is not the alveolar model, but rather a model involving crosscurrent gas exchange (Powell and Wagner, 1979).

Support of this concept comes from both anatomical studies of the arrangement of the bird lung and functional studies in which it has been demonstrated that expired P_{CO_2} can exceed that in the arterial blood by more than can be explained on the basis of mammalian lung structure. We have used the inert gas elimination technique in the lungs of normal geese and obtained retention and excretion data that have been fitted with both the standard alveolar least-squares analysis based on Eq. (1), and also a modified approach (also by least-squares criteria) in which Eq. (1) has been replaced by the appropriate equations for crosscurrent gas exchange (Scheid and Piiper, 1970; Powell and Wagner, 1979). We have found consistently that the normalized sum of squares obtained with the alveolar model is of the order of 40–100, whereas those obtained with the crosscurrent model have in all cases been considerably less than 10. While this result does not prove that crosscurrent gas exchange is the only possible mechanism operating in the goose, it supports the hypothesis of crosscurrent gas exchange, and certainly rules out a mammalian alveolar arrangement as being responsible for gas exchange in the goose.

2. *Other Equivalent Models in Mammalian Lungs*

While the sum of squares can be used to judge the ability of the model to fit the data even in the presence of experimental error, it is possible that other models of gas exchange will fit a set of data equally as well as the basic parallel alveolar model described in Eqs. (1)–(3).

A likely example in clinical respiratory disease is that of series ventilation. Although the standard inert gas elimination analysis is formulated on the basis of lung units ventilated only in parallel with one another, it may be that in certain disease states some lung units receive their inspiration ''second-hand'' from their neighboring units through the process of series or collateral ventilation. An important consideration is that of interpreting insert gas elimination data should such series or collateral ventilation be present. This question has been addressed on two levels. The first relates to *bulk* series or collateral ventilation in which gases move between lung units by bulk flow in a manner not dependent on diffusion processes and therefore independently of molecular weight (Wagner and Evans, 1977). However, it is possible that a second form of series ventilation exists. This is sometimes referred to as stratification (Chapter 5 of this volume) and from the functional standpoint it can be described as the existence of partial pressure differences due to incomplete diffusive gas mixing, an effect that would be dependent on molecular weight. Thus, gases of high molecular weight would be more vulnerable than gases of low molecular weight. The interpretation of elimination data when series bulk ventilation is present has been addressed at some length (Wagner and Evans, 1977). It has been found that for every individual quantitative arrangement of series ventilated lung units, there exists a purely parallel equivalent arrangement such that inert gas exchange for all gases is identical. This result has two major implications: (1) series bulk ventilation in the steady state cannot be identified by using the multiple inert gas elimination technique, and (2) by the same token, if such series inequality exists it can be interpreted as if it were a parallel problem. In other words, even if series ventilation is present, a purely parallel model will fit the data just as well and the resultant ventilation–perfusion inequality can be interpreted as if it were occurring on a parallel rather than series basis.

Two other physiologically reasonable departures from the basic parallel model have been examined in the same way. First, it is known that the anatomic dead space acts as a mixing chamber for the last expired gas in each breath. Thus, on each inspiration, the first inspired gas to each lung unit contains some mixture of gas expired from all lung units. This notion of shared or ''common'' dead space will clearly change the amount of gas that is transferred in each lung unit from that which would occur in the absence of common dead space. This problem was first addressed for the respiratory gases O_2 and CO_2 by Ross and Farhi (1960) and more recently and generally by Fortune and Wagner (1979) and Petrini and co-workers (1979). As with the series ventilation analysis, under most all conditions it was found that the presence of shared or common dead space does alter gas exchange, but that the perturbations that result can still be interpreted as if they were taking place in a lung with purely parallel pathways and no sharing of dead space. Both the analysis of Ross and Farhi and of Fortune and Wagner show that the presence of shared dead space improves gas exchange under most conditions. The latter study has shown that the changes in inert gas transfer that are likely to result from sharing of dead space are, however, minor and do not change the overall interpretation of patterns of ventilation–blood flow mismatching determined from the inert gas elimination technique, which ignores common dead space.

Finally, variation in hematocrit among different regions of the lung will affect gas exchange to some extent, as first suggested by Briscoe (1959). This is because the solubility of gases in red cells is different from that in plasma (Young and Wagner, 1979). We have studied the potential effects of maldistribution of hematocrit acting in addition to ventilation–perfusion mismatching and found that the possible effects are reasonably small. The perturbations produced result in slightly altered inert gas tensions, which can still be fitted by the fundamental parallel model, which ignores hematocrit inequality. The distributions of ventilation–perfusion ratios recovered under such conditions by the standard least-squares approach do not differ significantly through the added effect of hematocrit inequality.

Thus, in summary, we have found that the parallel alveolar model of ventilation–perfusion mismatching adequately fits observed inert gas elimination data under a wide variety of conditions in both man and experimental mammals. This supports the use of the parallel model as a framework for interpreting abnormalities in gas exchange. However, several extensions of this relatively simple model may well occur, particularily in disease states. The three most likely of these, namely, series ventilation, sharing anatomic dead space, and existence of hematocrit variations within the lung, will all perturb inert (and respiratory) gas exchange. These perturbations are generally small, but in all cases theoretical analysis shows that data obtained under such conditions can still be adequately fitted using the simple parallel alveolar model.

3. Resolution of Lung Units of Different Ventilation–Perfusion Ratio

As explained in the early sections of this chapter, much effort has been invested over the years in devising methods for quantitating the amount of ventilation–perfusion mismatching. Most such methods are limited in their resolution. Specifically, the separation of areas of low $\dot{V}_A/\dot{Q}$ from

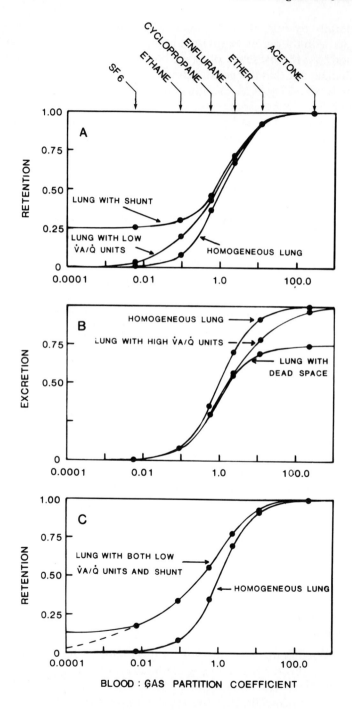

BLOOD : GAS PARTITION COEFFICIENT

areas of zero $\dot{V}_A/\dot{Q}$ (shunt) on the one hand, and the separation of areas of high $\dot{V}_A/\dot{Q}$ from areas of infinitely high $\dot{V}_A/\dot{Q}$ (unperfused lung or dead space) has long been a problem. The multiple inert gas elimination technique was devised with the primary intention of improving the resolution at the ends of the $\dot{V}_A/\dot{Q}$ spectrum as stated above. Although it is clear from Chapter 8 of this volume that no current method has perfect resolution, the multiple inert gas technique is able to resolve these problems considerably better than previous approaches. The reason for this improved resolution is straightforward and resides in the utilization of several gases of appropriate solubilities. This can be understood in terms of Eq. (1) in the following example. Figure 4A shows the retention–solubility curves (Wagner *et al.*, 1974c) of two lungs, one of which contains 25% shunt and the other of which contains 25% of the blood flow associated with the mode of low ventilation–perfusion ratio, $\dot{V}_A/\dot{Q} = 0.05$. The remaining 75% of the blood flow in each case is associated with lung units of normal ventilation–perfusion ratio, and the total ventilation and blood flow for the two lungs is the same. Although for gases of partition coefficient greater than about 1, the difference in the retention curves for the two lungs is not great, there is a marked difference between the retention curves of gases of low solubility. This is because no matter how insoluble a gas, if there is no ventilation (shunt), that gas cannot escape from the blood into the gas phase. On the other hand, for an extremely insoluble gas, even if the ventilation–perfusion ratio is as low as 0.05 as in this example, most of the gas does escape into alveolar gas and is eliminated. Because the retention–solubility curves are so different under these two conditions, it should be clear how it is possible to resolve between the presence of low $\dot{V}_A/\dot{Q}$ areas or shunt in these examples. In Fig. 4B, exactly the same concept is illustrated at the other end of the $\dot{V}_A/\dot{Q}$ spectrum, where excretion curves are illustrated for two lungs, one having

Fig. 4. Retention (arterial/mixed venous partial pressure ratio) and excretion (mixed expired/mixed venous partial pressure ratio) curves for different lungs. (A) The retention curve for a homogeneous lung is shown and compared with the retention curves of two abnormal lungs. In one, there is a 25% shunt, and in the other 25% of the cardiac output perfuses units of low $\dot{V}_A/\dot{Q}$ ratio. Notice the large differences in SF_6 and ethane retention in each case. (B) Excretion curves are shown for a homogeneous lung, a lung with 25% of the ventilation associated with units of high ventilation–perfusion ratio, and a lung with a dead-space. Notice the separation of the curves for gases of high solubility. (C) The retention curve is shown for a lung containing both low $\dot{V}_A/\dot{Q}$ units and shunt with a homogeneous curve for comparison. Although the solid line to the left of the SF_6 retention point is correct, it is possible that the retention curve could fall away more steeply, as shown by the dashed line. Uncertainty in the retention curve leads to uncertainty in the distribution of ventilation–perfusion ratios that would be recovered from such a curve, as described more fully in the text.

25% of the ventilation associated with completely unperfused units (dead space), the other having the same fraction of ventilation associated with units of high $\dot{V}_A/\dot{Q}$ ($\dot{V}_A/\dot{Q}$ = 30.0). While for gases of low solubility the excretion curves are very similar to one another, for gases of high solubility the excretion curves separate considerably according to whether the abnormal units are completely unperfused (dead space) or are units of high $\dot{V}_A/\dot{Q}$.

With the gases that are currently used in the multiple inert gas elimination technique (see Fig. 4A), a good resolution can be obtained in areas of $\dot{V}_A/\dot{Q}$ such as those illustrated, and many clinical examples are found to correspond to just these values of $\dot{V}_A/\dot{Q}$ (Wagner *et al.*, 1977b, 1978a). For example, some patients with asthma who appear to have a mode of low $\dot{V}_A/\dot{Q}$ units, but no shunts are found to have retention–solubility curves approaching zero for insoluble gases. We can be quite confident about the resolution in such cases. Some patients with chronic obstructive lung disease have areas of high $\dot{V}_A/\dot{Q}$ and their excretion curves look like those in Fig. 4B of the lung with 25% ventilation in unit of $\dot{V}_A/\dot{Q}$ = 30.

Some difficulty in resolution does arise in some instances, however. If areas of low and zero ventilation–perfusion ratio coexist, then a retention solubility curve as shown in Fig. 4C will be found. Notice that here the retention of the least soluble gas used, SF_6, is quite high, and, as is illustrated, it is not clear as to the fate of the retention curve to the left of this point. Thus, the curve could continue downward and eventually reach the abscissa at a sufficiently low solubility or the curve might flatten out and become horizontal well above the abscissa. In both cases, resolution would greatly improve if a gas 10 or 100 times less soluble than SF_6 could be used (but such a gas is not currently available). It would then be possible to differentiate between low $\dot{V}_A/\dot{Q}$ units and shunt with considerable reliability, even when both are present. Given that the least-soluble gas currently available is SF_6, the precise resolution between poorly ventilated and unventilated lung units when both exist together will be incomplete. These situations are recognizable by having a high retention for the least soluble gas *and* a high slope for the retention solubility curve passing through the retention value of that gas. The techniques outlined in Chapter 8 of this volume (particularly those of linear programming) can be used to define quantitatively just how much resolution is present in a given situation.

4. Modality of Distributions

Closely tied to the issue of resolution between different regions of the $\dot{V}_A/\dot{Q}$ spectrum, is the issue of modality of the distribution obtained from the multiple inert gas technique. One of the most important findings in a variety of these disease states to date has been that of bimodal and in some cases trimodal $\dot{V}_A/\dot{Q}$ distributions (as opposed to what could have been found, namely, the existence of broad unimodal distributions). It is clearly of major importance to know with certainty that a distribution indicated as bimodal by the inert gas analysis is, in fact, a bimodal distribution and not erroneously interpreted as bimodal because of limitations in the analysis. The use of enforced smoothing in the least-squares analysis as proposed by Evans and Wagner (1977) has been found to reflect modality quite reliably. Thus, while rigorous interpretation depends upon techniques such as linear programming described by Olszowka and Wagner in Chapter 8 of this volume, we have found repeatedly that such techniques have always confirmed the impression given when enforced smoothing is used. The reliability of the enforced smoothing technique in defining modality comes from the way in which smoothing is utilized. As described by Olszowka and Wagner, part of the term to be minimized in the least-squares approach contains the sum of squares of compartmental perfusions. Minimization of this component will always be accomplished best by unimodal rather than bimodal (and particularly trimodal) distributions, so that presence of more than one mode in the results is very likely to be a real finding.

Generally, distributions obtained with the inert gas method that do contain more than one mode show the modes as smoothly contoured and often separated by a region of the $\dot{V}_A/\dot{Q}$ spectrum devoid of ventilation and blood flow. It is important to interpret these patterns in the correct manner. The linear programming technique of Olszowka and Wagner can be used to make some generalizations regarding proper interpretation. First, the region between any pair of modes may be devoid of ventilation and blood flow as shown, but not necessarily in every case. However, whenever a clearly separated bimodal or trimodal pattern results, there can never be sufficient ventilation or blood flow between the modes to allow a unimodal curve to fit the data the adequately. However, bimodal distributions in which the modes are not completely separated cannot always be resolved as such. When intermodal distance is of the order of one decade of ventilation–perfusion ratios (or more), bimodal definition is generally possible, but if the two modes are separated by less than a decade of $\dot{V}_A/\dot{Q}$, then they may merge and not be separately identifiable using the current inert gas technique. It would take more inert gases and less experimental error to achieve the separation of modes under those conditions. In addition to proper interpretation of the region between modes, the shape of the mode requires some discussion. There is generally insufficient information from the inert gas technique to make precise statements about the height, width, and shape of a mode. This is not surprising since there are only six gases forming the data base. The potential variation in height and shape of a mode can be explored with the linear programming technique of Olszowka and Wagner. However, the total amount of ventilation and blood flow in a mode and its mean position along the $\dot{V}_A/\dot{Q}$ axis can be determined with considerable accuracy.

In summary, up to three modes of a $\dot{V}_A/\dot{Q}$ distribution can in theory be defined by the current inert gas elimination technique using six different inert gases. The least-squares approach using enforced smoothing (Evans and Wagner, 1977) reliably indicates the presence, location, and magnitude of such modes when they exist. This is supported by independent linear programming techniques, as discussed by Olszowka and Wagner. Although the existence and magnitude of such modes can generally be defined, there are some limitations regarding the amount of information that is available, particularly pertaining to the precise height and width of a mode on the one hand, and the presence or absence of ventilation and blood flow in the region between the modes on the other. Modes separated by less than about one decade of $\dot{V}_A/\dot{Q}$ may not be separable with the current technique.

5. Gas Diffusion: The Effects of Molecular Weight

Still further information can be obtained from application of the inert gas elimination technique. Recall that retention–solubility curves are interpreted on the assumption that inert gases are transferred in accordance with solubility and ventilation/perfusion ratio alone [Eq. (1)]. To the extent that diffusion processes are incomplete for inert gases, those gases of high molecular weight (SF_6 MW, 146, and halothane, MW, 197.5) will be retained to a relatively greater degree than would be expected on the basis of solubility alone as compared to the remaining four gases, whose molecular weights range from 30 (ethane) to 74 (ether). This concept can be exploited in the analysis of retention and excretion data, particularly using the gas halothane since it is bracketed (in terms of solubility) by two gases on each side, all of which have reasonably low molecular weights by comparison. Thus, the next gases of higher solubility are ether and acetone, of molecular weights 74 and 58, respectively, whereas the gases of lower solubility are ethane and cyclopropane, of molecular weights 30 and 42, respectively. With this particular arrangement of solubilities and molecular weights, the least-squares analysis would result in a poor fit (to retention data) that would be directionally opposite for halothane compared to the four surrounding gases (if halothane were sufficiently influenced by diffusion processes). This would be evident in examination of the sum of squares and the sign of the differences (or residuals) for each gas. Thus, the analysis of the residual sum of squares referred to earlier in this chapter is extended here to subdivide the components of the sum of squares, gas by gas, a particular pattern being expected if molecular weight is an important factor determining the elimination of the gas. Preferential interference to the exchange of high molecular weight gases has never been observed in our hands, in man or animals in normal or diseased states, including patients with chronic obstructive lung disease in whom parenchymal destruction leading to large gas spaces may well result in incompleteness of diffusive gas mixing. Adaro and Farhi (1971) reported in an abstract that a small reduction in elimination of freon 12 (MW, 86.5) occurred compared to acetylene (MW, 26) in a dog preparation.

Molecular weight dependency of gas exchange can also be explored graphically using retention or excretion data as follows. While the relationship between retention and solubility [Eq. (1)] is hyperbolic on a linear scale, the inverse relationship (that is, the plot of the reciprocal of retention against the reciprocal of solubility) is, in a homogeneous lung, a linear relationship [Eq. (1)]. Even in lungs with some degree of ventilation blood flow mismatching, one or other of the retention and excretion curves usually results in a fairly linear inverse relationship. Such a linear transformation is simply a convenient tool for comparing the retention and excretion values for different gases. Halothane would again be the appropriate gas to study and would lie below the straight line connecting acetane, ether, cyclopropane, and ethane. In this graphical manner, the behavior reflected by the above sum of squares analysis would be evident.

6. Diffusion of Gases between Alveolar Gas and Capillary Blood

While comparison of the inert gases one to the other gives information about diffusion in the gas phase, comparison of the inert gases as a group with oxygen gives information about the completeness of diffusion equilibration across the blood–gas barrier between capillary blood and alveolar gas. Although experimental verification is currently infeasible, calculations of the rate of attainment of partial pressure equilibrium for inert gases (Forster, 1957; Wagner, 1977b) suggest that all inert gases equilibrate very rapidly. As blood enters the gas exchange vessels from the mixed venous blood, all of the inert gas transfer takes place within the first few hundredths of a second and the remaining time spent in the gas exchange region does not result in further gas exchange. The rate of equilibration is independent of the blood–gas partition coefficient, but does depend on molecular weight. For a hypothetical inert gas of molecular weight 32, 99% of the gas exchange takes place within 0.04 sec (assuming a normal diffusing capacity). Similar calculations for oxygen reveal an approximately tenfold greater time required for the same degree of equilibration. The fundamental reason for this difference in behavior is that the diffusion of oxygen from alveolar gas to capillary blood depends upon the very low solubility of oxygen in the blood gas barrier, a solubility approximately equal to that in saline, namely, 0.0031 ml/100 ml/mm Hg. On the other hand, the rate of rise of partial pressure of oxygen in the blood depends to a large extent on the presence of hemoglobin. As oxygen reaches the blood, it diffuses into the red cell and combines rapidly with hemoglobin. This delays its rise in partial pressure. Variations in the rate of diffusion equilibration of inert gases (over the range of molecular weights encompassed in inert gas technique) are much smaller than the order of magnitude difference between oxygen and any such inert gas (Forster, 1957; Wagner, 1977b).

This fundamental difference in the rate of diffusion equilibration for inert gases on the one hand, and oxygen on the other, affords the potential for evaluating the role of alveolar–capillary diffusion impairment in O_2 exchange in diseased lungs. This has in the past been an essentially impossible task because the same pathological changes that lead to diffusion impairment produce ventilation–perfusion disturbances, and the two cannot usually be separated by traditional methods.

In a lung with ventilation–blood flow inequality, but no diffusion impairment for inert gases or oxygen, the $\dot{V}_A/\dot{Q}$ distribution recovered from the inert gas data can be used to calculate an expected value for arterial P_{O_2}. Such a calculation uses directly measured mixed venous P_{O_2} and P_{CO_2} values together with information concerning hemoglobin concentration, temperature, and acid–base balance. Such a calculation should statistically agree with directly measured values for arterial P_{O_2} since, after allowances are made for the nonlinear nature of the oxyhemoglobin dissociation curve, the rules of gas exchange are similar for inert gases and oxygen. However, when diffusion impairment becomes evident, oxygen will be affected to a much greater extent than inert gases and, in fact, most workers believe that situations in which diffusion impairment interferes with inert gas transfer would not be compatible with life. In a setting where oxygen is diffusion limited but inert gases are not, the measured arterial P_{O_2} will be lower than that calculated from the inert gas data since the calculation expressly assumes complete diffusion equilibration for all gases in the system. While small degrees of diffusion impairment may not be detectable because of the presence of random experimental error, if a significant fraction of the total alveolar–arterial P_{O_2} difference is caused by diffusion impairment, it will be detectable by this indirect comparison between inert gases and oxygen. Illustrations of this comparison will follow in the review of ventilation–perfusion inequality in disease states.

A question that might be raised is whether any other physiological phenomenon could cause a similar internal inconsistency between inert gas and oxygen transfer. A theoretical possibility is the contribution of what are known generally as postpulmonary shunts. Bronchial veins and thebesian veins carrying desaturated blood may empty into the arterial side of the circulation and thereby cause a depression of arterial P_{O_2}. Such a shunt, however, will not affect arterial inert gas levels since passage of inert gases through the bronchial and thebesian circulations does not result in modification of their concentrations. One way to resolve the uncertainty concerning these two possible mechanisms for inconsistency between inert gas and oxygen transfer is to compare them during both air breathing and oxygen breathing. If the inconsistency were produced by diffusion impairment, the breathing of 100% oxygen would abolish (or at least considerably reduce) the difference between inert gas and O_2 exchange. If, however, bronchial or thebesian venous shunts were responsible, the discrepancy between inert gas and oxygen exchange should increase upon oxygen breathing.

Factors such as series inequality of ventilation, intrapulmonary variation in hematocrit, and the reinspiration of shared deadspace are not potential causes of such inconsistency. As discussed earlier, these extensions of the basic parallel model all produce perturbations of inert gas exchange that can be interpreted on a parallel-model basis. We have found consistently that these parallel-model extensions and their "as if" parallel equivalents produce the same arterial P_{O_2} and P_{CO_2} as well.

7. Intrapulmonary and Extrapulmonary Factors in Hypoxemia

One of the most helpful analyses that can be made using $\dot{V}_A/\dot{Q}$ distributions obtained from inert gas data is to partition the causes of hypoxemia into intra- and extrapulmonary factors. This is of considerable clinical importance since understanding of a disease state in which both intra- and extrapulmonary factors play a role is essential for making rational therapeutic decisions. This is particularly likely to be the case in the intensive care setting, where intrapulmonary factors such as the distribution of ventilation–perfusion ratios, shunting, and dead space may rapidly change, while at the same time extrapulmonary factors such as cardiac output, total ventilation, hemoglobin concentration, and acid–base status may also change frequently. Understanding the net change in arterial P_{O_2} when several such variables are simultaneously altered is possible using the results of the inert gas approach. (This concept will also be illustrated in the discussion to follow concerning findings made using the method in patients with different cardiopulmonary diseases.)

The actual data (inert gas data, mixed venous P_{O_2}, cardiac output, hemoglobin, acid–base status, and so on) can be used to calculate the expected arterial P_{O_2}; this is done by using the principles enunciated in Chapter 8 of this volume. It is then a straightforward matter using the digital computer to change any one of the input variables such as cardiac output, hemoglobin, or acid–base status and to recalculate the expected arterial P_{O_2}. In this way, the net effect of any single-variable change can be estimated, leaving other variables at their real levels. Such an analysis adds considerably to insight into the mechanisms of hypoxemia, and particularly into the relative importance of intra- and extrapulmonary factors, the determination of which will often affect therapeutic decisions.

V. VENTILATION–PERFUSION INEQUALITY IN DISEASE

A. Specific Disease States

Previously published findings are briefly summarized and more recent data are presented in light of the preceding discussion concerning the quantity and quality of information that can be obtained by application of the inert gas procedure. While it is recognized that the number of patients studied is relatively small, and in particular that most patients studied were in advanced stages of their illness, analysis of individual results in the disease states to follow has provided considerably insight into the factors that determine abnormal gas exchange.

1. Chronic Obstructive Pulmonary Disease (COPD)

We have applied the inert gas technique to 23 patients with various clinical presentations of chronic obstructive pulmonary disease (Wagner et al., 1977b). All were in advanced stages of the disease with grossly reduced air-flow rates. We made an attempt to select two groups of patients. One exhibited the clinical characteristics of hyperinflation, chest X-ray changes showing attenuation of vascular markings, flattening of diaphragm, and normal or smaller than normal cardiac silhouettes. These patients had little or no sputum production and had relatively mild hypoxemia with essentially no hypercapnia. Those patients who fit the clinical criteria of Burrows and co-workers (1966) for type A can be contrasted with the second group (type B variety), who in general had moderately severe hypoxemia often with CO_2 retention and had evidence of present or past right heart failure, and whose chest X-ray findings did not reveal the attenuated vascular markings and hyperinflation characteristic of the type A patient.

In type A patients, an almost uniform finding was that, in addition to units of normal ventilation–perfusion ratio, a population of lung units of very high ventilation–perfusion ratio was present. In contrast there was rarely any shunt and no areas of extremely low ventilation–perfusion ratio ($\dot{V}_A/\dot{Q} < 0.1$). The reason for hypoxemia in these patients was that the mode of lung units that received most of the perfusion had a somewhat lower than normal average value of $\dot{V}_A/\dot{Q}$ (about 0.6 compared to the normal of 0.8–1.0). Statistical analysis confirmed bimodality of distributions, strongly supporting the conclusion that the units of relatively normal $\dot{V}_A/\dot{Q}$ and those of high $\dot{V}_A/\dot{Q}$ were not part of a continuous spectrum. The behavior of the high molecular weight gases was not found to be different from that of the low molecular weight gases, supporting the conclusion that gaseous diffusion processes were not a contributing factor to hypoxemia. This is thought to be an important result since it is just this group of patients that would be expected on anatomical grounds to be vulnerable to such a problem because of the development of large air spaces in the destructive emphysematous process. Measured arterial P_{O_2} values were statistically not different from those calculated on the basis of complete alveolar–capillary diffusion equilibration according to the rationale advanced earlier in this chapter. Thus, all of the hypoxemia was explained by the observed pattern of ventilation–perfusion mismatching, and diffusion impairment across the blood gas barrier does not appear to be detectable as a mechanism of hypoxemia in these patients. An important finding was the response to 100% oxygen breathing. These patients (even after 30 min of 100% oxygen breathing) rarely had an arterial P_{O_2} above 500 torr, which would suggest by classical analysis a reasonably large shunt (unventilated units). However, inert gas data were rarely compatible with more than 1 or 2% shunt since the retention of the least soluble gas used, sulfahexafluoride, rarely exceeded these values. This apparent inconsistency is probably best explained by the slow nitrogen wash-out of poorly ventilated lung units in this disease state. Even after 30 min of oxygen breathing, poorly ventilated lung units still have high alveolar nitrogen partial pressures and consequently fairly low alveolar oxygen partial pressures. Such units will contribute to the relatively low arterial P_{O_2} that was found.

On exercise, these patients generally dropped their arterial P_{O_2}. The three most likely physiological mechanisms to explain such a drop in arterial P_{O_2} on exercise are (1) worsening of ventilation–perfusion relationships, (2) a fall in mixed venous P_{O_2} (because oxygen uptake increases relatively more than cardiac output), and (3) the development of alveolar–end-capillary partial pressure differences because of incomplete diffusion equilibration across the blood–gas barrier. The third mechanism was ruled out in these patients since, as was found at rest, the arterial P_{O_2} calculated from the observed distributions measured during exercise agreed closely with directly measured P_{O_2} values. The first mechanism was also ruled out since the observed distributions during exercise were statistically no different from those seen during rest. This finding must be interpreted in light of the advanced stages of disease in these patients since they were not capable of increasing oxygen uptake to more than about 750 ml/min. In other words, patients able to perform higher levels of exercise, raising their cardiac output and minute ventilation to greater levels, might show changes in the distribution of ventilation and blood flow. The operative mechanism was, in fact, the fall in mixed venous P_{O_2}.

The type B patients showed much more variation in their $\dot{V}_A/\dot{Q}$ distributions. Some had patterns similar to those of type A, some had areas of low ventilation–perfusion ratio without areas of high ventilation–perfusion ratio, and some showed both patterns simultaneously (areas of low, normal, and high $\dot{V}_A/\dot{Q}$). This variability is difficult to interpret, but it is tempting to speculate that high $\dot{V}_A/\dot{Q}$ areas in type B patients still reflect "emphesymatous changes" as in the type A patients. It is well known that such changes are difficult to detect in patients of predominantly type B clinical presentation. It is also tempting to speculate that areas of low $\dot{V}_A/\dot{Q}$ observed in these patients are due to airway obstruction and inadequate ventilation of lung units probably because of retention of mucus in the smaller airways. This is certainly compatible with the results seen in patients with asthma (to be described later). All of the other analyses referred to above reveal the same operative mechanisms as in type A patients. Thus, there was no evidence of diffusion impairment either at rest or during exercise, and the apparently poor response to 100% oxygen breathing was again seen to be due to the failure of nitrogen wash-out from poorly ventilated lung units in the allotted period, and not to the presence of shunt. The fall in arterial P_{O_2} on exercise again was ascribed to the fall in mixed venous P_{O_2} rather than changes in the $\dot{V}_A/\dot{Q}$ distribution or to the development of alveolar–end-capillary differences due to diffusion impairment.

2. Interstitial Lung Disease

A total of ten patients with advanced interstitial lung disease of various etiologies were studied, both at rest and during exercise, as well as while breathing 100% oxygen. At rest, most of the lung is operating in the range of normal $\dot{V}_A/\dot{Q}$, but, in general, between 10 and 20% of the cardiac output is associated with essentially unventilated or completely unventilated units (Wagner *et al.*, 1976). Thus, in these patients there were no areas of moderately reduced ventilation–perfusion ratios; units were either normal or essentially unventilated. A surprisingly small fraction of the cardiac output was associated with these shuntlike areas in view of the large alveolar arterial gradient for oxygen. However, it was repeatedly found that inert gas and oxygen exchange were internally consistent, such that the observed shunt and $\dot{V}_A/\dot{Q}$ inequality completely accounted for the hypoxemia. The reason for the moderately severe hypoxemia in the face of relatively modest $\dot{V}_A/\dot{Q}$ inequality was the low value of the mixed venous P_{O_2}, which was uniformly 30 mm Hg or less even at rest. This is consistent with the pulmonary vascular involvement characteristically seen in advanced stages of interstitial lung disease, and, indeed, pulmonary vascular resistance was elevated in these patients. Thus, a somewhat lower than normal cardiac output resulted in a lower than normal venous P_{O_2}, which, when combined with only modest degrees of ventilation blood flow inequality, led to large alveolar–arterial P_{O_2} differences.

As in the patients with chronic obstructive lung disease, there was no evidence that failure of diffusion equilibration between alveolar gas and end-capillary blood played any role in the mechanism of hypoxemia. On exercise, there was a uniform decrease in arterial P_{O_2} in all patients. We again investigated the mechanism of this fall and found that changes in the $\dot{V}_A/\dot{Q}$ distribution were minor and could not account for the added hypoxemia. However, even though the mixed venous P_{O_2} fell and accounted for a considerable portion of the fall in arterial P_{O_2} on exercise, not all of the observed hypoxemia could be explained on this basis. About half of the drop in P_{O_2} could not be explained on the basis of inert gas exchange, suggesting a contribution by diffusion impairment. It is worth stressing that this is the only clinical state observed in which diffusion impairment appears to play a detectable role. Even then, it is only upon exercise in advanced disease and the amount of hypoxemia attributable to diffusion impairment is small. Thus, on the average, only about 15% of the total alveolar arterial P_{O_2} difference on exercise is attributable to this mechanism. As with the patients with chronic obstructive lung disease, no difference was observed in the behavior of low and high molecular weight inert gases. Upon oxygen breathing, there was no change in distribution of ventilation–perfusion ratios, and, in particular, those areas appearing as very poorly ventilated on room air remained poorly ventilated during oxygen breathing. This finding is in contrast with the findings made under other clinical conditions (Wagner *et al.*, 1974a,b) in which conversion of low $\dot{V}_A/\dot{Q}$ units into shunt (unventilated units) was seen to accompany the breathing of oxygen.

3. Asthma

The inert gas elimination technique has recently been used in patients with asthma. The initial study involved a small group of asymptomatic patients who by most clinical criteria would be judged to be essentially, but not completely in remission (Wagner et al., 1978a). Thus, these patients, in addition to being asymptomatic, had no dyspnea, no wheezing, no sputum production, and on pulmonary function testing had mild (or no) reduction in air flow rates. Chest X rays were normal. Arterial P_{O_2} was generally 80 or more with a normal arterial P_{CO_2}.

In spite of these normal or nearly normal findings, a consistent observation in the $\dot{V}_A/\dot{Q}$ distributions recovered from inert gas data was the presence of a mode of lung units of very low ventilation–perfusion ratios (mean $\dot{V}_A/\dot{Q} = 0.07$) (Wagner et al., 1978a). Equally consistently, no shunt was found. The mode of low $\dot{V}_A/\dot{Q}$ ratios received on the average about 20% of the cardiac output and less than 1% of the ventilation, the remainder of the ventilation and blood flow being associated with units in the normal range of $\dot{V}_A/\dot{Q}$. There was generally a clear-cut separation between these two populations of units, and statistical testing confirmed with a high degree of probability the existence of two modes in the distribution.

These patients were all given aerosolized isoproterenol and thereafter the distributions were measured at 5-min intervals for 20 min. Acute changes at 5 min were remarkably consistent and consisted of a doubling of the perfusion of the lung units of low $\dot{V}_A/\dot{Q}$. The distributions were otherwise little changed. By 10 min after bronchodilator therapy, the distributions had returned to their baseline configurations and remained so for the rest of the observation period without further change. Air flow rates uniformly improved after bronchodilator therapy and remained well above the baseline values throughout the 20-min observation period. Finally, four of the patients were given 100% oxygen to breathe and no change was found in their $\dot{V}_A/\dot{Q}$ distribution. The mode of low $\dot{V}_A/\dot{Q}$ units present while breathing room air lay within the $\dot{V}_A/\dot{Q}$ range known to be susceptible to oxygen-induced atelectasis (Dantzker et al., 1975), yet there was no conversion of these areas into shunt on oxygen breathing.

When all of these results are taken together, the following picture emerges.

1. There is a surprising amount of $\dot{V}_A/\dot{Q}$ inequality present in some asymptomatic asthmatics despite relatively normal results obtained by other techniques.

2. The reason for the nearly normal arterial P_{O_2} in the face of a modest amount of $\dot{V}_A/\dot{Q}$ inequality was the high mixed venous P_{O_2} observed in these patients. This can be seen to be the reverse of the situation observed in patients with interstitial lung disease described earlier. The mixed venous point was in turn due to high values for cardiac output, which in turn are explained by the anxiety of the experimental situation, and possibly by residual bronchodilator effects from earlier therapy.

3. The consistently bimodal pattern taken together with the absence of shunt strongly suggests that collateral ventilation plays an important role in this disease state. The low $\dot{V}_A/\dot{Q}$ units were undoubtedly caused by obstruction of distal airways [by bronchoconstriction, mucus, or edema (see below)], but it is hard to imagine diffuse obstruction of distal airways by any such means resulting in such a clear-cut mode of low $\dot{V}_A/\dot{Q}$ units without shunt. This is because one would expect complete obstruction of at least some distal airways and resulting shunt development, and a greater range of $\dot{V}_A/\dot{Q}$ values in the distribution. Ventilation of completely obstructed units by collateral pathways is an attractive explanation for the absence of shunt and for bimodality, and is more reasonable than postulating "almost, but not quite complete" obstruction in such a uniform manner. There is good anatomic evidence (Lambert, 1955; Loosli, 1937; Macklin, 1936; Martin, 1966) and physiological evidence to support the existence of collateral pathways in the peripheral regions of the lung.

4. The acute response to bronchodilator therapy, namely, the worsening of ventilation–perfusion relationships as manifested by the increase in perfusion of poorly ventilated lung units, explains the fall in arterial P_{O_2} seen not only in our patients, but also quite frequently in other patients with asthma (Chick et al., 1973; Ingram et al., 1970; Knudson and Constantine, 1967; Tai and Read, 1967).

As ventilation–perfusion relationships worsened acutely, cardiac output was also observed to increase by about 50%. The mechanism for worsening of $\dot{V}_A/\dot{Q}$ relationships may be in part (a) the rise in cardiac output itself altering the distribution of perfusion, and (b) preferential vasodilatation of the blood vessels associated with the poorly ventilated units. (Such units may have been subject to excessive vasoconstriction prior to therapy on the basis of either alveolar hypoxia or the effect of some mediator that was part of the asthmatic process.) Because the changes after bronchodilator involve an increase in perfusion of poorly ventilated units, the results are not compatible with the alternative theory of deterioration following bronchodilator therapy, namely, poorly ventilated lung units losing even more of their ventilation when the better ventilated pathways are dilated by the isoproterenol (Knudson and Constantine, 1967).

5. The failure of the $\dot{V}_A/\dot{Q}$ inequality to disappear after bronchodilator

therapy in the face of continued improvement in air flow rates suggests that the physical basis of reduced ventilation in these low $\dot{V}_A/\dot{Q}$ units is not bronchoconstriction, but rather the presence of mucus and/or edema in the appropriate airways. Although it could be argued that the low $\dot{V}_A/\dot{Q}$ units receive very little bronchodilator when delivered by aerosol, subsequent studies described below support the notion that the low $\dot{V}_A/\dot{Q}$ units are created by mucus and edema in the airways rather than bronchoconstriction.

6. Finally, the failure of units with low $\dot{V}_A/\dot{Q}$ areas to collapse during 100% oxygen breathing further supports the notion of collateral ventilation in that collateral pathways may have provided the means for lung units of low $\dot{V}_A/\dot{Q}$ to escape atelectasis by increasing their inspired ventilation.

Following this initial study, a number of relatively well-controlled asthmatics completely free of symptoms and with normal or nearly normal air flow rates were challenged with either methacholine or an antigen (to which they were naturally sensitive, as determined by prior challenging procedures). We then measured $\dot{V}_A/\dot{Q}$ distributions before and after inhalation challenge sufficient to reduce air flow rates by at least 30%, and in some cases as much as 80%. In some patients, we followed the time course of changes without further intervention, and in some we used bronchodilator therapy (either isoproterenol or metaproterenol) (Wagner et al., 1977a, 1978b).

The findings can be summarized as follows. Prior to challenge, most of the patients had essentially normal distributions of $\dot{V}_A/\dot{Q}$. Challenge with methacholine generally produced modest widening of the $\dot{V}_A/\dot{Q}$ distribution, but did not produce a bimodal pattern in any way similar to that described above for the spontaneous asthmatic group. This is despite relatively greater reduction in air flow rates than seen in the spontaneous asthmatics. Thus, in comparing the initial patients with those challenged with methacholine, less ventilation–perfusion inequality was seen despite more air flow obstruction, as judged by flow rates. We take this apparently paradoxical finding as further evidence that acute bronchoconstriction is not sufficient to produce a population of lung units of very low $\dot{V}_A/\dot{Q}$ as seen in spontaneous asthmatics. Administration of bronchodilator rapidly reversed the relatively minor increases in $\dot{V}_A/\dot{Q}$ inequality seen with methacholine and any arterial hypoxemia that followed challenge was also abolished. Challenge with antigenic substances by inhalation produced generally similar results as seen with metacholine. There was a tendency, however, for slightly more severe $\dot{V}_A/\dot{Q}$ disturbances to develop at a given degree of air flow rate reduction, but still antigenic challenge did not produce distinct population of low $\dot{V}_A/\dot{Q}$ units in the acute setting.

We feel that these studies are internally consistent with the notion that symptoms and reduction in expiratory air flow rates go hand in hand and are related primarily to bronchoconstriction (probably predominantly of the large, more central airways). Gas exchange disturbances, on the other hand, may well occur in asymptomatic patients and are related more to mucus retention and/or edema formation in peripheral airways, changes not easily identified in measurements of air flow rates. Evidence collected so far suggests that patients with spontaneously occurring low $\dot{V}_A/\dot{Q}$ areas will drop their arterial P_{O_2}, given certain bronchodilators, especially isoproterenol, whereas patients with mainly bronchoconstriction will have arterial hypoxemia abolished by bronchodilator therapy. Thus, even in those patients in whom the arterial P_{O_2} is relatively normal, a fall in arterial P_{O_2} following treatment with isoproterenol probably indicates the existence of a fair amount of ventilation–blood flow inequality and may well indicate the need for more aggressive therapy aimed at mobilizing secretions.

4. General Anesthesia

General anesthesia has long been known to be associated with abnormalities in gas exchange and many investigators have looked into this problem. The causes are undoubtedly many, as stressed by Rehder and co-workers (1975) (see also Volume II, Chapter 4), and a complete explanation of the mechanism of gas exchange disturbances in patients undergoing anesthesia will probably differ from patient to patient. However, a major stumbling block in the elucidation of such mechanisms has been the inability to characterize accurately the gas exchange disturbances themselves, first because elevated levels of inspired P_{O_2} are used, and, second, soluble gaseous anesthetic agents such as nitrous oxide are commonly employed as part of the anesthetic regime. The standard tools for quantitating gas exchange are related to analyzing the arterial P_{O_2} [for example, in terms of venous admixture according to the original concepts of Riley and Cournand (1951)]. However, in the presence of the raised inspired oxygen concentrations and the additional concentrating effect on alveolar P_{O_2} of soluble gas uptake (Farhi and Olszowka, 1968), venous admixture values may variably underestimate the true abnormality present. Thus, if all of the gas exchange abnormality is comprised of unventilated lung (shunt), venous admixture will accurately reflect the abnormality even under these conditions, but to the extent that areas of low $\dot{V}_A/\dot{Q}$ are present, quite large underestimates may result.

Without attempting to elucidate the mechanisms of abnormalities of gas exchange at this point, we have undertaken a pilot study in which 10 patients with mild abnormalities of gas exchange due to chronic obstructive lung disease were studied during general anesthesia for nonthoracic surgical indications (Dueck *et al.*, 1979). In every case, large changes in patterns of inert gas elimination were observed during anesthesia. These changes corresponded to the development of various combinations of shunt and of areas of low $\dot{V}_A/\dot{Q}$, often amounting to 40% of the cardiac output.

An example of the magnitude of these changes is shown in Fig. 5 where the inert gas retentions and associated $\dot{V}_A/\dot{Q}$ distribution are shown both before and after induction of anesthesia. Body position and total ventila-

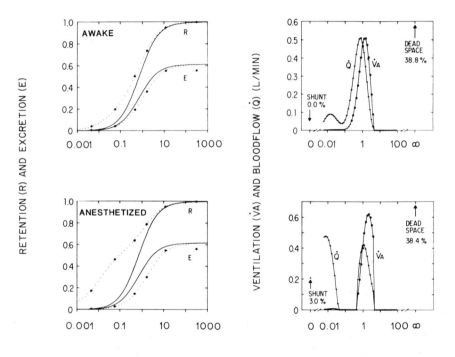

Fig. 5. Upper left: Retention and excretion points (●) obtained in a patient with mild chronic obstructive pulmonary disease lying supine prior to anesthesia. Solid lines are the retention and excretion curves of the corresponding homogeneous lung. Upper right: Associated $\dot{V}_A/\dot{Q}$ distribution showing areas of low ventilation–perfusion ratio, but no shunt. Lower left: Retention and excretion data obtained in the same patient in the same position at the same level of ventilation during anesthesia. The retentions of sulfahexafluoride, ethane, and cyclopropane are greatly elevated compared to the awake control values. Lower right: Associated $\dot{V}_A/\dot{Q}$ distribution showing a large increase in the perfusion of units with very low ventilation–perfusion ratio. This amounts to almost 50% of the cardiac output. Shunt remains very small.

tion were the same before and after induction, and ventilation was assisted without PEEP during anesthesia. Although the mechanism of these large changes is not evident from these measurements, several possibilities arise. The concentrating effect of nitrous oxide on alveolar gas tension and the rapid uptake of nitrous oxide itself could explain through reduction in expired ventilation (Dantzker *et al.*, 1975) some of the elevation of inert gas retention. Changes in the mechanical properties of the chest wall, particularly of the diaphragm (Froese and Bryan, 1977), could influence the distribution of ventilation and thus the distribution of ventilation–perfusion ratios. However, measurements made with radioactive gases in normal subjects by Landmark and co-workers (1977) do not confirm that the topographical changes are of sufficient magnitude to account for the gas exchange disturbances we observed here. Change in vascular tone because of chemical interference to hypoxic vasoconstriction by the anesthetic agents is another possible factor as yet not evaluated. Reduction in lung volume of some lung units for reasons that are not yet clear must have occurred (since FRC uniformly fell in these patients) and this may lead to interference with their ventilation. It is clearly the object of future studies in this setting to attempt to elucidate the relative roles of these, and possibly other factors in this important problem.

B. General Conclusions

Experience with the multiple inert gas elimination technique in both experimental and clinical disease states in animals and man over the last 6 years leads to some general conclusions about patterns of abnormal gas exchange.

1. The Shape of Distributions in Lung Disease

It has been our experience that when ventilation–blood flow inequality occurs in a wide variety of lung diseases (ranging from vascular obstruction in pulmonary embolism to airway obstruction in asthma and chronic obstructive lung disease) that the patterns of $\dot{V}_A/\dot{Q}$ maldistribution are multimodal in character rather than broad and unimodal. The latter would reflect a range of abnormalities continuously from the normal range to complete abolition of either ventilation or blood flow. To some extent, the clear-cut modality may reflect our choice of advanced disease states, and it may well be possible that milder forms of disease are associated with less clearly defined modality of distributions. This question remains to be resolved. It is important to stress, however, that the findings of multimodality are mathematically reliable. The very nature of enforced smoothing in the method tends to favor recovery of distributions of unimodal shape in an effort to minimize the residual sum of squares. Thus, the direction of error in a mathematical sense would be to recover unimodal distributions when, in fact, they are more than one mode is confirmed by the rigorous procedure of linear programming.

It is also important to consider the implications of multimodality as compared to the existence of broad unimodal distribution. We feel that this is particularly relevant to the discussion of patients with emphysema in which a mode of high $\dot{V}_A/\dot{Q}$ regions is present (presumably because of alveolar wall and hence alveolar capillary destruction of areas of lung that still remain ventilated). This is also important in the analysis of distributions in asthmatic subjects where the clear-cut bimodality seems more compatible with the notion of collateral ventilation than with some range of degrees of airway obstruction without collateral ventilation.

It is fortunate that the distributions recovered are in general bimodal in disease states. This is because broad unimodal distributions give rise to inert gas retention data that are subject to much "nonuniqueness," a notion discussed at length both in Chapter 8 of this volume and in previous publications (Olszowka, 1975; Evans and Wagner, 1977; Wagner, 1977a). Thus, a broad unimodal distribution gives rise to data that could be interpreted equally well as consisting of several modes of $\dot{V}_A/\dot{Q}$. On the other hand, a clearly bimodal distribution is not subject to such uncertainty in interpretation and, as stated, we have examined this question rigorously using the linear programming techniques of Chapter 8 of this volume.

2. Collateral Ventilation

$\dot{V}_A/\dot{Q}$ distributions and patterns of inert gas elimination cannot just by the numbers obtained reveal the existence of collateral ventilation. However, as discussed for patients with asthma, the $\dot{V}_A/\dot{Q}$ patterns observed do suggest the presence of collateral ventilation in that disease. Similar arguments apply to patients with chronic obstructive lung disease, and even patients with interstitial lung disease. The absence of very poorly ventilated units in patients with chronic obstructive lung disease of clinical type A may be due to the free collateral ventilatory channels that are known to exist in this disease state. The failure of low $\dot{V}_A/\dot{Q}$ areas to collapse and become transformed into shunt on oxygen breathing, both in patients with chronic obstructive lung disease having low $\dot{V}_A/\dot{Q}$ areas and in patients with interstitial lung disease, suggests the importance of collateral ventilation in stabilizing the gas exchange performance of those affected regions in chronic disease states.

In contrast, both normal subjects, and, in particular, patients with acute lung disease from trauma or edema, appear to be more susceptible to atelectasis as a consequence of oxygen breathing. This is consistent with the idea that fluid in the peripheral airways prevents collateral ventilation channels from effectively maintaining ventilation to obstructed lung units.

Further support of the importance of collateral ventilation comes from comparative physiological studies of the effects of anesthesia in dogs and sheep. Dogs are well known to have extensive collateral ventilation (Van Allen *et al.*, 1930), but sheep, on the other hand, are known to have very little collateral ventilation. Anesthesia affects these two species somewhat differently in that dogs tolerate general anesthesia very well. Thus, dogs can be anesthetized and mechanically ventilated for a period of several hours without the development of much shunt, whereas sheep treated similarly may develop severe hypoxemia and considerable atelectasis fairly rapidly (R. Dueck, personal communication). Although it is premature to ascribe these differences to the presence or absence of collateral ventilation, all of these studies taken together certainly offer strong evidence that collateral ventilation is an important mechanism for preventing more serious development of gas exchange abnormalities in diseased lungs. The severe hypoxemia and poor response to high oxygen concentration breathing frequently seen in the intensive care setting may reflect the inability of collateral ventilation to be effective when there is fluid in the airways.

3. Intrapulmonary and Extrapulmonary Factors in the Mechanism of Hypoxemia

Most medical students are taught that the four causes of hypoxemia are hypoventilation, shunt, ventilation–perfusion inequality, and diffusion impairment. Each of these causes undoubtedly can produce hypoxemia, but one of the more important results of studies of gas exchange over the last few years has been experimental verification of the important role played by other predominantly extrapulmonary factors in determining the absolute level of the arterial P_{O_2}. Studies have been cited earlier in which patients with interstitial lung disease usually have severe hypoxemia, while patients with asthma may have little hypoxemia. We find that, in fact, patients with asthma may have more ventilation–blood flow inequality than patients with interstitial lung disease and yet have less severe hypoxemia. It is important to recognize the important role of the mixed venous P_{O_2}, which in turn reflects the cardiac output (in relation to oxygen uptake) in explaining these apparently inconsistent results. Another setting where the interaction between intra- and extrapulmonary factors is important is in the intensive care ward. Here, in patients with heart failure following myocardial infarction, the level of hypoxemia can be severe. This is usually due to a very low cardiac output combined with mild to modest ventilation–blood flow inequality rather than to severe ventilation–blood flow inequality alone. In other situations in the intensive care setting in acute respiratory failure, the cardiac output may be inordinately high so that the degree of hypoxemia does not accurately reflect the amount of ventilation–blood flow inequality.

The interpretation of the arterial P_{O_2} in terms of its determinants (intrapulmonary versus extrapulmonary factors) is therefore of major practical importance in the understanding of patients with various cardiopulmonary diseases. This is particularly so because therapeutic implications are major. In a patient in the intensive care setting it is important to know whether alterations in arterial P_{O_2} take place because the lungs are getting better (or worse) on the one hand, or because cardiac output, hemoglobin concentration, acid–base status, etc., are changing, on the other. This knowledge will clearly affect the type of therapy.

4. The Role of Diffusion Impairment in Hypoxemia

In various forms of clinical cardiopulmonary disease, including chronic obstructive pulmonary disease, diffuse interstitial lung disease, asthma, and pulmonary edema of various kinds, we have found very little evidence that failure of diffusion equilibration between alveolar gas and end-capillary blood contributes significantly to hypoxemia. The only condition under which this may be a factor in our experience is during exercise in patients with advanced interstitial lung disease. Although it appears not to matter what the etiology of the interstitial process is, the quantitative effect remains relatively small. Thus, only some 15% of the total alveolar–arterial P_{O_2} difference is on the average due to failure of alveolar–end-capillary diffusion equilibration, while the remaining 85% is due to the combination of ventilation–blood flow mismatching and shunt.

Moreover, we have never observed any difference in the degree of elimination of inert gases that can be related to differences in molecular weight. In this regard, the range of molecular weights among the six inert gases is from 30 to 197.5, that is, a sixfold range. This result applies to all of the clinical conditions listed above and provides strong evidence that diffusion within the gas phase of the lungs is never sufficiently impaired to contribute measurably to hypoxemia.

5. Changes Induced by Breathing 100% Oxygen

Ever since Briscoe first suggested that the breathing of 100% oxygen could induce atelectasis (Briscoe *et al.*, 1960), there has been interest in whether this is likely to be of clinical significance. This has always been a difficult question to answer since the development of shunt by 100% oxygen breathing cannot usually be sorted out using conventional tools (because shunt is calculated from the measurement of arterial P_{O_2} breathing

100% oxygen). Our accumulated experimental evidence in both normal subjects and patients with a variety of cardiopulmonary diseases suggests that oxygen-induced atelectasis does, in fact, occur. Experimental data agree with theoretical predictions that only lung units of $\dot{V}_A/\dot{Q}$ less than about 0.1 are susceptible to collapse during 100% oxygen breathing. Moreover, we have found that patients with chronic lung diseases such as interstitial lung disease, asthma, and chronic obstructive pulmonary disease do not appear to be vulnerable to this process, even when lung units of $\dot{V}_A/\dot{Q}$ less than 0.1 are present, and we have tentatively attributed this to the existence of collateral ventilatory pathways in such lungs. Oxygen-induced atelectasis appears to occur in normal subjects when they have such areas of low $\dot{V}_A/\dot{Q}$ (older subjects) (Wagner *et al.*, 1974b), and particularly in the intensive care setting in patients with posttraumatic respiratory failure ("adult respiratory distress syndrome") and pulmonary edema. Under these conditions, areas of low $\dot{V}_A/\dot{Q}$ that are present breathing room air appear to be largely converted to unventilated lung upon breathing 100% oxygen. These changes generally appear to occur within 30 min of oxygen breathing. While we suspect that such atelectasis could be reversed and possibly prevented by judicious use of positive pressure ventilation, this remains to be demonstrated.

REFERENCES

Adaro, F., and Farhi, L. E. (1971). Effects of intralobular gas diffusion on alveolar gas exchange. *Fed. Proc., Fed. Am. Soc. Exp. Biol.* **30**, 437. (Abstr.)

Arndt, H., King, T. K. C., and Briscoe, W. A. (1970). Diffusing capacities and ventilation : perfusion ratios in patients with the clinical syndrome of alveolar capillary block. *J. Clin. Invest.* **49**, 408–422.

Briscoe, W. A. (1959). A method for dealing with data concerning uneven ventilation of the lung and its effect on gas transfer. *J. Appl. Physiol.* **14**, 291–298.

Briscoe, W. A., Cree, E. M., Filler, J., Houssay, H. E. J., and Cournand, A. (1960). Lung volume, alveolar ventilation and perfusion interrelationships in chronic pulmonary emphysema. *J. Appl. Physiol.* **15**, 785–795.

Burrows, B., Fletcher, C. M., Heard, B. E., Jones, N. L., and Wootliff, J. S. (1966). The emphazematous and bronchial types of chronic airways obstruction. A clinicopathological study of patients in London and Chicago. *Lancet* **9**, 830–935.

Canfield, R. E., and Rahn, H. (1957). Arterial–alveolar N_a gas pressure differences due to ventilation–perfusion variations. *J. Appl. Physiol.* **10**, 165–172.

Chick, T. W., Nicholson, D. P., and Johnson, R. L., Jr. (1973). Effects of isoproterenol on distribution of ventilation and perfusion in asthma. *Am. Rev. Respir. Dis.* **107**, 869–870.

Corbet, A. J. S., Ross, J. A., Beaudry, P. H., and Stern, L. (1974). Ventilation–perfusion relationships as assessed by a ADN_2 in hyaline membrane disease. *J. Appl. Physiol.* **36**, 74–81.

Corbet, A. J. S., Ross, J., Popkin, J., and Beaudry, P. (1975). Relationship of arterial–alveolar nitrogen tension to alveolar–arterial oxygen tension, lung volume, flow measurements, and diffusing capacity in cystic fibrosis. *Am. Rev. Respir. Dis.* **112**, 513–519.

Dantzker, D. R., Wagner, P. D., and West, J. B. (1975). Instability of lung units with low $\dot{V}_A/\dot{Q}$ ratios during O_2 breathing. *J. Appl. Physiol.* **38**, 886–895.

Dueck, R., Young, I., Clausen, J., and Wagner, P. D. (1980). Altered distribution of pulmonary ventilation and blood flow in human subjects following induction of inhalation anesthesia. *Anesthesiology* (in press).

Evans, J. W., and Wagner, P. D. (1977). Limits on $\dot{V}_A/\dot{Q}$ distribution from analysis of experimental inert gas elimination. *J. Appl. Physiol.* **42**, 889–898.

Farhi, L. E. (1967). Elimination of inert gas by the lung. *Respir. Physiol.* **3**, 1–11.

Farhi, L. E., and Olszowka, J. A. (1968). Analysis of alveolar gas exchange in the presence of soluble inert gases. *Respir. Physiol.* **5**, 53–67.

Farhi, L. E., and Rahn, H. (1955). A theoretical analysis of the alveolar–arterial O_2 difference with special reference to the distribution effect. *J. Appl. Physiol.* **7**, 799–703.

Farhi, L. E., and Yokoyama, T. (1967). Effects of ventilation–perfusion inequality on elimination of inert gases. *Respir. Physiol.* **3**, 12–20.

Forster, R. E. (1957). Exchange of gases between alveolar air and pulmonary capillary blood: Pulmonary diffusing capacity. *Physiol. Rev.* **37**, 391–452.

Fortune, J. B., and Wagner, P. D. (1979). Effects of common deadspace on inert gas exchange in mathematical models of the lung. *J. Appl. Physiol.* **47**(4):896–906.

Froese, A. B., and Bryan, A. C. (1977). Effects of anesthesia and paralysis on diaphragmatic mechanics in man. *Anesthesiology* **41**, 242–255.

Ingram, R. H., Jr., Krumpe, P. E., Duffell, G. M., and Maniscalco, B. (1970). Ventilation-perfusion changes after aerosolized isoproterenol in asthma. *Am. Rev. Respir. Dis.* **101**, 364.

Kety, S. (1951). The theory and applications of the exchange of inert gas at the lungs and tissues. *Pharmacol. Rev.* **3**, 1–41.

King, T. C., and Briscoe, W. A. (1967). Bohr integral isopleths in the study of blood gas exchange in the lung. *J. Appl. Physiol.* **22**, 659–674.

King, T. C., Ali, N., and Briscoe, W. A. (1973). Treatment of hypoxia with 24 percent oxygen. *Am. Rev. Respir. Dis.* **108**, 19–29.

Knudson, R. J., and Constantine, H. P. (1967). An effect of isoproterenol on ventilation–perfusion in asthmatic versus normal subjects. *J. Appl. Physiol.* **22**, 402–403.

Lambert, M. W. (1955). Accessory bronchiole–alveolar communications. *J. Pathol. Bacteriol.* **70**, 311–312.

Landmark, S. J., Knopp, T. J., Rehder, K., and Sessler, A. D. (1977). Regional pulmonary perfusion and $\dot{V}/\dot{Q}$ in awake and anesthetized–paralyzed man. *J. Appl. Physiol.: Respir. Environ. Exercise Physiol.* **43**, 993–1000.

Lenfant, C. (1963). Measurement of ventilation–perfusion distribution with alveolar–arterial differences. *J. Appl. Physiol.* **18**, 1090–1094.

Lenfant, C. (1964). Measurement of factors impairing gas exchange in man with hyperbaric pressure. *J. Appl. Physiol.* **19**, 189–194.

Lenfant, C. (1965). Effect of high F_I of measurement of ventilation–perfusion distribution in man at sea level. *Ann. N.Y. Acad. Sci.* **21**, 797–808.

Lenfant, C., and Aucutt, C. (1966). Measurement of blood gases by gas chromatography. *Respir. Physiol.* **1**, 398–407.

Lenfant, C., and Okubo, T. (1969). Distribution function of pulmonary blood flow and ventilation–perfusion ratio in man. *J. Appl. Physiol.* **24**, 668–677.

Loosli, C. G. (1937). Interalveolar communications in normal and pathologic mammalian lungs. Review of literature. *Arch. Pathol.* **24**, 734–744.

Macklin, C. C. (1936). Alveolar pores and their significance in the lung. *Arch. Pathol.* **21**, 202–203.

Markello, R., Winter, P., and Olszowka, A. (1972). Assessment of ventilation–perfusion inequalities by arterial–alveolar nitrogen differences in intensive-care patients. *Anesthesiology* **37**, 4–15.

Markello, R., Olszowka, A., Winter, P., and Farhi, L. (1973). An updated method for determining $\dot{V}_A/\dot{Q}$ inequalities and direct shunt using O_2, CO_2 and N_2. *Respir. Physiol.* **19**, 221–232.

Martin, J. B. (1966). Respiratory bronchioles as the pathway for collateral ventilation. *J. Appl. Physiol.* **21**, 1443–1444.

Olszowka, A. J. (1975). Can $\dot{V}_A/\dot{Q}$ distributions in the lung be recovered from inert gas retention data? *Respir. Physiol.* **25**, 191–198.

Peslin, R., Dawson, S., and Mead, J. (1971). Analysis of multicomponent exponential curves by the Post-Widder's equation. *J. Appl. Physiol.* **30**, 462–472.

Petrini, M. F., Robertson, H. T., and Hlastala, M. P. (1979). Separation of respiratory deadspace into its series and parallel components. *Fed. Proc., Fed. Am. Soc. Exp. Biol.* **38**, 949. (Abstr.)

Powell, F. L., and Wagner, P. D. (1979). Inert gas transfer in the goose. *Fed. Proc., Fed. Am. Soc. Exp. Biol.* **38**, 965. (Abstr.)

Rahn, H. (1949). A concept of mean alveolar air and the ventilation–blood flow relationship during pulmonary gas exchange. *Am. J. Physiol.* **158**, 21–30.

Rahn, H., and Fenn, W. O. (1955). "A Graphical Analysis of the Respiratory Gas Exchange." Am. Physiol. Soc., Washington, D.C.

Rehder, K., Sessler, A. D., and Marsh, H. M. (1975). General anesthesia and the lung. *Am. Rev. Respir. Dis.* **112**, 541–563.

Riley, R. L., and Cournand, A. (1949). "Ideal" alveolar air and the analysis of ventilation–perfusion relationships in the lung. *J. Appl. Physiol.* **1**, 825–847.

Riley, R. L., and Cournand, A. (1951). Analysis of factors affecting partial pressures of oxygen and carbon dioxide in gas and blood of lungs: Theory. *J. Appl. Physiol.* **4**, 77–101.

Ross, B. B., and Farhi, L. E. (1960). Deadspace ventilation as a determinant in the ventilation–perfusion concept. *J. Appl. Physiol.* **15**, 363–371.

Scheid, P., and Piiper, J. (1970). Analysis of gas exchange in the avian lung: Theory and experiments in the domestic fowl. *Respir. Physiol.* **9**, 246–262.

Tai, E., and Read, J. (1967). Response of blood gas tensions to aminophylline and isoprenaline in patients with asthma. *Thorax* **22**, 543–544.

Van Allen, C. M., Lindskog, G. E., and Richter, H. G. (1930). Gaseous interchange between adjacent lung lobules. *Yale J. Biol. Med.* **2**, 297–298.

Wagner, P. D. (1977a). A general approach to the evaluation of ventilation–perfusion ratios in normal and abnormal lungs. *Physiologist* **20**, 18–25.

Wagner, P. D. (1977b). Diffusion and chemical reaction in pulmonary gas exchange. *Physiol. Rev.* **57**, 257–313.

Wagner, P. D., and Evans, J. W. (1977). Conditions for equivalence of gas exchange in series and parallel models of the lung. *Respir. Physiol.* **31**, 117–138.

Wagner, P. D., Dantzker, D. R., Dueck, R., Uhl, R. R., Virgilio, R., and West, J. B. (1974a). Continuous distributions of ventilation–perfusion ratios in acute and chronic lung disease. *Clin. Res.* **22**, 134A. (Abstr.)

Wagner, P. D., Laravuso, R. B., Uhl, R. R., and West, J. B. (1974b). Continuous distributions of ventilation–perfusion ratios in normal subjects breathing air and 100% O_2. *J. Clin. Invest.* **54**, 54–68.

Wagner, P. D., Saltzman, H. A., and West, J. B. (1974c). Measurement of continuous distributions of ventilation–perfusion ratios: Theory. *J. Appl. Physiol.* **36**, 588–599.

Wagner, P. D., Dantzker, D. R., Dueck, R., dePolo, J. L., Wasserman, K., and West, J. B. (1976). Distribution of ventilation–perfusion ratios in patients with interstitial lung disease. *Chest* **69**, 256–257.

Wagner, P. D., Allen, D. H., Mathison, D. A., Metcalf, J. F., Rubinfeld, A. R. (1977a). Gas exchange following bronchial challenge in patients with extrinsic asthma. *Am. Rev. Respir. Dis.* **115**, 387. (Abstr.)

Wagner, P. D., Dantzker, D. R., Dueck, R., Clausen, J. L., and West, J. B. (1977b). Ventilation–perfusion inequality in chronic obstructive pulmonary disease. *J. Clin. Invest.* **59**, 203–216.

Wagner, P. D., Dantzker, D. R., Iacovoni, V. E., Tomlin, W. C., and West, J. B. (1978a). Ventilation–perfusion inequality in asymptomatic asthma. *Am. Rev. Respir. Dis.* **118**, 511–524.

Wagner, P. D., Ramsdell, J. W., Incaudo, G. A., Rubinfeld, A. R., and Young, I. H. (1978b). Gas exchange following bronchial challenge with antigen in patients with extrinsic asthma. *Am. Rev. Respir. Dis.* **117**, 409. (Abstr.)

West, J. B. (1969–1970). Effect of slope and shape of dissociation curve on pulmonary gas exchange. *Respir. Physiol.* **8**, 66–85.

Yokoyama, T., and Farhi, L. E. (1967). The study of ventilation-perfusion ratio distribution in the anesthetized dog by multiple inert gas washout. *Respir. Physiol.* **3**, 166–176.

Young, I. H., and Wagner, P. D. (1979). Effect of intrapulmonary hematocrit maldistribution on O_2, CO_2 and inert gas exchange. *J. Appl. Physiol.* **46**, 240–278.

8

Numerical Analysis of Gas Exchange

Albert J. Olszowka and Peter D. Wagner

I. NUMERICAL ANALYSIS IN STEADY STATE GAS EXCHANGE

A. Introduction

Of all the organs, the lungs are possibly the most amenable to mathematical modeling and a major part of this is related to gas exchange. There are both structural and functional reasons behind the rational applicability of such modeling. The lung is made (structure) up of a large number of anatomical units, each of which is qualitatively similar. In each unit, ventilation via the airways and perfusion via the blood vessels lead to exchange of gases between blood and gas phases that are separated by a tissue sheet of an average thickness of less than 1 μm. It is possible to calculate with relatively few assumptions how gas exchange occurs in such units (function) and to determine the factors that influence such gas exchange. As is well known (and as will be discussed in this chapter at some length), the principal determinants of gas exchange in such a lung unit are the relative amounts of ventilation and perfusion, but the relationships that dictate how ventilation and perfusion determine gas exchange involve several other factors as well. Important among these are the quantitative relationships between blood gas concentration and partial pressure, that is, the dissociation curves of the gases under consideration.

Once calculations of gas exchange in a single lung unit are performed, a logical next step is to examine gas exchange in all such single lung units of a given lung. Such units may differ from each other in their ventilation and perfusion, but will generally otherwise obey the same principles of gas exchange. Such a collection of lung units of different quantitative, but similar qualitative characteristics is termed a distribution of lung units with respect to some particular variable (such as their relative ventilation and perfusion).

These two principal concepts, namely, the behavior of a single unit of lung and the behavior of a distribution of such single units, are the keys to understanding gas exchange of the lungs as a whole organ, and the application of these concepts requires techniques of numerical analysis.

Behavior of the single lung units and of distributions is studied by first establishing the appropriate *algebraic equations* in each case and by then finding *methods for their quantitative solution*. This approach in general requires techniques of numerical analysis because most of the relevant equations are implicit rather than explicit in nature and cannot be solved directly. Rather they require a trial and error approach. To illustrate this important notion further, consider two algebraic equations:

$$Y = 3X^2 - X + 4 \tag{1}$$

$$5XY = \log_{10}(X + Y) \tag{2}$$

In Eq. (1), Y is a variable that can be computed directly given a value of X: Suppose $X = 1$; then Eq. (1) states that $Y = 6$. This is clearly the only correct value of Y given $X = 1$, and Eq. (1) is called an *explicit* equation. Now examine Eq. (2). If $X = 1$ is substituted into this equation, an equation in only Y remains, as for Eq. (1). One way to solve Eq. (2) for $X = 1$ is to try a value for Y, say $Y = 1$, and to evaluate both sides of Eq. (2). For this example, the left-hand side is 5 and the right-hand side $\log_{10} 2$, which are clearly not equal, proving that $Y = 1$ is not a correct solution. Using some structured sequence of "guesses" (i.e., numerical analysis) at Y, one would finally come to the conclusion that for $X = 1$, $Y = 0$ was a correct solution. Equation (2) is said to be an *implicit* equation. It further illustrates another difficulty that may arise in the solution of such implicit equations: Is $Y = 0$ the only correct solution for Eq. (2) for $X = 1$? In this case, there is one other value for Y, namely, $Y = -0.999991$, that satisfies Eq. (2).

Even before the availability of computers, methods for solving the implicit equations that quantitated the relationships between $\dot{V}_A/\dot{Q}$ and gas exchange were developed (Riley and Cournand, 1949; Rahn and Fenn, 1955). Moreover, the graphical approach represented by the O_2–CO_2 diagram of Rahn and Fenn was readily applicable when computers arrived on the scene. Thus the initial computer programs for solving the implicit equations of gas exchange indeed used it with minimal modification (Kelman, 1968; Olszowka and Farhi, 1968; West, 1969).

In time this approach was supplanted by numerical techniques more particularly suited to digital computers. In this chapter we describe the most widely used of such "structured guessing" approaches, which solve by computer the implicit relationships important to gas exchange. We do not provide any rigorous development of the procedures used, but attempt to give the reader a feeling for why they work and show him how they have been used in both research and medical practice. Our hope, then, is to provide enough insight into the numerical procedures in common usage in the field so that the average reader can use the programs with the mystery removed.

At the outset, it is useful to return to the physiological concepts referred to above, that is, the behavior of single lung units and the behavior of distributions of such units. Two kinds of questions are generally posed in this context, as illustrated in Figs. 1A and 1B. In Fig. 1A, the idea is to calculate how the overall performance of the lung results from some im-

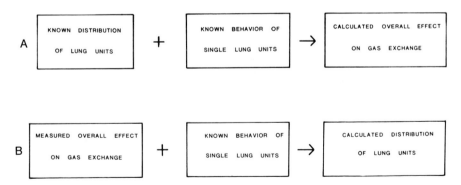

Fig. 1. The two general classes of problems seen in numerical analysis of gas exchange. (A) A known distribution of lung units (theoretically assumed or experimentally measured) is used to calculate the overall effect on gas exchange. This requires an understanding of gas exchange in each of the lung units. (B) By measuring overall gas exchange for one or more gases and analyzing these data on the basis of the known behavior of single lung units, estimates of the distribution of these lung units can be made.

posed distribution of lung units based on predictable response of single lung units. For example, one could pose the following question: Given that the lung contains only two types of lung units [normal units and unventilated (shunt) units each of calculable P_{O_2}], how does a given distribution of such units (that is, allocation of perfusion to these units) affect the overall performance of the lung characterized by, say, the arterial P_{O_2}? The second type of question, illustrated in Fig. 1B, is what distribution of lung units must be present in the lung so as to explain measurable overall indexes of gas exchange given the predictable behavior of single units. The corresponding example would be to calculate the distribution of perfusion between normal units and unventilated (shunt) units given a measured arterial P_{O_2} value and the predictable P_{O_2} of both normal and unventilated units. This question is, of course, recognizable as the determination of venous admixture by the classical Riley analysis (Riley and Cournand, 1949).

In this section of the chapter we discuss both types of questions in the above order.

B. Steady State Equations for Gas Exchange

1. Explicit Equations for Inert Gases

Analysis of gas exchange in a single lung unit may involve the use of either explicit or implicit relationships as referred to above. As an example of the former, consider the case of an ''inert'' gas (i.e., one obeying Henry's law) being infused into the venous side of the systemic circulation, but not contained in the inspirate. By inert we do not mean pharmacologically inert; we use this term as traditionally applied by physiologists to gases for which the relationship between partial pressure and concentration in blood is linear.

If $\dot{V}_A$ and $\dot{Q}$ are the alveolar expired ventilation and blood flow of the lung unit (liters/min), α_G the solubility of the gas [(vol/vol/torr)] $P_{\bar{v}_G}$, P_A and $P_{c'_G}$, respectively, its mixed venous, alveolar, and end-capillary partial pressures (torr), and $C_{\bar{v}_G}$ and C_{c_G}, its mixed venous and end-capillary concentrations (vol/vol), then application of Dalton's law and the principle of conservation of matter yield

$$\dot{V}_A P_{A_G} = k\dot{Q}(C_{\bar{v}_G} - C_{c'_G})$$
$$= k\dot{Q}\alpha_G(P_{\bar{v}_G} - P_{c'_G}) \tag{3}$$

The left-hand side of this equation expresses mass transfer of gas out of the mouth in expiration, while the right-hand side gives net transfer of gas out of the blood into alveolar gas over the same time period. Setting these two terms equal to one another implies conservation of matter under steady state conditions. The equation can be rearranged:

$$(\dot{V}_A/\dot{Q})P_{A_G} = k\alpha_G(P_{\bar{v}_G} - P_{c'_G}) \tag{4}$$

The constant k makes the units consistent and corrects for the convention that gas concentrations arc expressed at STPD while ventilation volumes are expressed at BTPS. It has torr units and is computed using the relation

$$k = 760(T + 273)/273$$

where T is temperature (°C). At 37°C, $k = 863$.

If it is now assumed that the diffusion process across the blood : gas barrier is complete, alveolar and end-capillary partial pressures are the same so that $P_A = P_{c'}$. Equation (4) then becomes

$$(\dot{V}_A/\dot{Q})P_{A_G} = k\alpha_G(P_{\bar{v}_G} - P_{A_G})$$

Calling $k\alpha_G = \lambda_G$, the blood : gas partition coefficient, and rearranging terms:

$$P_{A_G}/P_{v_G} = P_{c'_G}/P_{v_G} = \lambda_G/(\lambda_G + \dot{V}_A/\dot{Q}) \tag{5}$$

which is the well-known expression defining inert gas elimination (Farhi, 1967). Note that in this simple case the alveolar gas tension is defined *explicitly* as a function of only two variables, the ventilation–perfusion ratio of the lung unit and the blood : gas partition coefficient of the gas. Equation (5) may now be used to calculate alveolar (and end-capillary) gas tensions, all that is required being values for $\dot{V}_A/\dot{Q}$ and λ_G. Such calculations are clearly trivial.

2. Implicit Equations for the Respiratory Gases O_2 and CO_2

Exactly the same reasoning can be applied to O_2 and CO_2, the only addition to the scheme being the delivery of oxygen in inspired gas necessitating the definition of another variable, $\dot{V}_I$, the inspired alveolar ventilation (liters/min). Equations (6) and (7) thus define the mass balance relationships for O_2 and CO_2:

$$(\dot{V}_I/\dot{Q})P_{I_{O_2}} - (\dot{V}_A/\dot{Q})P_{A_{O_2}} = k(C_{c'_{O_2}} - C_{\bar{v}_{O_2}}) \tag{6}$$

$$(\dot{V}_A/\dot{Q})P_{A_{CO_2}} = k(C_{v_{CO_2}} - C_{c'_{CO_2}}) \tag{7}$$

The terminology is the same as that used for inert gases except that the inert gas subscript G is replaced by O_2 and CO_2, respectively. To complete the analysis for the respiratory gases, nitrogen (N_2) must also be considered:

$$(\dot{V}_I/\dot{Q})P_{I_{N_2}} - (\dot{V}_A/\dot{Q})P_{A_{N_2}} = \lambda_{N_2}(P_{c'_{N_2}} - P_{\bar{v}_{N_2}}) \tag{8}$$

and, finally, the sum of all partial pressures in alveolar gas, including water vapor (P_{H_2O}), must sum to barometric pressure P_B:

$$P_{A_{O_2}} + P_{A_{CO_2}} + P_{A_{N_2}} = P_B - P_{H_2O} \tag{9}$$

If we again assume that diffusion equilibrium between blood and gas is achieved, $P_{A_{N_2}} = P_{c'_{N_2}}$ and for O_2 and CO_2 the blood–gas concentrations can be computed from $P_{A_{O_2}}$ and $P_{A_{O_2}}$ knowing the equilibrium O_2 and CO_2 dissociation curves. This means that for any given composition of inspired gas and mixed venous blood and any desired value of $\dot{V}_A/\dot{Q}$, Eqs. (6)–(9) form a system of four equations in four unknown variables ($\dot{V}_I/\dot{Q}$, $P_{A_{N_2}}$, $P_{A_{O_2}}$, and $P_{A_{CO_2}}$). Note that we take $\dot{V}_A/\dot{Q}$ as the specified and $\dot{V}_I/\dot{Q}$ as the unspecified variable to be determined, but one may treat $\dot{V}_I/\dot{Q}$ as the specified variable instead (Dantzker *et al.*, 1975).

The requirement that a system of equations be solved certainly makes the analysis of the exchange of the respiratory gases more difficult than the analysis of inert gas elimination given above. However, what truly sets this analysis apart is the nonlinearity and interdependence of the oxygen and CO_2 dissociation curves, which contrast with the simple linear relationship between gas concentration and equilibrium partial pressure exhibited by the inert gases.

Indeed, if O_2 and CO_2 did exhibit such simple behavior, one could with a little effort modify Eqs. (6)–(9) to form a system linear in the unknown variables $\dot{V}_I/\dot{Q}$, $P_{A_{O_2}}$, $P_{A_{CO_2}}$, and $P_{A_{N_2}}$, and by an appropriate combination of multiplying through by suitable constants and subtracting of one equation from another, explicit expressions for each of these unknowns could be obtained. The principles of the procedures involved are illustrated in the example below, where for the sake of simplicity a linear system of equations with only two unknowns is considered:

$$ax + by = c \tag{10}$$

$$dx + ey = f \tag{11}$$

Here the unknowns are x and y, and a, b, c, d, e, and f are given constants.

Multiplying (10) and (11) by $1/a$ and $1/d$, respectively, gives

$$x + b(y/a) = c/a \tag{12}$$

$$x + e(y/d) = f/d \tag{13}$$

and subtracting (13) from (12) and solving for y yields

$$y = (c/a - f/d)/(b/a - e/d)$$
$$= (cd - fa)/(bd - ae) \tag{14}$$

To return to the physiological setting, we must solve Eqs. (6)–(9). We can simplify the problem to some extent by reducing the number of equations and unknowns to two by a procedure analogous to that just given in Eqs. (10)–(14). This is possible because while Eqs. (6) and (7) remain nonlinear equations, (8) and (9), are, in fact, linear. Thus from (9)

$$P_{A_{N_2}} = P_B - P_{H_2O} - P_{A_{O_2}} - P_{A_{CO_2}} \tag{15}$$

Taking as stated above that $P_{c'_{N_2}} = P_{A_{N_2}}$, this value of $P_{A_{N_2}}$ is substituted into Eq. (8), and the variable $\dot{V}_I/\dot{Q}$ is isolated to give

$$\dot{V}_I/\dot{Q} = (\lambda_{N_2} + \dot{V}_A/\dot{Q})(P_B - P_{H_2O} - P_{A_{O_2}} - P_{A_{N_2}})/P_{I_{N_2}}$$
$$- \lambda_{N_2}(P_v/P_{I_{N_2}}) \tag{16}$$

Next, this expression for $\dot{V}_I/\dot{Q}$ (which contains only the two unknowns, $P_{A_{O_2}}$ and $P_{A_{CO_2}}$) is itself substituted into Eq. (6), which, after gathering terms with common coefficients and substituting $F_{I_{O_2}}$ (the dry gas fraction of oxygen in the inspirate) for the ratio $(P_{I_{O_2}}/[P_B - P_{H_2O}])$ and $(1 - F_{I_{O_2}})$ for the ratio $(P_{I_{O_2}}/[P_B - P_{H_2O}])$ yields

$$(\dot{V}_A/\dot{Q})[(P_{I_{O_2}} - F_{I_{O_2}}P_{A_{CO_2}} - P_{A_{O_2}})]/(1 - F_{I_{O_2}}) + \lambda_{N_2}(P_B - P_{H_2O}$$
$$- P_{A_{O_2}} - P_{A_{CO_2}} - P_{\bar{v}_{N_2}}) = k(C_{c'_{O_2}} - C_{v_{O_2}}) \tag{17}$$

Thus the original system of four equations that defines the alveolar exchange of the respiratory gases can be modified to give a system of two equations [Eqs. (7) and (17)] in two unknowns ($P_{A_{O_2}}$ and $P_{A_{CO_2}}$) on the continued assumption that the blood–gas contents are determined from the alveolar pressures and equilibrium dissociation curves.

We are still left with the problem of solving these two equations to obtain the unknown values of $P_{A_{O_2}}$ and $P_{A_{CO_2}}$. In the graphical methods that antedate the use of computers, a significant simplification of Eq. (17) is required to facilitate the solution, namely, the second term on the left-hand side of Eq. (17) is ignored. In effect this is equivalent to ignoring N_2 exchange and setting the right-hand side of Eq. (8) to zero, thus defining $\dot{V}_I/\dot{Q}$ more simply in terms of $\dot{V}_A/\dot{Q}$:

$$\dot{V}_I/\dot{Q} = (\dot{V}_A/\dot{Q})(P_{A_{N_2}}/P_{I_{N_2}})$$

Dividing the simplified form of Eq. (17) into Eq. (7) gives two forms for the respiratory exchange ratio R of the lung unit in question. In so doing, the variable $\dot{V}_A/\dot{Q}$ is neatly cancelled from the system so that rather than directly specifying $\dot{V}_A/\dot{Q}$, we specify a value of R for which the $P_{A_{O_2}}$ and $P_{A_{CO_2}}$ are to be determined, where

$$R = \frac{P_{A_{CO_2}}(1 - F_{I_{O_2}})}{(P_{I_{O_2}} - F_{I_{O_2}}P_{A_{CO_2}} - P_{A_{O_2}})} \tag{18}$$

and

$$R = \frac{(C_{\bar{v}_{O_2}} - C_{c'_{CO_2}})}{(C_{c'_{O_2}} - C_{\bar{v}_{O_2}})} \tag{19}$$

For such an R value one can plot on an O_2–CO_2 diagram the straight "gas R" line defining the pair of $P_{A_{O_2}}$, $P_{A_{CO_2}}$ values that satisfy the first of these two expressions for R. Similarly, by use of a suitable nomogram (Dill *et al.*, 1937), one can construct on the curved blood R line satisfying the second expression for R. The alveolar gas pressures and corresponding gas concentrations at the point of intersection of these two lines satisfy Eqs. (7) and (17) as well as (18) and (19) since the latter were derived from the former.

In fact, in this method, Eq. (7) is used to compute $\dot{V}_A/\dot{Q}$ (with the help of a nomogram) once $P_{A_{O_2}}$ and $P_{A_{CO_2}}$ are determined. Figure 2 illustrates such a calculation for $R = 0.6$, $P_{\bar{v}_{O_2}} = 40$, $P_{\bar{v}_{CO_2}} = 46$, $P_{I_{O_2}} = 150$. At the point of intersection of the two R lines, $P_{A_{O_2}} = 84.4$, $P_{A_{CO_2}} = 42.9$, and the corresponding $\dot{V}_A/\dot{Q} = 0.58$.

When computer programs that performed $\dot{V}_A/\dot{Q}$ computations first appeared (Kelman, 1968; Olszowka and Farhi, 1968), they followed a strategy very similar to the graphical method, namely, the equations were solved to match a chosen value of R.

Step a: Chose an R value.
Step b: Assume an arbitrary $P_{A_{O_2}}$.

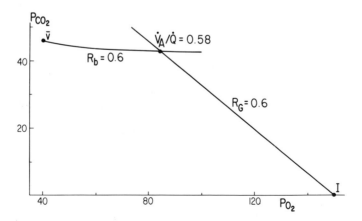

Fig. 2. O_2–CO_2 diagram. The intersection of the straight line gas R line and the curved blood R line labeled R_G and R_b, respectively, determines the gas composition in a respiratory unit having the corresponding gas exchange ratio. Once that composition is known, the $\dot{V}_A/\dot{Q}$ of the unit is computed using Eq. (7).

Step c: Determine the value of $P_{A_{CO_2}}$ that together with the chosen $P_{A_{O_2}}$ value corresponds to values for $C_{c'_{O_2}}$ and $C_{c'_{CO_2}}$ such that Eq. (19) is satisfied.

Step d: Rearranging Eq. (18), set

$$P^*_{A_{O_2}} = P_{I_{O_2}} - \left(\frac{(1 - F_{I_{O_2}}) + RF_{I_{O_2}}}{R}\right) P_{A_{CO_2}}$$

Step e: If $P^*_{A_{O_2}} \simeq P_{A_{O_2}}$ to go to step g.

Step f: Otherwise set $P_{A_{O_2}} = P^*_{A_{O_2}}$ and go back to step c.

Step g: Set

$$\dot{V}_A/\dot{Q} = k\frac{C_{\bar{v}_{CO_2}} - C_{c'_{CO_2}}}{P_{A_{CO_2}}}$$

Step h: Save $\dot{V}_A/\dot{Q}, P_A, P_{A_{CO_2}}$, etc.

Step i: Choose another value of R and go back to step c.

Step j: Continue on with the rest of the program.

Step c of the above strategy involves the computation of the blood concentration of oxygen and carbon dioxide, which are associated with the corresponding set of partial pressures. A number of programs exist for such computations (Kelman, 1968; Olszowka and Farhi, 1968; Thomas, 1972). Each uses slightly different formulas for quantitating the Bohr and Haldane effects, the Donnan equilibrium, etc. Rather than discuss their relative merits, we refer to an algorithm that selecting useful features from each, uses pH, the plasma pH, and P_{O_2}, the oxygen partial pressure, to compute S, the fraction of hemoglobin bound to oxygen; C_{O_2}, the oxygen concentration of blood; as well as P_{CO_2} and C_{CO_2}, the carbon dioxide partial pressure and concentration of blood, respectively.

Although the reader might feel that in the light of the discussion up to now it might seem more natural to devise an algorithm which uses P_{O_2} and P_{CO_2} rather than P_{O_2} and pH as inputs, the empirical relationships available are such that one cannot explicitly relate the concentrations of O_2 and CO_2 to the corresponding partial pressures. Thus in computing blood–gas concentrations, determining a point on the blood R line, performing $\dot{V}_A/\dot{Q}$ calculations, etc., it is more efficient to iterate pH and P_{O_2} rather than P_{CO_2} and P_{O_2}.

3. Computer Algorithms for the O_2 and CO_2 Dissociation Curves

Because of space limitations, the description and FORTRAN listing of these subroutines, coded as GAS1 and GAS2, cannot be given here. They have been deposited with the National Auxiliary Publications Service and can be obtained from that source.* A corresponding description of the programs of Kelman for the O_2 and CO_2 dissociation curves appears elsewhere (West and Wagner, 1977).

4. Solution of Equations of Gas Exchange by Iteration

We now describe the two methods for performing these tasks that we have found to be particularly useful.

The first solves the implicit function in one variable:

$$F(x) = 0 \tag{20}$$

The second solves the pair of implicit functions in two variables:

$$F(x, y) = 0 \tag{21}$$

$$G(x, y) = 0 \tag{22}$$

For illustrative purposes we refer to the variables pH and P_{O_2} instead of x and y. The methods are quite general, however, and can be used to solve problems involving other variables. Therefore, the FORTRAN code (subroutines FINDX and FINDXY, deposited with the National Auxiliary Publications Service, see footnote on p. 272) uses the variables x and y rather than pH and P_{O_2}.

We develop the strategy utilized in the first routine (coded as FINDX) by considering the problem of executing step c in the computerization of the graphical analysis of (Rahn and Fenn, 1955) outlined earlier. Specifically, for a given $P_{A_{O_2}}$ one must solve Eq. (19). An equivalent form of this equation is

$$R - \frac{C_{\bar{v}_{CO_2}} - C_{c'_{CO_2}}}{C_{c'_{O_2}} - C_{\bar{v}_{O_2}}} = 0 \tag{23}$$

If we set P_{O_2} to $P_{A_{O_2}}$ and guess at a value for pH, the gas subroutines described above can be used to compute the corresponding O_2 and CO_2 concentrations. These concentrations can be tentatively assigned to $C_{c'}$ and $C_{c'}$, respectively, to evaluate the function $F(\text{pH})$ defined by

$$F(\text{pH}) = R - \frac{C_{\bar{v}_{CO_2}} - C_{c'_{CO_2}}}{C_{c'_{O_2}} - C_{\bar{v}_{O_2}}} \tag{24}$$

It is now important to realize that finding the value of pH such that $F(\text{pH}) = 0$ is equivalent to solving Eq. (23) and in turn Eq. (19), for once

---

* See NAPS document No. 03460 for 29 pages of supplementary material. Order from NAPS % Microfiche Publications, P. O. Box 3513, Grand Central Station, New York, New York 10017.

the proper pH is determined, the P_{CO_2} corresponding to that pH may be assigned to $P_{A_{CO_2}}$.

In general, the first guess at pH will not be the correct one and thus $F(pH)$ will be nonzero. A second guess at pH is then used in a similar manner to obtain a second determination of $F(pH)$, which in general will also be nonzero. If we let pH_1 and pH_2 be the first two guesses at pH, and F_1 and F_2 the corresponding values of $F(pH)$, we can plot F_1 and F_2 on the ordinate against the respective values of pH_1 and pH_2 on the abscissa. These two points labeled 1 and 2 in Fig. 3A represent two evaluations of $F(pH)$. Although at this point in time we may not have actually computed any other points on the curve, we might imagine that the continuous curved line drawn through these two points is, in fact, a plot of Eq. (24). Our goal, solving Eq. (23), becomes that of finding the value of pH where this curve crosses the abscissa (that is, point A in the figure). We now invoke the secant or false position method by approximating the curve with a straight "secant" line drawn through points 1 and 2 and determining where this line intercepts the abscissa. From geometric considerations we may write

$$\frac{pH_2 - pH}{pH_1 - pH_2} = \frac{-F_2}{F_1 + F_2}$$

and solving for pH we get

$$pH = pH_2 + (pH_2 - pH_1)F_2/(F_1 - F_2) \tag{25}$$

as the value of pH at that point. The first point on $F(pH)$ may now be discarded, the second relabeled 1, the point corresponding to the new trial pH labeled 2, and the processes repeated again (see Fig. 3B). These repetitive computations ("iterations") are continued and it can be seen that a value of pH is reached that is very close to the value at A. In practice, some "tolerance" is chosen ahead of time, such that when this procedure gives values to F that are closer to zero than the tolerance specified, the process is halted and the result accepted as a solution.

It is worth commenting here that this strategy is not foolproof. Indeed, if the function F has several maxima, minima, or sharp peaks or if it crosses the abscissa at more than one point, *the above strategy will likely fail unless the initial trial values for the variable being iterated are close to the desired solution.*

On the other hand, if F is monotone (i.e., has a derivative or slope that does not change sign), a solution is virtually guaranteed. Moreover, even if the function is not monotone over the whole range of values that can be assigned to the iterated variable, there generally is a range over which it is monotone. If the solution exists in this range, restricting the search to this

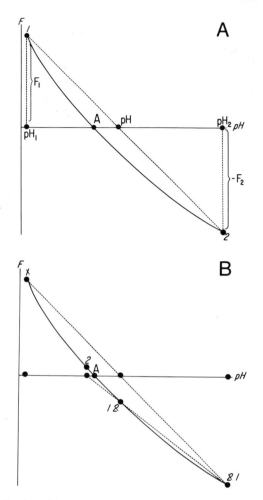

Fig. 3. (A) Application of the secant method to obtain each new value of pH as a trial solution to the problem $F(\text{pH}) = 0$. The trial value is obtained by approximating the function F
with a secant line passing the points on F (labeled 1 and 2) associated with the two previous
trial values of pH. (B) After each new trial value is obtained, one of the previous points is
discarded, the others relabeled, and the procedure outlined in Fig. 4A is repeated.

range will generally guarantee success. Hence, subroutine FINDX, which
contains the code for the above algorithm, will discard any value for pH
computed by Eq. (25) that is outside a range set by the user. In practice,
the range is usually determined by physiologic considerations, e.g., 6.8 to
8.0 if pH is being iterated.

Application of FINDX to solving the $\dot{V}_A/\dot{Q}$ problem is not confined to finding a point on the Blood R line. To evaluate Eq. (23), the mixed venous O_2 and CO_2 concentrations must be determined from knowledge of the mixed venous equilibrium pressures. In this case, FINDX is used to determine the value of pH such that the function

$$F(\text{pH}) = P_{CO_2} - P_{\bar{v}_{CO_2}} \tag{26}$$

has a value arbitrarily close to zero. In this case, P_{CO_2} is determined by subroutine GAS1 with P_{O_2} assigned the value of $P_{\bar{v}_{O_2}}$ and pH assigned values by subroutine FINDX using the above described strategy. Once the derived pH is found, subroutine GAS2 can then be utilized to determine $C_{\bar{v}_{O_2}}$ and $C_{\bar{v}_{O_2}}$.

Although the computerized form of the graphical approach to solving the $\dot{V}_A/\dot{Q}$ problem is relatively fast compared to the graphical method, it is not very efficient since $P_{A_{O_2}}$ itself is being iterated independently of pH. Furthermore, this approach reverses the roles of the independent $(\dot{V}_A/\dot{Q})$ and dependent (R) variables—a useful fiction necessary to get the job done when computers were not available, but no longer needed. Finally, the graphical method ignores the exchange of nitrogen. Examination of Eq. (17) indicates that if $\dot{V}_A/\dot{Q}$ is very small, the term reflecting nitrogen exchange might not be sufficiently negligible to do so. All these objections are dealt with by using a second algorithm for solving implicit equations—one that iterates two variables to solve two simultaneous implicit equations.

In solving the respiratory gas exchange problem with this algorithm, it is recommended that Eq. (9) be used instead of (17) as one of the pair of equations to be solved. To do so, the mass balance equation for oxygen instead of that for nitrogen can be used to get an expression for $\dot{V}_I/\dot{Q}$. Thus from Eq. (6) we have

$$\dot{V}_I/\dot{Q} = \frac{(\dot{V}_A/\dot{Q})P_{A_{O_2}} + k(C_{c'_{O_2}} - C_{\bar{v}_{O_2}})}{P_{I_{O_2}}} \tag{27}$$

Equation (8) can also be rearranged to give

$$P_{A_{N_2}} = \frac{(\dot{V}_I/\dot{Q})P_{I_{N_2}} + \lambda_{N_2}P_{\bar{v}}}{\dot{V}_A/\dot{Q} + \lambda_{N_2}} \tag{28}$$

Using Eqs. (27) and (28) to determine the value assigned to $P_{A_{N_2}}$, the $\dot{V}_A/\dot{Q}$ problem can be reduced to solving Eqs. (7) and (9), which can be put into the following form:

$$(\dot{V}_A/\dot{Q})P_{A_{CO_2}} = k(C_{\bar{v}_{CO_2}} - C_{c'_{CO_2}}) = 0 \tag{29}$$

$$P_B - P_{H_2O} - P_{A_{O_2}} - P_{A_{CO_2}} - P_{A_{N_2}} = 0 \tag{30}$$

For an arbitrary pH and equilibrium oxygen pressure, $P_{A_{O_2}}$ (assuming equilibrium exists) as well as the oxygen and carbon dioxide blood concentrations can be computed by the blood gas subroutines described earlier. Defining functions $F(\text{pH}, P_A)$ and $G(\text{pH}, P_{A_{O_2}})$ to be

$$F(\text{pH}, P_{A_{O_2}}) = (\dot{V}_A/\dot{Q})P_{A_{CO_2}} - k(C_{\bar{v}_{CO_2}} - C_{c'_{CO_2}}) \tag{31}$$

$$G(\text{pH}, P_{A_{O_2}}) = P_B - P_{H_2O} - (P_{A_{O_2}} + P_{A_{N_2}} + P_{A_{N_2}}) \tag{32}$$

where $P_{A_{N_2}}$ is determined by Eq. (28), the problem is to determine the value of pH and $P_{A_{O_2}}$ such that simultaneously

$$F(\text{pH}, P_{A_{O_2}}) = 0 \tag{33}$$

$$G(\text{pH}, P_{A_{O_2}}) = 0 \tag{34}$$

One additional advantage of using this approach is that the analysis of gas exchange in the presence of additional gases can easily be dealt with by using an expression similar to Eq. (28) to compute its partial pressure and then adding the result to the sum in Eq. (32) (Farhi and Olszowka, 1968). Furthermore, if $\dot{V}_I/\dot{Q}$ instead of $\dot{V}_A/\dot{Q}$ is to be treated as the independent variable, the only modification required in the algorithm is to replace Eq. (27) with the following:

$$\dot{V}_A/\dot{Q} = [(\dot{V}_I/\dot{Q})P_{I_{O_2}} - k(C_{c'_{O_2}} - C_{\bar{v}_{O_2}})]/P_{A_{O_2}}$$

To get a feel for the strategy that will choose the trial values for pH and P_{O_2} needed to solve Eqs. (33) and (34), consider Fig. 4A, which contains a three-dimensional plot of the function $F(\text{pH}, P_{O_2})$. The surface representing this function intersects the $\text{pH}-P_{O_2}$ plane along the line labeled $F = 0$. At the points labeled 1, 2, and 3 the function has values corresponding to the first three trial pairs of pH and P_{O_2} values. Extending the principle of the iteration scheme used when only one equation had to be solved (Fig. 3), the curved surface F can be approximated by passing a secant plane labeled F^* through points 1, 2, and 3. This plane surface in turn intersects the $\text{pH}-P_{O_2}$ plane along the straight line labeled $F^* = 0$. Although not shown here, one can also imagine a curved surface representing the function $G(\text{pH}, P_{O_2})$ intersecting the $\text{pH}-P_{O_2}$ plane along a line $G = 0$ and that this surface can also be approximated by a secant plane intersecting the $\text{pH}-P_{O_2}$ plane along a straight line $G^* = 0$. In Fig. 4B, the lines $G = 0$, $G^* = 0$, $F = 0$, and $F^* = 0$ are plotted on a $\text{pH}-P_{O_2}$ axis system. The point where $G = 0$ and $F = 0$ intersect corresponds to the solution of the system defined by Eqs. (33) and (34) and is labeled A. The intersection of the lines $F^* = 0$ and $G^* = 0$ provides the next pair of trial values for pH and P_{O_2} and is labeled A^*. Evaluating F and G at this point and discarding the value of F and G corresponding to one of the other trial values, one can repeat the procedure again and again until both F and G are arbitrarily small.

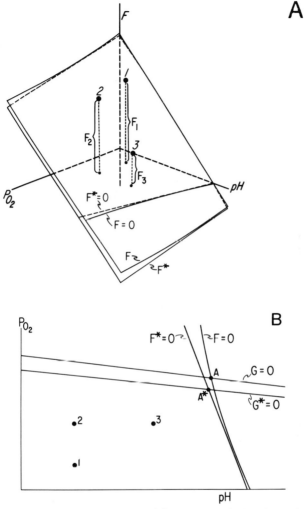

Fig. 4. Graphical description of the use of the secant method to determine trial pH and P_{O_2} values to solve the pair of equations $F(pH, P_{O_2}) = 0$ and $G(pH, P_{O_2}) = 0$. (See text for details.)

To compute each new pair of trial values the following set of calculations must be performed (Ostrowski, 1969):

$$T_1 = F_2 G_3 - G_2 F_3$$

$$T_2 = F_1 G_3 - G_1 F_3$$

$$T_3 = F_1 G_2 - G_1 F_2$$

$$D = T_1 - T_2 + T_3$$

$$\text{pH} = (\text{pH}_1 T_2 - \text{pH}_2 T_2 + \text{pH}_3 T_3)/D \tag{35}$$

$$p_{O_2} = (p_{O_2,} T_2 - P_{O_2,} T_2 + P_{O_2,} T_3)/D \tag{36}$$

The earlier discussion about the possible failure of the algorithm used to solve implicit equations with one unknown also applies to this algorithm. The subroutine that implements it (FINDXY) also uses a similar strategy to minimize the chance of failure, namely, it immediately discards any value of pH and P_{O_2} value not within a preset range. In practice, this is usually determined by physiologic considerations, e.g., 6.8–8.0 for pH and 0 to $P_{I_{O_2}}$ for P_{O_2}.

It must be noted that in using the algorithm described above the first three trial pairs of unknown variables must not be in a straight line. For then planes F^* and G^* would be coplanar and the lines $F^* = 0$ and $G^* = 0$ colinear. The practical effect is that these lines are therefore parallel and intersect at infinity, or in algebraic terms the denominator in Eqs. (35) and (36) would be zero—and most FORTRAN systems would stop the program at the point where those expressions are evaluated.

Iterating both pH and P_{O_2} in the above manner, one can compute the alveolar gas concentrations consistent with a given $\dot{V}_A/\dot{Q}$ and set of inspired and mixed venous gas concentrations without ignoring inert gas exchange. The significance of ignoring that exchange can also be quantitated by comparing the alveolar tensions computed when λ_{N_2} is set to zero with those computed when it is set to its actual value. Such a comparison is shown in Table I, where $P_{A_{O_2}}$ is tabulated for a given set of $\dot{V}_A/\dot{Q}$ values and different inspired oxygen tensions. Note that if room air is inspired, consideration of N_2 exchange has little effect on the oxygen tension computed, but at low $\dot{V}_A/\dot{Q}$ values neglect of such exchange can significantly effect the alveolar $P_{A_{O_2}}$ values computed when oxygen-enriched mixtures are inspired.

One can also iterate pH and P_{O_2} to solve other problems involving blood–gas exchange. For example, given arterial oxygen and carbon dioxide concentrations $C_{a_{O_2}}$ and $C_{a_{CO_2}}$, one can find the corresponding arterial gas tension $P_{a_{O_2}}$ and $P_{a_{CO_2}}$ by iterating pH_a and $P_{a_{O_2}}$ to solve the equations

$$F(\text{pH}_a, P_{a_{O_2}}) = C_{a_{O_2}} - C_{O_2} = 0 \tag{37}$$

$$G(\text{pH}_a, P_{a_{O_2}}) = C_{a_{CO_2}} - C_{CO_2} = 0 \tag{38}$$

where C_{O_2}, C_{CO_2}, and $P_{a_{CO_2}}$ are computed by subroutines GAS1 and GAS2.

5. Behavior of Distributions of Lung Units

The scheme described above for solving the equations that quantify gas exchange in a single unit is especially useful for handling questions that

TABLE I

Effect of N_2 Exchange on Alveolar P_{O_2}

	$P_{A_{O_2}}^{*a}$					
	$F_{I_{O_2}} = 0.21$		$F_{I_{O_2}} = 0.40$		$F_{I_{O_2}} = 0.60$	
$\dot{V}_A/\dot{Q}$	I	II	I	II	I	II
0.00	40.1	40.0	40.8	40.0	43.6	40.0
0.02	41.2	41.1	44.5	43.5	55.0	49.6
0.04	42.3	42.2	48.7	47.5	77.3	65.5
0.06	43.5	43.3	53.6	52.2	127.7	104.5
0.08	44.6	44.5	59.7	57.9	176.7	158.6
0.10	45.9	45.7	67.5	65.3	212.3	199.5
0.15	49.1	48.9	97.8	94.3	266.7	260.6
0.20	52.5	52.4	129.9	127.3	297.0	293.5
0.26	56.3	56.2	153.4	151.7	316.2	314.1
0.30	60.3	60.2	170.5	169.3	329.6	328.1
0.35	64.7	64.5	183.2	182.4	339.5	338.4
0.40	69.2	69.0	193.1	192.5	347.1	346.3

[a] Nitrogen exchange considered in computing $P_{A_{O_2}}$ values in columns I and ignored in computing $P_{A_{O_2}}$ values in columns II. In all cases, $P_{v_{O_2}} = 40$, $P_{v_{CO_2}} = 46$, $P_{v_{N_2}} = P_{I_{N_2}} = 713 - P_{I_{O_2}}$.

deal with a distribution of such units. Consider first the problem posed in Fig. 1A. Given some distribution of lung units, what is the effect on overall gas exchange (e.g., Wagner 1979a, West, 1969–70, 1971)?

Generally, the way such distributions are quantitated are to assign to each respiratory unit an alveolar ventilation–perfusion ratio $(\dot{V}/\dot{Q})_i$ and bloodflow of q_i. Provided that the mixed venous as well as inspired gas composition is known, the oxygen concentrations $C_{c'_{O_{2i}}}$ and carbon dioxide concentrations $C_{c'_{CO_{2i}}}$ in the blood leaving such unit can be determined by solving Eqs. (33) and (34). Then, using the Fick principle, the arterial and oxygen carbon dioxide concentration can be computed using the relationship

$$C_{a_{O_2}} = \Sigma q_i C_{c'_{O_{2i}}} / \Sigma q_i \qquad (39)$$

$$C_{a_{CO_2}} = \Sigma q_i C_{c'_{CO_{2i}}} / \Sigma q_i \qquad (40)$$

and the corresponding arterial gas tensions determined by solving Eqs. (37) and (38). While one can assume that the mixed venous composition is normal and then study the effect that a given distribution has on the arterial gas composition, the venous composition itself depends in part on the $\dot{V}_A/\dot{Q}$ distribution, and is not an independent variable. For if the individual is to survive with a specific $\dot{V}_A/\dot{Q}$ maldistribution, the venous composition has to be such that the transfer of oxygen and carbon dioxide across the lungs match the metabolic needs of the body. If $\dot{V}_{O_2}$ and $\dot{V}_{CO_2}$ represent tissue oxygen consumption and carbon dioxide production, then we may write the following set of implicit equations in $C_{\bar{v}_{O_2}}$ and $C_{\bar{v}_{O_2}}$:

$$U(C_{\bar{v}_{O_2}}, C_{\bar{v}_{O_2}}) = \dot{V}_{O_2} - \Sigma q_i(C_{c'_{O_{2_i}}} - C_{\bar{v}_{O_2}}) \tag{41}$$

$$V(C_{\bar{v}_{O_2}}, C_{\bar{v}_{CO_2}}) = \dot{V}_{CO_2} - \Sigma \dot{q}_i(C_{\bar{v}_{CO_2}} - C_{c'_{CO_{2_i}}}) \tag{42}$$

The sums in both the above expressions represent the oxygen and CO_2 transfer in the lungs and are dependent on $C_{\bar{v}_{O_2}}$ and $C_{\bar{v}_{CO_2}}$ not only because these variables appear explicitly, but also because the blood concentrations $C_{c'_{O_{2_i}}}$ and $C_{c'_{O_{2_i}}}$ in each unit themselves depend on $C_{\bar{v}_{O_2}}$ and $C_{\bar{v}_{CO_2}}$.

To determine the mixed venous composition that satisfies Eqs. (41) and (42) a trial and error approach is necessary. To choose the trial values for $C_{\bar{v}_{O_2}}$ and $C_{\bar{v}_{CO_2}}$ the strategy used in determining the trial value of pH and P_{O_2} to solve Eqs. (33) and (34) is also applicable. The only practical difficulty in implementing that strategy is that most computer languages do not permit recursion. If recursion were permitted, subroutine FINDXY could be used to solve Eqs. (41) and (42), which in order to get the values of $C_{c'_{O_{2_i}}}$ and $C_{c'_{CO_{2_i}}}$ requires the FINDXY be called to solve Eqs. (33) and (34). Since FORTRAN does not permit a subroutine to call itself, a subroutine that, except for its name, is identical in appearance to FINDXY would have to be included in any program that solves Eqs. (41) and (42).

Though we have treated the $\dot{V}_A/\dot{Q}$ distribution as an independent variable in the above discussion, in reality the increase in stimulation of the peripheral and central chemoreceptors that results from the effect of maldistribution of blood composition may lead to a compensatory increase in ventilation.

Indeed, West, using a discrete approximation of the log normal distribution as a model for $\dot{V}_A/\dot{Q}$ maldistribution, explored this matter (West, 1969). The log normal distribution has the form

$$f(\dot{V}/\dot{Q}) = \frac{1}{(2\pi)^{1/2}\sigma} \frac{1}{\dot{V}/\dot{Q}} \exp\{-[\ln(\dot{V}/\dot{Q}) - \ln(\mu)]^2/2\sigma^2\}$$

where $f(\dot{V}/\dot{Q}) \cdot d(\dot{V}/\dot{Q})$ represents the fraction of the total blood flow $\dot{Q}_T$ going to lung units with ventilation–perfusion ratios between $\dot{V}/\dot{Q}$ and $\dot{V}/\dot{Q} + d(\dot{V}/\dot{Q})$. It can formally be shown that

$$\dot{V}_{A_T}/\dot{Q}_T = \mu \exp(\sigma^2/2)$$

where $\dot{V}_{A_T}$ and $\dot{Q}_T$ represent the total alveolar ventilation and lung perfusion. If we assume a value for $\dot{Q}_T$ one can independently model the effect of either changes in total ventilation or maldistribution by varying $\dot{V}_{A_T}$ or

σ. For example, using a specific value of σ to quantitate the degree of maldistribution, one can determine the magnitude of ventilation that will maintain a particular $P_{a_{CO_2}}$ as well as a rate of gas transfer that satisfies the metabolic requirements of the tissues. To solve this problem, it is convenient to treat the $P_{a_{O_2}}$ as the variable that is iterated along with the total alveolar ventilation. For with the specified $P_{a_{CO_2}}$ and trial value of $P_{a_{O_2}}$ one can, with methods described earlier, compute the corresponding arterial concentrations, and in turn by applying the Fick principle determine the mixed venous composition. Then with the given value of σ and $\dot{Q}_T$ as well as the trial value of $\dot{V}_{A_T}$ defining the $\dot{V}_A/\dot{Q}$ distribution, we can, using Eqs. (39) and (40), determine an arterial gas composition that would agree with the values of $C_{a_{O_2}}$ and $C_{a_{CO_2}}$ calculated above, if the trial values of $\dot{V}_{A_T}$ and $P_{a_{O_2}}$ were correct. In effect, solving this problem is equivalent to solving the pair of equations

$$U(P_{a_{O_2}}, \dot{V}_{A_T}) = (\Sigma f_i C_{c'_{O_{2i}}}) - C_{a_{O_2}}$$

$$V(P_{a_{O_2}}, \dot{V}_{A_T}) = (\Sigma f_i C_{c'_{CO_{2i}}}) - C_{a_{CO_2}}$$

where the fractional flows f_i represent a discrete approximation to the log normal distribution and consequently are functions of $\dot{V}_{A_T}$.

Although the variables to be iterated are $P_{a_{O_2}}$ and $\dot{V}_{A_T}$ instead of $C_{\bar{v}_{O_2}}$ and $C_{\bar{v}_{CO_2}}$, the subroutine that solves Eqs. (41) and (42) can be used here also.

Since the overall effect on gas exchange as well as the lung distribution are only partially defined—$P_{a_{O_2}}$ and $\dot{V}_{A_T}$ being unknown—this last application straddles the two major types of problems that deal with overall gas exchange in the lung (Figs. 1A and 1B).

C. Estimation of Distributions from Steady State Gas Exchange Data

Using the algorithms discussed above, calculating the overall effect of a given distribution of lung units ventilating in parallel on the basis of our knowledge of the behavior of a single unit (Fig. 1A) is not difficult. Doing the reverse, i.e., determining the distribution of ventilation and perfusion among those units on the basis of the measured effect of that distribution on gas exchange (Fig. 1B) is another matter. In fact, since the number of respiratory units is very large and the likelihood that they all have the same ventilation–perfusion ratio is small, one can never obtain enough gas exchange data to produce a detailed and unique description of the distribution of ventilation–perfusion ratios among those respiratory units. Nevertheless, two philosophically different approaches that provide partial solutions to this gas exchange problem are available.

1. Measurement of Distributions Characterized by Few (1–3) Parameters

In the first, one assumes that the lung can be represented by a specific $\dot{V}_A/\dot{Q}$ distribution whose parameters—which are relatively few in number—are to be determined. For example, if one assumes that the $\dot{V}_A/\dot{Q}$ distribution is log normal and the cardiac output $\dot{Q}_T$, O_2 consumption $\dot{V}_{O_2}$, CO_2 production $\dot{V}_{CO_2}$, and arterial blood composition are known, then by a sequence of steps similar to those just outlined, $\dot{V}_{A_T}$ and σ can be iterated until the arterial blood composition predicted by the distribution agreed with the measured values.

On the other hand, one is also free to interpret the above set of data in terms of the more familiar Riley model of the lung (Riley and Cournand, 1949). Here, instead of assuming a continuous $\dot{V}_A/\dot{Q}$ distribution, a discrete one representing just three respiratory units or compartments is used. The first is perfused, but not ventilated; the second is both ventilated and perfused; and the third is ventilated, but not perfused. In clinical applications the emphasis is on obtaining the fraction of the cardiac output going to the first compartment, and we do so here also.

Since gas exchange occurs only in the second compartment, it can be assigned the gas exchange ratio of the whole lung. Thus the composition of the blood draining that compartment can be determined by using the computerized version of the graphical method described earlier. In doing so, the only modification required is that Eq. (24) can be replaced by the following:

$$F(\text{pH}) = R - \frac{C_{\bar{v}CO_2} - C_{c'CO_2}}{C_{c'O_2} - C_{\bar{v}O_2}}$$

where $C_{c'O_2}$ and $C_{c'CO_2}$ are the computed concentrations of O_2 and CO_2 in the blood draining the second compartment.

Since no exchange occurs in the blood perfusing the first compartment, the O_2 and CO_2 concentrations in the blood perfusing, they will stay at the mixed venous levels. Applying the Fick principle to oxygen exchange, we may then write

$$\dot{Q}_T C_{a_{O_2}} = \dot{Q}_s C_{\bar{v}_{O_2}} + (\dot{Q}_T - \dot{Q}_s) C_{c'_{O_2}}$$

where $\dot{Q}_T$ and $\dot{Q}_s$ are the respective blood flows through the whole lung and the first compartment. Solving for $\dot{Q}_s/\dot{Q}_T$ gives

$$\dot{Q}_s/\dot{Q}_T = \frac{C_{c'_{O_2}} - C_{a_{O_2}}}{C_{c'_{O_2}} - C_{\bar{v}_{O_2}}}$$

In using such specific continuous distributions or simple compartmental models to represent the lung, two kinds of uncertainty arise: that due to measurement error and that due to uniqueness.

The effect of measurement error can easily be estimated by repeating the calculations outlined above after altering in some systematic fashion the measured cardiac output, arterial gas composition, gas exchange, etc., by amounts dependent on the known measurement error.

Although one can uniquely define the parameters of the above models if the data are error free, or at least precisely bound them if measurement error is considered, there still is an element of nonuniqueness present. For a number of different types of continuous distributions or simple compartmental models which fit the gas exchange data equally as well can always be found (Wagner, 1977a).

In the next section, the other approach to the problem of determining the $\dot{V}_A/\dot{Q}$ distribution in the lung is described. Here, the problem of uniqueness arises not in the choice of model used, for the distribution used is sufficiently general to encompass all possible combinations of respiratory units ventilating in parallel. Instead, the parameters themselves, because they are too numerous, cannot be uniquely determined.

2. Measurement of Multicompartment Distributions

a. Introduction. In contrast to the above approach in which the lung is described by a *small number of parameters* (such as venous admixture or a log normal distribution of a particular dispersion) equal in number to the number of data inputs, the measurement of multicompartment distributions uses a lung model consisting of parameters *whose number greatly exceeds the number of measured variables*. At first sight, this seems irrational since whenever the number of unknowns in a system exceeds the number of data points, no unique solution to the problem is generally obtainable. However, it was pointed out above that such "nonuniqueness" is not confined to the multicompartment approach—it is just as evident in the first kind of approach described, even though it is disguised. In the first approach the parameters of a particular model may be unique, *but the model itself is not*. For example, given a particular arterial and venous P_{O_2}, the calculation of venous admixture gives a unique solution. However, (1) there may be no actual shunt so that the venous admixture calculated really may reflect regions of low $\dot{V}_A/\dot{Q}$, or (2) on the other hand, the venous admixture may indeed reflect true shunt.

The philosophy of the multicompartment approach is to generalize the model to the extent that the problem of model uniqueness is greatly reduced, and to accept some uncertainty about the parameter values obtained. In general, the multicompartment approach exploits a particular set of data more fully than does the approach based on a small number of parameters. The cost of this advantage is that the user of such a method must learn to interpret the result properly, keeping in mind the uncertainty of the determined parameters. Treatment of such uncertainty is covered more completely in Section II on linear programming.

b. Numerical Analytical Techniques for Measurement of Multicompartment Distributions. Suppose we specify a model of the lung consisting of a large number (N) of compartments ventilated and perfused in parallel, each characterized by its own value of ventilation–perfusion ratio, $\dot{V}_A/\dot{Q}_j, j = 1, \ldots, N$. Values for $\dot{V}_A/\dot{Q}$ of 0 and ∞ are fully acceptable for two of these compartments, thus allowing the existence of shunt ($\dot{V}_A/\dot{Q} = 0$) and dead space ($\dot{V}_A/\dot{Q} = \infty$; unperfused lung). As long as N exceeds about 20, its value is of little importance. We generally use $N = 50$ as a compromise between economy in computing and fine discretization of the $\dot{V}_A/\dot{Q}$ domain. Thus 48 compartments having $\dot{V}_A/\dot{Q}$ ratios greater than zero and less than infinity are specified with $\dot{V}_A/\dot{Q}$ values equally spaced on a logarithmic scale. Choice of scale (log, linear, or other) is mostly a matter of convenience. Log scales have long been used (West, 1969) in this setting and appear to be the most appropriate.

The problem involved in determining multicompartment distributions is then to allocate perfusion (and thus ventilation) properly among the various compartments, so as to be compatible with the measured set of data.

The principles outlined in Fig. 1B are applied by equations analogous to Eqs. (39) and (40). Stated in words, the concentration of any gas in mixed arterial blood can be expressed as the perfusion-weighted average of the concentrations of the gas in the individual lung units. Such equations are called mixing equations, and fundamentally are just statements of conservation of matter.

Any gas may be used to exploit equations such as (39) and (40) in order to obtain multicompartment estimates of the $\dot{V}_A/\dot{Q}$ distribution. In principle, the greater the number of gases, the more detailed and precise is the resulting estimate of the $\dot{V}_A/\dot{Q}$ distribution. Inert gases are the tracer gases of choice because (1) many suitable gases are available, chosen on the basis of differing blood: gas partition coefficients λ [Eq. (5)]; (2) the "known behavior of single lung units" exchanging inert gases (Fig. 1B) is particularly simple [Eq. (5)] and is thus well suited to mathematical analysis; (3) they can be fruitfully studied under varying physiologic conditions (such as different $F_{I_{O_2}}$ values) without affecting gas exchange themselves, in contrast to, for example, O_2; and (4) they provide an important basis for detection of incomplete diffusion equilibration of O_2 between alveolar gas and end-capillary blood because of their order of magnitude greater rate of diffusion equilibration (Forster, 1957; Wagner, 1977c).

The appropriate mixing equation for an inert gas is

$$P_a = \sum_{j=1}^{j=N} P_{c'_j} \dot{q}_j \left/ \sum_{j=1}^{j=N} \dot{q}_j \right. \tag{43}$$

where P_a is mixed arterial inert gas tension, $P_{c'_j}$ is end-capillary inert gas tension in compartment j having blood flow $\dot{q}_j$, and N is the number of compartments in the model (usually 50). This is analogous to Eqs. (39) and (40).

Since from Eq. (5), $P_{c'_j} = P_{\bar{v}}[\lambda/(\lambda + \dot{V}_A/\dot{Q}_j)]$ for a gas being eliminated $(P_I = 0)$, Eq. (5) becomes

$$R \equiv \frac{P_a}{P_{\bar{v}}} = \sum_{j=1}^{j=N} \frac{\lambda \dot{q}_j}{(\lambda + \dot{V}_A/\dot{Q}_j)} \left/ \sum_{j=1}^{j=N} \dot{q}_j \right. \tag{44}$$

where $R(\equiv P_a/P_{\bar{v}})$ is termed the retention of the gas.

In fact, if $\dot{q}_j$ is defined as fractional blood flow

$$\sum_{j=1}^{j=N} \dot{q}_j = 1.0$$

and a simpler result appears:

$$R = \sum_{j=1}^{j=N} \frac{\lambda \dot{q}_j}{\lambda + \dot{V}_A/\dot{Q}_j} \tag{45}$$

For the case of $N = 50$, with the specified set of 50 $\dot{V}_A/\dot{Q}$ values and a gas of known λ, Eq. (45) gives a *single equation in* 50 unknowns [actually 49 since $\dot{q}_{50}$ ($\dot{V}_A/\dot{Q} = \infty$) must be zero]. Suitable choice of the set of 49 $\dot{q}_j$ [so as to make the R.H.S. of Eq. (45) equal to the measured value of R] is the task at hand. If such a choice can be made, the plot, compartment by compartment of paired values of $\dot{q}_j$ and $\dot{V}_A/\dot{Q}_j$, gives the desired $\dot{V}_A/\dot{Q}$ distribution.

Clearly, 1 equation in 49 unknowns borders on the absurd, but if several (say six) gases with widely differing blood : gas partition coefficients λ are measured simultaneously, six equations may now be written. Each has the form of Eq. (45), differing only in the values of R and λ in each case. It is important to realize that the set of $\dot{q}_j$ and $\dot{V}_A/\dot{Q}_j$ is common to all six equations, so that this set of six equations constitutes a system of six simultaneous linear equations in 49 unknowns.

Following is an account of how this equation system is solved to give a meaningful $\dot{V}_A/\dot{Q}$ distribution. A complete technical description of the actual algorithm with listing is given in the material deposited with the National Auxiliary Publications Service (NAPS) (see footnote on page 272). That algorithm differs from the following account in one detail, namely, the constraint that in the solution the fractional perfusions $\dot{q}_j$ sum to 1.0. In the listing deposited with NAPS, the use of a Lagrange multiplier for enforcing this constraint is described, but for simplicity this aspect is omitted here to clarify the logic of the solution process.

First, the six equations will be written in matrix notation:

$$\mathbf{R} = A\mathbf{q} \qquad (46)$$

Here, $\mathbf{R}$ is the set ("vector") of six measured retentions; A is the set ("matrix") of alveolar inert gas tensions so that for compartment j ($j = 1, 50$) and gas i ($i = 1, 6$):

$$A_{i,j} = \frac{\lambda_i}{\lambda_i + \dot{V}_A/\dot{Q}_j} \qquad \text{[from Eq. (5)]}$$

and $\mathbf{q}$ is the vector containing the 50 perfusions (49 unknown) of the $\dot{V}_A/\dot{Q}$ compartments.

A least-squares best fit by a set of $\mathbf{q}$ to the retentions $\mathbf{R}$ is then performed. Because of random error in the data, the fit will not in general be perfect so that a residual sum of squares S will exist. This may be expressed in matrix notation as follows:

$$S = \|\mathbf{R} - A\mathbf{q}\|^2 \qquad (47)$$

When S is minimized with respect to $\mathbf{q}$, the least-squares best fit to the data will have been obtained.

For a variety of reasons, we choose to introduce a smoothing parameter Z into this system. Smoothing stabilizes the resulting distribution in the presence of random error; the closeness of fit to the measured data turns out to have useful statistical meaning (Evans and Wagner, 1977); the practical effect of smoothing is to permit useful classifying criteria to be applied to resulting distributions. We have found through rigorous evaluation by linear programming (see Section II) that the smoothed distributions reliably reflect major features of the real $\dot{V}_A/\dot{Q}$ distribution. We do not rationalize the use of smoothing on the argument that real distributions are likely to be smooth functions, even though in many cases this might be a reasonable expectation. Finally, introduction of smoothing greatly facilitates the numerical analytical procedure used to obtain the least-squares solution to Eq. (47).

Smoothing is introduced in a standard manner (Hoerl and Kennard, 1970) by adding to Eq. (47) a term in squared blood flows:

$$S = \|\mathbf{R} - A\mathbf{q}\|^2 + Z\|\mathbf{q}\|^2 \qquad (48)$$

The term Z is a scalar number, the magnitude of which determines the amount of smoothing. Our approach is to use just enough smoothing to stabilize visually the $\dot{V}_A/\dot{Q}$ distributions in the presence of error. Dawson and co-workers, on the other hand, have found a way to set Z objectively to an appropriate value (Dawson *et al.*, 1978), although the application of this concept is not yet widespread.

How the addition of the term in the squared blood flows produces smoothing is illustrated by considering a two-compartment lung having fractional perfusions of $\dot{q}$ and $1 - \dot{q}$: If we write $S = \dot{q}^2 + (1 - \dot{q})^2$, which is the nonmatrix equivalent to the smoothing term in Eq. (48), it is easy to see that S is a parabola with respect to $\dot{q}$, having a single minimum at $\dot{q} = 0.5$. In other words, the sum of squares of the two perfusions is minimized when they are equal. Thus in Eq. (48) the smoothing term tends to equalize the distribution of perfusion among the compartments, a procedure that is equivalent to smoothing.

Returning to Eq. (48), the desired set of $\mathbf{q}$ (i.e., the desired $\dot{V}_A/\dot{Q}$ distribution) is that set which satisfies the requirement that $\partial s/\partial \dot{q} = 0$. This is the least-squares criterion. For each $\dot{q}_j$, S is a parabola with a single minimum [see Eq. (48)]. Thus if $\partial s/\partial \dot{q}$ is simultaneously zero when evaluated for all 50 values of $\mathbf{q}$, these values of $\mathbf{q}$ form the desired distribution. The task is to compute the desired set of $\mathbf{q}$. Appropriate differentiation of Eq. (48) (continuing in matrix notation and setting the derivative to zero) gives

$$A'(\mathbf{R} - A\mathbf{q}) = Z\mathbf{q} \tag{49}$$

where A^t is the transpose of the matrix A.

Now, define the residual

$$\mathbf{r} = \mathbf{R} - A\mathbf{q} \tag{50}$$

This residual $\mathbf{r}$ is by inspection the difference between the data $\mathbf{R}$ and the fit to the data $A\mathbf{q}$.

Substituting (50) into (49) gives

$$A^t\mathbf{r} = Z\mathbf{q} \quad \text{or} \quad \mathbf{q} = A^t\mathbf{r}/Z \tag{51}$$

and substitution of (51) into (50) gives

$$\mathbf{r} = \mathbf{R} - (AA^t\mathbf{r}/Z) \quad \text{or} \quad \mathbf{r}[I + (AA^t/Z)] = \mathbf{R} \tag{52}$$

where I is the identity matrix.

Notice that Eq. (49) contains the vector $\mathbf{q}$ consisting of 49 unknowns, but that Eq. (52), expressing the identical relationships, contains the vector $\mathbf{r}$ consisting of only six unknowns. In fact, this substitution of $\mathbf{r}$ for $\mathbf{q}$ has transformed the system into a simple set of six simultaneous linear equations in six unknowns, $\mathbf{r}$ (I, Z, A^t, A, and R are all known). Thus the problem is identical in nature to that of the two equations in two unknowns described in Eqs. (10) and (11), and the simple method of solution by elimination of variables described in the text accompanying these equations is directly applicable.

Therefore, the entire problem of finding a $\dot{V}_A/\dot{Q}$ distribution compatible with a given set of inert gas retention comes down to a straightforward task of solution of six simultaneous equations in six unknowns. Once the six unknown $\mathbf{r}$'s are computed, the 49 unknown values of q are directly calculated from Eq. (51).

There is, however, one remaining aspect of the problem so far neglected: the *positivity constraint*. In other words, the set of 49 values of $\mathbf{q}$ so determined are only acceptable if all are greater than or equal to zero. Notice that this is a physiological rather than a mathematical requirement, and it raises a concept of fundamental importance—application of mathematical methods in physiology must be done in a manner allowing both mathematical and physiological constraints to be incorporated, or else the efforts may be in vain. The importance of the positivity constraint is well documented in the present application (Pimmel *et al.*, 1977).

Enforcement of the positivity constraint is the most difficult part of the entire least-squares analysis. It is done by a trial and error procedure, an outline of which follows.

In essence, Eq. (52) is solved for $\mathbf{r}$ as described above, but repetitively using different subsets of the original 50 compartments each iteration. In Eq. (52), this means that AA^t changes with each iteration since different subsets of $A_{i,j}$ are used each time. With each iteration, however, the data (R) and the value of Z are kept constant. Choice of subset is made according to the following logic (described in technical detail in the deposited material):

Step a: Solve Eq. (52) using all 50 compartments in the calculation of AA^t. Calculate $\dot{Q}_j$, $j = 1, \ldots, 50$, from Eq. (51).

Step b: Inspect the solution $\dot{q}_j$, $j = 1, \ldots, 50$. If all $\dot{q}_j \geq 0$, the problem has been solved and the program ends. If for at least one compartment k, $\dot{q}_k < 0$, the algorithm proceeds to step c.

Step c: Discard (temporarily) compartments with $\dot{q} < 0$, reducing the number of compartments, to say M, and hence altering the matrix AA^t. Proceed to step d.

Step d: Using just this number of compartments, solve Eq. (52) completely anew for $\mathbf{r}$, and then (51) for $\dot{q}$. Proceed to step e.

Step e: Inspect the solution $\dot{q}_j$, $j = 1, \ldots, M$ ($M < 50$). If any of the $\dot{q}_j \leq 0$, go to step c. However, if all of the compartments now have $\dot{q}_j \geq 0$, $j = 1, \ldots, M$, go to step f.

Step f: For each of the compartments discarded in the above process, evaluate $\partial s/\partial \dot{q}_j$ at $\dot{q}_j = 0$, one compartment at a time using the differential of Eq. (48). Locate which compartments *if any* are associated with a *negative* value of $\partial s/\partial \dot{q}$. Any one such compartment would lead to a smaller sum of squares if reintroduced into the system and given the appropriate positive value of $\dot{q}$; this is the meaning of a negative derivative $\partial s/\partial \dot{q}$. Expand the number of compartments (M from step e) to include such compartments and proceed to step d. If, however, $\partial s/\partial \dot{q}$ (at $\dot{q} = 0$) for all discarded compartments ≥ 0, reintroduction of such compartments would only worsen the fit, so that the problem is now finished.

In this manner, not only is the least-squares criterion met, but also the solution contains only nonnegative compartmental bloodflows.

An important practical point in the proper execution of this approach concerns weighting factors. Two kinds of weighting are used. The first accounts for differences in the variance of retention **R** among the six gases, and thus weights the six equations each relative to the other. The second is a compartmental weight designed to provide uniform smoothing over the whole $\dot{V}_A/\dot{Q}$ range. These weights appear in the algorithm (deposited with NAPS) and are described in more detail elsewhere (Evans and Wagner, 1977).

We generally couple the algorithms described for least-squares analysis of inert gas retentions with algorithms presented earlier in this chapter, which compute overall O_2 and CO_2 exchange based on the derived distribution and associated data concerning mixed venous and inspired P_{O_2} and P_{CO_2}. In this way, a value of arterial P_{O_2} can be computed ("predicted" P_{O_2}) and compared to actual arterial P_{O_2} values as measured. Systematic differences between the two with the measured P_{O_2} being less than the predicted value strongly suggest failure of diffusion equilibration between alveolar gas and end-capillary blood (Wagner, 1977c). Such differences have been found only rarely, even in advanced pulmonary disease (Wagner, 1977b; Wagner et al., 1977).

II. LINEAR PROGRAMMING IN PULMONARY GAS EXCHANGE

A. Introduction

The previous section dealt with the question of analysis of real data in various ways so as to come up with a distribution of lung units compatible with a given set of data. Implicit in these types of approaches is the understanding that more than one distribution of lung units is generally compatible with a given set of data. Thus the result obtained is one of many compatible distributions and its interpretation is consequently limited. On the other hand, the methods described do not require extensive computer time and can provide exceedingly useful qualitative and quantitative information in research and in clinical situations.

This section describes an approach that is complementary to those mentioned above and is based on a numerical analytical procedure known as linear programming. This approach is used to investigate the variation within the many distributions compatible with a given set of data. By examining the extent of this variability, one can make rigorous statements about those features of a distribution which can be defined, and to what extent this can be done. Thus linear programming is a tool which can examine a set of data and provide the information upon which is based the interpretation of single distributions obtained with the previously described approaches. Its disadvantage is the lengthy nature of the computations (because of their repetitiveness), which makes the approach impractical on a day-to-day basis. For example, the least-squares analysis of inert gas retention data takes 2 sec on a Burroughs 6700 computer, but on the same machine, a full linear programming evaluation of these data (taking account of error) takes more than 30 min. Thus linear programming is usually reserved for occasional analysis of data when specific questions concerning interpretation of distributions obtained from least-squares analysis arise.

Two kinds of questions have to date been investigated by linear programming. The first is that of computing the absolute upper bound on compatible distributions. The second is that of determining whether a single population of lung units (that is, a *unimodal distribution*) is compatible with the data or whether the distribution contains more than one mode. Each of these problems and their solutions by linear programming will now be explained.

B. Absolute Upper Bounds on Compatible Distributions

To illustrate the meaning of this term, consider a distribution determined from a set of inert gas retention data by a least squares approach in which 5% of the cardiac output is found in lung units with a ventilation–perfusion ratio of 0.1. The issue addressed here is the following: Is 5% the greatest amount of blood flow that could be present in units of $\dot{V}_A/\dot{Q} = 0.1$, or is there another distribution also compatible with the data in which 10% or even 20% (etc.) of the cardiac output is associated with units of $\dot{V}_A/\dot{Q} = 0.1$? In other words, what is the greatest possible fraction of cardiac output that could perfuse units of $\dot{V}_A/\dot{Q} = 0.1$? The greatest possible perfusion of such a unit is referred to here as the absolute upper bound. Linear programming will provide the value of this absolute upper bound. This is a powerful approach because no other distribution whatsoever can still fit the original data and have more perfusion in units of $\dot{V}_A/\dot{Q} = 0.1$.

Suppose in a particular instance the absolute upper bound was 20% of the cardiac output in units of $\dot{V}_A/\dot{Q} = 0.1$. The linear program not only determines this value, but simultaneously decrees the way in which the remaining 80% of the blood flow *must* be distributed to the other lung units in order that this maximum of 20% can occur.

Running the linear program once will give the absolute upper bound on the blood flow for lung units of, in the above example, $\dot{V}_A/\dot{Q} = 0.1$. Running it a second time (*de novo*) will permit the (independent) absolute upper bound on perfusion to be determined for another lung unit of any one desired $\dot{V}_A/\dot{Q}$. Continued independent repetitive execution of the program using a given data set will result in the absolute upper bound perfusion for as many $\dot{V}_A/\dot{Q}$ values as desired.

The interpretation of the absolute upper bound is generally straightforward. If for a given lung unit of specified $\dot{V}_A/\dot{Q}$ the bound is low (say less than 1–2% of the cardiac output), then for physiologic purposes there can be essentially no such lung units present in the lung under study. Conversely, regions of $\dot{V}_A/\dot{Q}$ spectrum in which the upper bound is high are regions that could have large amounts of perfusion. A good example of the application of these principles is given in (Wagner et al., 1977).

Linear programs for calculation of absolute upper bounds are extremely general in their application. Within the realm of pulmonary gas exchange, almost identical computer codes will determine (1) the absolute upper bound ventilation for lung units of various ratios of ventilation to volume in the multibreath N_2 wash-out test (Wagner, 1979b); (2) the absolute upper bound perfusion in lung units of different ventilation–perfusion ratios based on data consisting of the arterial P_{O_2} at various levels of inspired P_{O_2}; and (3) the absolute upper bound perfusion in lung units of different ventilation–perfusion ratios based on data consisting of inert gas retentions for several gases (Evans and Wagner, 1977), to name the three most common situations where the approaches might be used.

The principles of linear programming are best illustrated geometrically. This illustration will be based on the multibreath N_2 wash-out, but the principles are identical for other situations such as those mentioned above. To use linear programming effectively, the spectrum of ventilation/volume ratios from zero to infinity is specified by a representative sampling of values equally spaced between reasonable physiological bounds (0.005–100) on a logarithmic scale. We generally work with some

50 such values, but both the bounds and number of values can be altered at will. Many N_2 wash-outs concentrate on the first 20 or so breaths, so the problem in practice generates a "matrix" of lung units × breaths of respective dimension (50 × 20). Again, a greater number of breaths can be analyzed. While effective use of linear programming does, in fact, involve these dimensions, it is clearly impossible to illustrate geometrically the approach with more than three ventilation/volume ratio "compartments" since the geometric representation of each different compartment corresponds to an axis. Even so, with three compartments, the representation must be three dimensional.

The premise behind linear programming is that there are in principle more potential compartments (50) than pieces of information (20 breaths; 50 > 20). Since nobody can know how many actual lung units of definable ventilation/volume ratio are present in any given case, and since there are millions of alveoli in the lung, the potential number of units is enormous and much greater than the relatively small number of breaths that are measured. Thus in the geometric example of three specified lung units we shall examine what happens when there are only two "pieces" of data available. One of these pieces of data is simply the constraint that the fractional ventilations of the three specified compartments add up to 1.0. The other is the mixed expired N_2 concentration at the end of the first breath of the multibreath wash-out. Any other one breath of the wash-out could equally well have been chosen.

For this example, we specify three lung units only be present, having ventilation/volume ratios of 0.02, 0.2, and 2.0 liters/breath per liter, respectively. Suppose that prior to the wash-out, each unit has a N_2 concentration of 1.0 units and that the mixed expired N_2 concentration after the first breath is 0.6771 in the same arbitrary unit. In keeping with the concepts presented in Section I,A (see Fig. 1B), we need first to examine the predictable wash-out behavior of the three lung units. If the ventilation/volume ratio is designated $\dot{V}_A/VOL$, then the individual unit N_2 concentration after the nth breath, $C_{(N)}$, is given by

$$C_{(N)} = \left(\frac{1}{1 + \dot{V}_A/VOL}\right)^{+N} \tag{53}$$

This formula is based on simple dilution and is well known as the basis of the many approaches to studying the N_2 wash-out.

For the current example, $N = 1$, and $\dot{V}_A/VOL = 0.02, 0.2$, and 2.0, so that for three compartments

$$C_1 = 0.980, \quad 0.833, \quad 0.333$$

respectively. If $\dot{V}_{A_1}$, $\dot{V}_{A_2}$ and $\dot{V}_{A_3}$ are, respectively, the three compartmental ventilations (in fractional terms), Eqs. (54) and (55) embody the two "pieces" of data for this example:

$$(0.980\,\dot{V}_{A_1}) + (0.833\,\dot{V}_{A_2}) + (0.333\,\dot{V}_{A_3}) = 0.6771 \tag{54}$$

$$\dot{V}_{A_1} + \dot{V}_{A_2} + \dot{V}_{A_3} = 1.0 \tag{55}$$

With one more compartment than equation, an infinitely large set of values of $\dot{V}_{A_1}$, $\dot{V}_{A_2}$, and $\dot{V}_{A_3}$ can be found to satisfy the above two equations, even when the additional implicit positivity constraint is enforced. This constraint reflects the physiological requirement that none of the compartmental ventilations are negative.

Equations (54) and (55) can be represented graphically in a three-dimensional diagram in which the unknowns $\dot{V}_{A_1}$, $\dot{V}_{A_2}$, and $\dot{V}_{A_3}$ form the axes (Fig. 5). Equation (54) is that of a plane which when limited to the positive domain is given by the triangle ABC. The solution to Eqs. (54) and (55), (that is, the set of values of $\dot{V}_{A_1}$, $\dot{V}_{A_2}$, and $\dot{V}_{A_3}$ that satisfy both equations simultaneously) is given geometrically in Fig. 5 by the straight-line interval H–I. In other words, all sets of values lying along that line are equally correct solutions to the two N_2 wash-out Eqs. (54) and (55).

So far, all that has been described is the graphical solution to Eqs. (54) and (55) without reference to the absolute upper bounds on compartmental ventilation that are given by linear programming. Recall that the absolute upper bound is just the maximum possible ventilation of the specified $\dot{V}_A/VOL$ compartments still compatible with the given data (known more generally as "constraints" than "data"). Inspection of Fig. 5 and of the straight-line interval H–I in particular, reveals that the maximum value of $\dot{V}_{A_1}$ must occur at the *end point* I of the interval H–I. Maximum value of $\dot{V}_{A_3}$ also occurs at I, while the maximum value of $\dot{V}_{A_2}$ occurs at the other end of the interval at point H. That these *are* the respective maximum compatible (or absolute upper bound) ventilations is evident just from inspection of the interval H–I when it is remembered that H–I is a *straight line*.

Linear programming is the generic name of the mathematical procedure that exploits the concept just described, finding in essence the end points of intervals as in Fig. 5. Note that in Fig. 5 that the maximum of all three ventilations occurs at the interval end points, but to know which end requires a search of the various end points and comparison of the values at the end point. There will always be one end point that gives the maximum value as in the example discussed. Thus the algorithm in common usage (the simplex algorithm of Dantzig) (Dantzig, 1963) looks through such "end points" until the end point coinciding with maximal ventilation is found. Unlike the geometric illustration, the algorithm (which has been

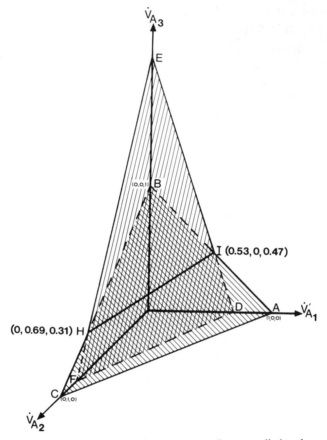

Fig. 5. Geometric representation of linear programming as applied to the multibreath N_2 wash-out. The analysis assumes that three compartments (with ventilations $\dot{V}_{A_1}$, $\dot{V}_{A_2}$, and $\dot{V}_{A_3}$) make up the lung, and that the sum of these ventilations is 1.0. The nitrogen wash-out data in this example come from the expired nitrogen concentration at the end of the first breath. The requirement that the ventilations sum to 1 results in the plane ABC. The requirement that the mixed expired concentration at the end of the first breath match the measured value (given the ventilation/volume ratios of the three compartments) results in plane DEF (see text for more details). The interval H–I, the line of intersection of the two planes within the positive octant, represents all possible compartmental ventilations that satisfy both of the above requirements. End points H and I give maximum possible ventilation in each of the three compartments. Linear programming is a method for evaluating such end points for any number of dimensions.

deposited with NAPS) is not limited to three compartments and two constraints. In some engineering applications, there are literally thousands of
compartments and constraints.

The description of linear programming given above has used data that
are completely free of error. In the real world, experimental error is ines-
capable, and for linear programming to be useful in analysis of real data,
some allowance for error must be made. Returning to Fig. 5, and Eqs. (54)
and (55), if the measured mixed expired N_2 concentrations were recorded
erroneously as 0.65 rather than the true value of 0.6771, the plane DEF
defined by Eq. (54) would be displaced and would intersect along a different interval (say, H'–I') than the correct interval H–I. It is clear that
the greater error in measured mixed expired N_2 concentration, the greater
the difference between the intervals H–I and H'–I', and in particular, the
greater the differences in the coordinates of H, H', and I, I' that give the
maximum possible compartmental ventilations.

Thus the value of the calculated upper bound ventilation will depend on
the magnitude and direction of experimental error. In the present example, if the variance of the measurement of mixed expired N_2 concentration is known, a library of values of this concentration can be calculated
by repeatedly adding random error of that variance to the experimental
value. This procedure, called a Monte Carlo simulation, will statistically
sample mixed expired N_2 levels that through random error could have
given rise to the actual measured value. For each set used in the library,
intervals H–I can be constructed and the corresponding values of maximum ventilation of a specific compartment determined. The mean and
standard deviation of this set of maximum values describe in a complete
statistical manner the absolute upper bound on compartmental ventilation, allowing for experimental error.

There is one problem with this approach, however. Consider the plane
DEF if the error in mixed expired N_2 concentration were very large, so
that the measured mixed expired N_2 concentration were 0.20 (instead of
0.6771). In this example, the planes ABC and DEF do not intersect in the
positive domain. In other words, no combination of values of $\dot{V}_{A_1}$, $\dot{V}_{A_2}$,
and $\dot{V}_{A_3}$, which are all positive, can be found to satisfy Eqs. (54) and (55).
It is therefore concluded that allowance for error can only be made in the
present scheme if the error is sufficiently small that the planes do intersect
in the positive domain of Fig. 5. In Fig. 5, quite large errors in measured
N_2 concentrations could occur and still permit intersection in the positive
domain (that is, provide a *feasible solution*). This is because of the low di-
mensionality of the problem—three compartments and two equations. In
the appropriate physiologic setting, the number of equations equals the
number of breaths followed and could reach 75–100 (5–7 min). The

chances of now obtaining a feasible solution when there is even a very small amount of error become very small. Thus in these highly dimensioned cases, not only is the Monte Carlo simulation an impractical device for examining effects of error, but also there is no currently feasible approach to this difficult problem.

C. Linear Programming in the Evaluation of the Minimum Number of Modes in a Distribution

A slightly different linear program to that described above can be used to determine whether for a particular set of error-free data a unimodal distribution will fit those data. If the answer is yes, the data could also be compatible with more than one mode, but only one mode is necessary to explain the results. On the other hand, if the answer is no, it may be concluded that more than one population of units must exist in order to explain the data. This issue is perceived as fundamental to the interpretation of distributions obtained using least-squares approaches discussed earlier since important mechanistic interpretations depend on such concepts.

The principles of using a linear program to test the unimodality are now given. First, recall (from the earlier description of the use of linear programming in determining upper bounds on distributions) that an important step is to determine feasibility. That is, the planes of Fig. 5 must intersect in the positive domain for physiologically feasible and meaningful results. If they do, the process is feasible; if not, it is infeasible. Once feasibility is established, the upper bounds can be calculated as described. In the unimodality evaluation, we are only concerned with the feasibility portion of the analysis. In other words, do the appropriate planes of Fig. 5 intersect in the positive domain or not? If so, a unimodal distribution will be compatible with the data; if not, then more than one population of units must exist.

The issue here, therefore, is how to build the unimodal requirement into a linear program. Figure 6A shows a unimodal distribution of ventilation (ordinate) as a function of ventilation/volume ratio (abscissa) as might be obtained from a multibreath N_2 wash-out. The cardinal feature of unimodality is a single maximum P from which compartmental ventilations decrease monotonically away from P on either side. Compartmental fractional ventilations $\dot{V}_{1-9}$ in Fig. 6A are all greater than 0. The distribution in Fig. 6A is related to the N_2 wash-out by the well-known expression

$$C_N = \dot{V}_1 C_{1,N} + \dot{V}_2 C_{2,N} + \cdots + \dot{V}_9 C_{9,N} \tag{56}$$

where from Eq. (53)

$$C_{j,N} = \left(\frac{1}{1 + \dot{V}_A/VOL_j}\right)^{+N}$$

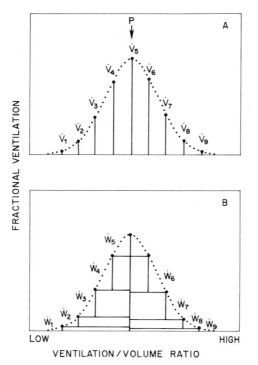

Fig. 6. Determination of minimum number of modes in a distribution. Compartmental ventilations ($\dot{V}_1 - \dot{V}_9$) (A) are replaced by incremental ventilations ($\dot{W}_1 - \dot{W}_9$) (B). This simple reformulation of the linear program allows the modality issue to be resolved (see text for further details).

[Recall that Eq. (54) is a specific example of (56) for just three compartments.] Turning to Fig. 6B, Eq. (56) can be reexpressed in terms of the *increments* in ventilation $\dot{W}_{1-9}$. Equation (56) becomes

$$C_N = \dot{W}_1 C_{1,N} + (\dot{W}_1 + \dot{W}_2)C_{2,N}$$
$$+ (\dot{W}_1 + \dot{W}_2 + \dot{W}_3)C_{3,N} + \cdots + (\dot{W}_8 + \dot{W}_9)C_{8,N} + \dot{W}_9 C_{9,N}$$

Terms in $\dot{W}_1$, $\dot{W}_2$, etc., are collected:

$$C_N = \dot{W}_1 \sum_{i=1}^{i=5} C_{i,N} + \dot{W}_2 \sum_{i=2}^{i=5} C_{i,N}$$
$$+ \dot{W}_3 \sum_{i=3}^{i=5} C_{i,N} + \cdots + \dot{W}_8 \sum_{i=6}^{i=8} + \dot{W}_9 \sum_{i=6}^{i=9} C_{i,N} \tag{57}$$

In this way, the nine ventilations $\dot{V}_{1-9}$ are replaced by the nine increments $\dot{W}_{1-9}$.

It is this reformulated version of Eq. (56) where the compartmental ventilations $\dot{V}_j$ have been replaced by incremental ventilations $\dot{W}_j$ that is now analyzed for feasibility by linear programming. The fundamental concept is that feasibility implies existence of a distribution with *all-positive increments* $\dot{W}_j$. Then, since $\dot{W}_j \geq 0$, the distribution of ventilation $\dot{V}_j$ *must* be unimodal, as can be appreciated from inspection of Fig. 6B.

Implementation of the test of unimodality thus requires only a minor modification of the fundamental program code — replacement of compartmental ventilations by incremental values. One issue remains, however. In order to execute this replacement, some choice of the $\dot{V}_A/VOL$ ratio for the peak P (Fig. 6A) has to be made, and the result of the unimodal test pertains only to this choice of P. To complete the analysis, the location of P must therefore be varied up and down the $\dot{V}_A/VOL$ axis. It is only after P has been moved over the entire extent of the $\dot{V}_A/VOL$ axis with no feasible result at any of the locations that one may conclude that a unimodal distribution is incompatible with the data.

Finally, the practicality of this test must be discussed. Its usefulness parallels that of the first linear program used for explaining upper bounds — it requires error-free data and can be coupled to the Monte Carlo simulations under the same conditions. Thus the same data analyzed for upper bounds can be separately analyzed for unimodality. As with the upper bound analysis, its practicality is limited when many real data points are collected because of the failure of the Monte Carlo approach under these conditions, but for small numbers of measurements, real error-containing data can be analyzed by the inclusion of the Monte Carlo simulation (Evans and Wagner, 1977).

D. Other Formulations of the Linear Program

The two applications of linear programming described above constitute the most general and informative analyses. However, it is quite feasible to pose other questions if desired. Thus relatively minor modifications would allow upper bounds to be determined on the cumulative distribution (of ventilation in the N_2 wash-out test, for example). Another question might be to determine the upper bound on ventilation of a string of adjacent units lumped together in a particular manner (e.g., a log-normal mode) as opposed to what we have illustrated, namely, upper bounds on ventilation of a single unit. A third question might be to determine feasibility of *excluding* certain regions of the $\dot{V}_A/VOL$ domain altogether. In other words, can a particular range of $\dot{V}_A/VOL$ ratios be absent from a distribution, or must there be some ventilation in this range?

E. Summary

Linear programming is thus a practical and useful technique for evaluating variability among distributions compatible with any given set of error-free data obtained from any of several different kinds of tests. Its basis is well established in spheres of mathematics and industry. In systems containing relatively few data points (less than about 10) such as the steady state inert gas elimination technique, linear programming can be combined with statistical methods (Monte Carlo simulation), which allows the effects of random errors in the data to be included. This makes the analysis appropriate for real data. Because these kinds of statistical approaches become impractical when there are many data points, linear programming approaches are currently only useful in such cases for the analysis of error-free data.

Many questions may be posed within the framework of linear programming. A major conclusion from work already done using these techniques is that the definability of important physiological features of a distribution depends on the particular set of data being analyzed (Evans and Wagner, 1977; Wagner, 1977a). This prevents general statements from being made concerning the potential resolution (or lack of resolution) of a particular test and emphasizes the need for individual analysis of data before such conclusions are reached. A second major conclusion is that in several of the currently used tests of distributions of ventilation and blood flow, the more traditional two- or three-compartment analyses of the data do not make the most use of the information available. Two- or three-compartment analyses do not give information about definable features of a distribution such as shape or number of modes—the use of linear programming does offer this possibility.

III. NONSTEADY STATE GAS EXCHANGE

A feature common to all of the preceding discussion is that the governing equations are steady state expressions and do not require integration using calculus for their solution. However, there exists a class of problems in respiratory physiology where the appropriate expressions to be solved are differential equations. Such equations do require integration for their solution. Common physiological situations requiring these procedures include (1) the modeling of tidal breathing (and rebreathing) as an inspiration–expiration process, and (2) the modeling of diffusion processes within the lung.

To illustrate the numerical analytical principles and procedures that are appropriate in these cases, an example of diffusion of gases between alveolar gas and capillary blood will be given. In keeping with tradition, the following simplifying assumptions are made. The lung unit has a well-mixed alveolar gas phase, a homogeneous blood gas barrier, and a capillary in which blood is flowing uniformly with no axial diffusion permitted. Consider a gas that is being taken up by the blood so that alveolar partial pressure P_A exceeds venous partial pressure $P_{\bar{v}}$. Then, as a small element of blood moves along the capillary, gas will diffuse into the blood from alveolar gas so that the partial pressure in the blood rises from $P_{\bar{v}}$ at time 0 to some value approaching P_A by the end of the capillary transit.

The problem is to determine how quickly gas is transferred into the blood, what the partial pressure–time profile looks like, and whether diffusion equilibrium exists such that at the end of the capillary there is no alveolar–end-capillary partial pressure difference.

The appropriate equation under the simplifying assumptions stated above is

$$\dot{V}_{gas(t)} = D[P_A - P_{(t)}] \tag{58}$$

This equation expresses Ficks' first law of diffusion and states that the instantaneous net flux of gas ($\dot{V}_{gas(t)}$) into the blood at time t, is proportional to the instantaneous partial pressure difference between the blood ($P_{(t)}$) and the alveolar gas (P_A). The constant D is the conductance of the system and is itself a complicated term composed of many variables (Forster, 1957; Wagner, 1977c). For inert gases, D is reasonably assumed to be constant in time, but for O_2, CO_2, and CO, D, in fact, varies with time. This is because one element of the "diffusion" resistance is chemical reaction (Roughton and Forster, 1957), the rates of which depend on the instantaneous partial pressures of these gases (Staub et al., 1962), which in turn are varying with time.

Equation (58) is a differential equation whose successful solution will answer the questions posed above. However, little can be achieved with this expression without further simplification. Consider the term $\dot{V}_{gas(t)}$. This is the net flux, say in milliliters of gas per minute at time (t). Since the gas in question is transported in the blood in physical solution (and, in some cases, chemically bound forms), $\dot{V}_{gas(t)}$ can be expressed in terms of the concentration of the gas in the blood at time (t):

$$\dot{V}_{gas(t)} = \frac{V_c}{100} \frac{dC_{(t)}}{dt} \tag{59}$$

where $C_{(t)}$ is the instantaneous concentration of the gas in the blood, ml/100 ml, and V_c is the capillary blood volume in ml. Equation (58) can now be written

$$\frac{dC_{(t)}}{dt} = \frac{100}{V_c} D[P_A - P_{(t)}] \tag{60}$$

Now the elements of Eq. (60) can be examined. The variables D, V_c, and P_A must have known values that can be inserted into (60). This equation then simply relates the rate of change of content $C_{(t)}$ to partial pressure $P_{(t)}$. However, content and partial pressure are related by the dissociation curve of the gas in question, so that knowledge of $P_{(t)}$ implies knowledge of $C_{(t)}$ and vice versa.

Two mathematical possibilities now arise. First, if the dissociation curve is suitably simple, e.g., as for an inert gas where $C_{(t)} = \beta P_{(t)}$, β being the (constant) solubility of the gas in blood, Eq. (60) can be directly integrated:

$$\frac{dC_{(t)}}{dt} = \beta \frac{dP_{(t)}}{dt} = \frac{100}{V_c} D(P_A - P_{(t)})$$

and by rearranging terms,

$$\frac{dP_{(t)}}{P_A - P_{(t)}} = \frac{100}{V_c} \frac{D}{\beta} dt \tag{61}$$

Direct integration of (61) is straightforward:

$$-\ln(P_A - P_{(t)}) = \frac{100}{V_c} \frac{D}{\beta} + K \tag{62}$$

where K is the constant of integration and is determined from the initial conditions knowing that when $t = 0$, $P_{(t)} = P_{\bar{v}}$. Thus from Eq. (62),

$$-\ln(P_A - P_{\bar{v}}) = K$$

Incorporating this result into Eq. (62),

$$-\ln(P_A - P_{(t)}) + \ln(P_A - P_{\bar{v}}) = \frac{100}{V_c} \frac{D}{\beta} t \tag{63}$$

Numerical evaluation of (63) for the given choice of P_A, $P_{\bar{v}}$, V_c, D, and β at various times t gives the required partial pressure time course of diffusion equilibration. Direct substitution also allows calculation of the length of time to achieve any desired degree of equilibration.

The second possibility stemming from Eq. (60) occurs when the relationship between content $C_{(t)}$ and partial pressure $P_{(t)}$ is sufficiently complex that direct integration of (60) is not feasible. This is the case for O_2,

CO_2, and CO. In such cases, it is possible to obtain the same information as in the more direct case [Eq. (63)], but a more cumbersome approach is required—the integration of Eq. (60) is performed numerically by what is generally known as a stepwise forward integration procedure. Two methods are discussed here, namely, Euler's method and the fourth-order Runge–Kutta procedure (Scheid, 1968), the latter being just a more sophisticated extension of the former.

To use Euler's method in Eq. (60) the derivative term $dC_{(t)}/dt$ is replaced by an approximation $\Delta C_{(t)}/\Delta t$. In other words, instead of using the true time derivative at any time t, the average slope of $C_{(t)}$ over a small finite time interval Δt is used. It should be immediately apparent that the greater the curvature in $C_{(t)}$, the smaller the time interval Δt must be to reflect accurately the derivative. Equation (60) then becomes

$$\Delta C_{(t)} = \frac{100}{V_c} D(P_A - P_{(t)}) \, \Delta t \qquad (64)$$

One begins at the point where $t = 0$, $P(t) = P_{\bar{v}}$, and $C_{(t)} = C_{\bar{v}}$, the venous content of the gas in question. Thus the initial calculation begins at the venous point and computes by (64) an approximate increment in content that will occur over the small interval Δt, the content is now

$$C_{(\Delta t)} = C_{\bar{v}} + \frac{100}{V_c} D(P_A - P_{\bar{v}}) \, \Delta t$$

Next, knowing the dissociation curve, this increment in content is used to calculate the corresponding increment in partial pressure. Equation (64) is now reevaluated over a *second* interval Δt, substituting this new partial pressure into the equation and subsequently calculating the new increment in content from Eq. (64). This procedure is repeated until the allocated total transit time is reached (summing all the Δt values).

Euler's method is well suited to the digital computer, but it is important to determine the optimal time interval Δt. If Δt is chosen too large, the numerical result will be in error; if Δt is taken to be too small, unnecessary computer time is wasted. The appropriate time interval is usually found by trial and error, beginning with a large value and decreasing it (say, by factors of 2) until the time course profile does not change with further reductions in Δt.

In Euler's method, the increment in content is determined simply from Eq. (64), as stated. The fourth-order Runge–Kutta method is more often used on the grounds that a more accurate time course can be obtained without the need for excessively small time steps. It calculates four different slopes over the time interval Δt (Scheid, 1968) and uses a weighted

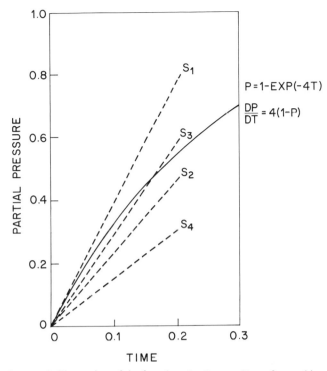

Fig. 7. Geometric illustration of the fourth-order Runge–Kutta forward integration procedure. Refer to Table II and the text. The solid curved line is the function to be approximated $P = 1 - \exp(-4t)$. Dashed lines S1–S4 represent for four slopes used in the forward integration.

average of these from which to calculate the content increment. Details of these slopes appear in textbooks of numerical analyses (such as in Scheid, 1968), and an example is given in Fig. 7 and Table II. This procedure is particularly useful when more than one gas is exchanging and when these gases interact, as is the case for O_2 and CO_2 (Hill *et al.*, 1973; Wagner and West, 1972).

Finally, for sufficiently small time intervals (in which the slope of the dissociation curve can be assumed to be constant throughout), an alternative to the numerical approach just discussed is to determine the slope of the dissociation curve, and directly integrate Eq. (66) as in Eqs. (61)–(63). This is in essence no different from Euler's method, but it does allow one to determine intermediate points in any such time interval without the further need for the time-consuming analysis required in the Euler method. As with Euler's method, the result is only as good as the assumption of a dissociation curve of constant slope throughout the time interval.

TABLE II

Example of Scheme for Fourth-Order Runge–Kutta Procedure[a]

Step	Instruction	Slope $(dP/dt) = 4(1 - P)$	$\Delta P = 0.2(dP/dt)$
1	Calculate slope S_1 at $P = 0$ from function expression	4.000 ⟶	0.800
2	Calculate slope S_2 at $P = \frac{1}{2}$ ΔP from function expression	2.400 ⟶	0.480
3	Calculate slope S_3 at $P = \frac{1}{2}$ new ΔP from function expression	3.040 ⟶	0.608
4	Calculate slope S_4 at $P = $ new ΔP from function expression	1.568 ⟶	0.314
5	Estimate ΔP at $t = 0.2$ from weighted average of slopes: $\Delta P = 0.2(S_1 + 2S_2 + 2S_3 + S_4)/6$ $= 0.2(4.000 + 4.800 + 6.080 + 1.568)/6$ $= 0.548$		

[a] Given function $dP/dt = 4(1 - P)$ with $P = 0$ when $t = 0$. Procedure begins at $t = 0$; time step size $= 0.2$. Direct integration of $dP/dt = 4(1 - P)$ gives $P = 1 - e^{-4t}$. Evaluation at $t = 0.2$ gives $P = 0.551$.

ACKNOWLEDGMENTS

This work was supported by NIH Grants HL 23190 (Olszowka) and HL 17731 and HL 00111 (Wagner). The major contributions of Dr. John W. Evans of the UCSD Department of Mathematics in the development of the computer programs for inert gas analysis and linear programming are gratefully acknowledged.

REFERENCES

Dantzig, G. B. (1963). "Linear Programming and Extensions," pp. 94–108. Princeton Univ. Press, Princeton, New Jersey.

Dantzker, D. R., Wagner, P. D., and West, J. B. (1975). Instability of lung units with low $\dot{V}_A/\dot{Q}$ ratios during O_2 breathing. J. Appl. Physiol. **38**(5), 886–895.

Dawson, S. V., Butler, J. P., and Reeds, J. (1978). Indirect estimation of physiological distribution functions. Fed. Proc., Fed. Am. Soc. Exp. Biol. **37**, 2903–2810.

Dill, D. B., Edwards, H. T., and Consolazio, W. V. (1937). Blood as a physio-chemical system. Man at rest. J. Biol. Chem. **118**, 635–648.

Evans, J. W., and Wagner, P. D. (1977). Limits on $\dot{V}_A/\dot{Q}$ distributions from analysis of experimental inert gas elimination. J. Appl. Physiol. **42**, 889–898.

Farhi, L. E. (1967). Elimination of inert gas by the lung. Respir. Physiol. **3**, 1–11.

Farhi, L. E., and Olszowka, A. J. (1968). Analysis of alveolar gas exchange in the presence of soluble inert gases. *Respir. Physiol.* **5**, 53–67.

Forster, R. E. (1957). Exchange of gases between alveolar air and pulmonary capillary blood: Pulmonary diffusing capacity. *Physiol. Rev.* **37**, 391–452.

Hill, E. P., Power, G. G., and Longo, L. D. (1973). Mathematical simulation of pulmonary O_2 and CO_2 exchange. *Am. J. Physiol.* **224**, 904–917.

Hoerl, A. E., and Kennard, R. W. (1970). Ridge regression: Biased estimation for non-orthogonal problems. *Technometrics* **12**, 55–67.

Kelman, G. R. (1965). Digital computer subroutine for the conversion of oxygen tension into saturation. *J. Appl. Physiol.* **21**, 1375–1376.

Kelman, G. R. (1968). Computer programs for the production of O_2–CO_2 diagrams. *Respir. Physiol.* **4**, 260–269.

Olszowka, A. J., and Farhi, L. E. (1968). A system of digital computer subroutines for blood gas calculations. *Respir. Physiol.* **4**, 270–280.

Ostrowski, A. M. (1969). "Solutions of Equations and Systems of Equations." Academic Press, New York.

Pimmel, R. L., Tsai, M. J., and Bromberg, P. A. (1977). Estimating $\dot{V}_A/\dot{Q}$ distributions from inert gas data with an enforced smoothing algorithm. *J. Appl. Physiol.* **43**, 1106–1110.

Rahn, H., and Fenn, W. O. (1955). "Graphical Analysis of the Respiratory Gas Exchange." Am. Physiol. Soc., Washington, D.C.

Riley, R. L., and Cournand, A. (1949). Ideal alveolar air and the analysis of ventilation–perfusion relationships in the lung. *J. Appl. Physiol.* **1**, 825–847.

Roughton, R. J. W., and Forster, R. E. (1957). Relative importance of diffusion and chemical reaction rates in determining rate of exchange of gases in the human lung, with special reference to true diffusing capacity of pulmonary membrane and volume of blood in the lung capillaries. *J. Appl. Physiol.* **11**, 290–302.

Scheid, R. (1968). "Theory and Problems of Numerical Analysis," pp. 198–225. Schaum's Outline Series, McGraw-Hill, New York.

Staub, N. C., Bishop, J. M., and Forster, R. E. (1962). Importance of diffusion and chemical reactions in O_2 uptake in the lung. *J. Appl. Physiol.* **17**, 21–27.

Thomas, L. J. (1972). Algorithms for selected blood acid–base and blood gas calculations. *J. Appl. Physiol.* **33**(1), 154–158.

Wagner, P. D. (1977a). A general approach to the evaluation of ventilation–perfusion ratios in normal and abnormal lungs. *Physiologist* **20**, 18–25.

Wagner, P. D. (1977b). Ventilation–perfusion inequality and gas exchange during exercise in lung disease. *In* "Muscular Exercise and the Lung" (J. A. Dempsey and C. E. Reed, eds.), pp. 345–356. Univ. of Wisconsin Press, Madison.

Wagner, P. D. (1977c). Diffusion and chemical reaction in pulmonary gas exchange. *Physiol. Rev.* **57**, 257–312.

Wagner, P. D. (1979a). Susceptibility of different gases to ventilation–perfusion inequality. *J. Appl. Physiol.* **46**(2), 372–386.

Wagner, P. D. (1979b). Information content of the multibreath nitrogen washout. *J. Appl. Physiol.* **46**(3), 579–587.

Wagner, P. D., and West, J. B. (1972). Effects of diffusion impairment on O_2 and CO_2 time courses in pulmonary capillaries. *J. Appl. Physiol.* **33**, 62–71.

Wagner, P. D., Dantzker, D. R., Dueck, R., Clausen, J. L., and West, J. B. (1977). Ventilation–perfusion inequality in chronic obstructive pulmonary disease. *J. Clin. Invest.* **59**, 203–216.

West, J. B. (1969). Ventilation–perfusion inequality and overall gas exchange in computer models of the lung. *Respir. Physiol.* **7**, 88–110.

West, J. B. (1969–1970). Effect of slope and shape of dissociation curve on pulmonary gas exchange. *Respir. Physiol.* **8,** 66–85.

West, J. B. (1971). Gas exchange when one lung region inspires from another. *J. Appl. Physiol.* **30,** 479–487.

West, J. B., and Wagner, P. D. (1977). Pulmonary gas exchange. *In* "Bioengineering Aspects of the Lung" (J. B. West, ed.), pp. 361–457. Dekker, New York.

9

Mathematical Analysis of Compartmental Lung Models

John W. Evans

PULMONARY GAS EXCHANGE, VOL. I

307

I. INTRODUCTION

In this chapter some results from the mathematical analysis of compartmental models of the lungs are given.

After this introduction there are six sections. Sections II–V deal with steady state gas exchange and sections VI and VII treat transient gas exchange. A summary of these sections is now given.

Section II treats steady state inert gas exchange where the inert gas is assumed to be present in trace amounts as is usual in retention–solubility studies (Evans and Wagner, 1977; Jaliwala *et al.*, 1975; Olszowska, 1975; Wagner *et al.*, 1974a,b,c, 1975, 1977, 1978). The model used is an extension of the compartmental model of Farhi (1967; Farhi and Yokoyama, 1967). It is assumed that the lung is composed of a number of compartments receiving continuous ventilation and perfusion at fixed rates and that there is complete equilibrium of the inert test gas (no diffusion impairment) within each compartment. The topic investigated is the form of the dependence of the retention of the inert test gas on solubility, the retention–solubility relation, under various restrictions on intercompartmental blood and air flow. The retention of an inert test gas is defined as usual as the fraction retained in the blood after passage through the lungs at steady state when there is no test gas in the inspired air. Specifically, conditions are sought that ensure that the retention–solubility relation is identical to that of some model in which there is no intercompartmental communication so that all compartments are perfused and ventilated in parallel. This is the problem of parallel equivalence (Wagner and Evans, 1977). Results are stated which show that the problem of parallel equivalence in these models is closely related to a well-known mathematical problem, the generalized eigenvalue problem (Wilkinson, 1965). The principal finding is that if the flow of blood and air between compartments is symmetric then there is parallel equivalence. Various examples with non-symmetric intercompartmental flows are given to show that the departure from parallel equivalence is possible. The proofs of these results are found in Evans (1979a).

In Section III the steady state exchange of an inert gas is considered in parallel ventilation and perfusion models. The amount of the inert gas is not restricted but it is assumed that the net exchange of other (carrier) gases is zero in each compartment. The exchange of the test gas is then compared to the exchange of the gas in a homogeneous (one-compartment) model with the same total alveolar ventilation and perfusion and the same inspiratory and venous partial pressures of the inert gas. The ratio of the exchange in the nonhomogeneous (multicompartmental) lung to the exchange in the homogeneous lung as a function of the solubility of the inert gas is seen to exhibit a stereotyped behavior in that it drops from one at zero solubility to a unique minimum and then approaches one again as the solubility tends to infinity. These results are proved in Colburn *et al.* (1974).

Section IV continues the investigation of Section III when the gas under consideration has a nonlinear dissociation curve. Conditions are described for the dissociation curve that are necessary and sufficient for there to be an impairment of gas exchange in any nonhomogeneous model with the gas at arbitrary fixed venous and inspiratory partial pressures. These results are proved in Evans *et al.* (1974).

Section V explores the amount of information that can be gained in theory from a reduced inert gas elimination test in which mixed venous partial pressures are not measured. It is seen that if the ratio of expired partial pressure to mixed arterial partial pressure as a function of solubility is known then only the ratio of total ventilation to total perfusion is needed to give the usual retention–solubility relation. In the absence of this knowledge all the parameters of a parallel ventilation and perfusion model can be given as functions of the total ventilation to total perfusion ratio and it is possible to represent all possible parallel ventilation and perfusion models with a given expiratory to mixed arterial-solubility relation. These results are proved in Evans (1979c).

Section VI is the first section dealing with transient gas exchange. The wash-out of gases of negligible solubility is considered (Lewis *et al.*, 1978). This allows a treatment which ignores blood flow and is not restricted to assumptions of continuous ventilation. First, general expressions are presented which give the transition from full inspiration to full expiration and back, and then results are stated from Evans (1970) showing that the output of an insoluble gas wash-out is equivalent to that of a model with parallel ventilation provided a symmetry condition similar to the earlier symmetry conditions is met. Next a specific compartmental model with a conducting airway compartment (dead space) is considered. It is seen that the effect of the dead space on the wash-out can be calculated through a set of equations and that the model parameters can be calculated from the coefficients and time constants of the wash-out values. These results are proved in Evans *et al.* (1967; see also Cantor and Evans, 1970).

Finally, Section VII deals with transient inert gas exchange. The compartmental description of Section II is augmented by parameters which give the storage capacity of each compartment and some ordinary differential equations and their solutions describing transient exchange are presented. Parallel ventilation and perfusion models are viewed as consisting of a distribution of lung volume over a parameter space of three ratios: fluid to volume, perfusion to volume, and ventilation to volume. In this setting, information including lung air and fluid volume gained in theory from a transient inert gas transfer study is outlined. Finally, examples are presented of models that are not equivalent to parallel ventilation and perfusion models in their transient gas exchange properties despite the presence of parallel perfusion and symmetric air flow between compartments. These results are proved in Evans (1979b).

Standard matrix notation (Gantmacher, 1959) is used throughout the remainder of the chapter and a background in linear algebra is often assumed.

II. STEADY STATE INERT GAS ELIMINATION: THE PROBLEM OF PARALLEL EQUIVALENCE

We now give the assumptions (Evans, 1979a) underlying a class of n-compartmental lung models where transport by air and/or blood is allowed between any two compartments. It is assumed that there is an inert soluble test gas with blood–gas partition coefficient λ present in trace amounts. The fluctuations due to cyclical breathing (Nye, 1970) and pulsatile blood flow are taken as having been averaged out.

A. Modeling Assumptions

1. Finite Compartmental Model. There are n compartments with $n \geq 1$.

2. Blood transport system. There is a *blood transport system.* A flow rate $\dot{Q}_{ij} \geq 0$ gives the blood flow from the jth to the ith compartment for $i \neq j$ with $1 \leq i, j \leq n$. A flow rate $\dot{Q}_{i0} \geq 0$ gives the input flow (from mixed venous blood) to the ith compartment and a flow rate $\dot{Q}_{0i} \geq 0$ gives the output flow (to mixed arterial blood) for $1 \leq i \leq n$.

3. *Air transport system.* There is an *air transport system.* A flow rate $\dot{V}_{ij} \geq 0$ gives the air flow from the jth to the ith compartment for $i \neq j$ with $1 \leq i, j \leq n$. A flow rate $\dot{V}_{i0}$ gives the input flow (inspiratory ventilation) and a flow rate $\dot{V}_{0i}$ gives the output flow (alveolar ventilation) for the ith compartment for $1 \leq i \leq n$.

4. *Test gas equilibrium.* There is complete *equilibrium of test gas* between the blood phase and the air phase of each compartment (no diffusion impairment), resulting in identical partial pressures of test gas in all channels leaving the compartment.

5. *Mass balance of test substance.* There is local *mass balance of test substance* in that for each compartment the amount of test substance entering is equal to the amount leaving.

6. *Mass balance of blood flow.* There is local *mass balance of blood flow* in that

$$\sum_{\substack{j=0 \\ j\neq i}}^{n} \dot{Q}_{ij} = \sum_{\substack{j=0 \\ j\neq i}}^{n} \dot{Q}_{ji}, \qquad \text{for} \quad 1 \leq i \leq n$$

With these assumptions the equations of steady state exchange can be stated in matrix form using the following:

1. The Air Transport Matrix A

Let A be the $n \times n$ matrix with entries A_{ij}, where

$$A_{ij} \stackrel{\text{def}}{\equiv} \begin{cases} -\dot{V}_{ij}, & \text{for} \quad i \neq j \\ \sum_{\substack{k=0 \\ k\neq i}}^{n} \dot{V}_{ki}, & \text{for} \quad i = j \end{cases}$$

so that for the ith row of A the off-diagonal entries give the air flow into the ith compartment from other compartments with negative sign, while the diagonal entry gives the total air flow out of the ith compartment.

2. The Blood Transport Matrix B

Let B be $n \times n$ with entries

$$B_{ij} \stackrel{\text{def}}{\equiv} \begin{cases} -\dot{Q}_{ij}, & \text{for} \quad i \neq j \\ \sum_{\substack{k=0 \\ k\neq i}}^{n} \dot{Q}_{ki} & \text{for} \quad i = j \end{cases}$$

The matrix B has an analogous interpretation of the diagonal and off-diagonal entries.

3. The Inspiratory Air Flow Vector a

Let **a** be the vector of inspiratory air flows whose ith entry is $\dot{V}_{i0}$ for $i = 1, \ldots, n$.

4. The Incoming Blood Flow Vector b

Let **b** be the corresponding vector for blood flow whose ith entry is $\dot{Q}_{i0}$ for $i = 1, \ldots, n$.

In addition let **e** be the n-column vector with all entries identically 1 and let a superscript T denote transpose so that $\mathbf{e}^\mathsf{T}$ is an n-row vector.

Before proceeding further we note that the ith entry of $\mathbf{e}^\mathsf{T}A$ (of $\mathbf{e}^\mathsf{T}B$) is $\dot{V}_{0i}$ (is $\dot{Q}_{0i}$) for $i = 1, \ldots, n$ and that by assumption (6) we have that the ith entry $B\mathbf{e}$ is

$$\sum_{\substack{k=0 \\ k \neq i}}^{n} Q_{ki} - \sum_{\substack{j=1 \\ j \neq i}}^{n} Q_{ij} = \dot{Q}_{i0}$$

for $i = 1, \ldots, n$ so that $\mathbf{b} = B\mathbf{e}$. The balance equations can now be given.

5. The Balance Equation in Matrix Form

Let P_I, P_E, $P_{\bar{v}}$, and P_a give the respective inspiratory, expiratory, mixed venous, and mixed arterial partial pressures of the test gas and let the n-column vector **P** have its ith entry the equilibrium partial pressure of the test gas in the ith compartment. The mass balance assumption (5) at equilibrium (4) is given simply as

$$(A + \lambda B)\mathbf{P} = P_I\mathbf{a} + \lambda P_{\bar{v}}\mathbf{b} \tag{1}$$

since the amount of test substance per unit time carried in an air channel is equal to the partial pressure times the flow rate and the amount in a blood channel is λ times the partial pressure times the flow rate with suitable normalization.

6. Solving for P

Except in degenerate cases discussed in Evans (1979a) the matrix $A + \lambda B$ has an inverse for $\lambda > 0$; thus we have

$$\mathbf{P} = P_I(A + \lambda B)^{-1}\mathbf{a} + \lambda P_{\bar{v}}(A + \lambda B)^{-1}\mathbf{b} \tag{2}$$

7. Solving for P_a and P_E

The arterial partial pressure P_a is just the result of mixing the amount $\sum_{i=1}^{n} \lambda \dot{Q}_{0i}P_i$ in the volume $\sum_{i=1}^{n} \dot{Q}_{0i}$ and is $\mathbf{e}^\mathsf{T}B\mathbf{P}/\mathbf{e}^\mathsf{T}B\mathbf{e}$. In the same way the expiratory partial pressure P_E is $\mathbf{e}^\mathsf{T}A\mathbf{P}/\mathbf{e}^\mathsf{T}A\mathbf{e}$. The results are the expressions

$$P_a = \frac{P_I \mathbf{e}^\mathsf{T} B(A + \lambda B)^{-1}\mathbf{a} + \lambda P_{\bar{v}}\mathbf{e}^\mathsf{T} B(A + \lambda B)^{-1}\mathbf{b}}{\mathbf{e}^\mathsf{T} B \mathbf{e}} \tag{3}$$

$$P_E = \frac{P_I \mathbf{e}^\mathsf{T} A(A + \lambda B)^{-1}\mathbf{a} + P_{\bar{v}}\mathbf{e}^\mathsf{T} A(A + \lambda B)^{-1}\mathbf{b}}{\mathbf{e}^\mathsf{T} A \mathbf{e}} \tag{4}$$

We are ready to state the retention–solubility relation in matrix form.

B. The Retention–Solubility Relation

When $P_I = 0$ expressions (3) and (4) simplify. The fraction of test gas retained in the blood (with $P_I = 0$) after a pass through the lungs as a function of solubility λ is called the retention $R(\lambda)$. This is equal to $P_a/P_{\bar{v}}$ and we have

$$R(\lambda) = \lambda \mathbf{e}^\mathsf{T} B(A + \lambda B)^{-1} B \mathbf{e}/\mathbf{e}^\mathsf{T} B \mathbf{e} \tag{5'}$$

where we have used the fact that $\mathbf{b} = B\mathbf{e}$.

We are now ready to specialize the above equation and consider parallel ventilation and perfusion models.

C. Equivalence to Parallel Ventilation and Perfusion Models

The n compartments are said to be ventilated (perfused) in parallel if the off-diagonal terms of A (of B) are zero. When both ventilation and perfusion are parallel we have $A = \mathrm{diag}(\dot{V}_{0i}, \ldots, \dot{V}_{0n})$ and $B = \mathrm{diag}(\dot{Q}_i, \ldots, \dot{Q}_n)$, where $\dot{Q}_i \overset{\mathrm{def}}{=} \dot{Q}_{i0} = \dot{Q}_{0i}$ for $i = 1, \ldots, n$. Also $\mathbf{b} = (\dot{Q}_i, \ldots, \dot{Q}_n)^\mathsf{T}$ and $\mathbf{a} = (\dot{V}_{i0}, \ldots, \dot{V}_{n0})^\mathsf{T}$ as usual.

Equation (5) then becomes (Farhi, 1967; Farhi and Yokoyama, 1967)

$$R(\lambda) = \frac{\lambda \sum\limits_{i=1}^{n} \dot{Q}_i^2/(\dot{V}_{0i} + \lambda \dot{Q}_i)}{\sum\limits_{i=1}^{n} \dot{Q}_i} = \lambda \sum\limits_{i=1}^{n} F_i/(\lambda + x_i) \tag{5}$$

where $F_i = \dot{Q}_i/\sum_{j=1}^{n}\dot{Q}_j$ and $x_i = \dot{V}_{0i}/\dot{Q}_i$ for $i = 1, \ldots, n$. In writing $R(\lambda)$ in this form, a compartment with $\dot{Q}_i = 0$ has $F_i = 0$ and $x_i = \infty$ and is taken as contributing nothing to the sum. The quantity F_i is called the fractional perfusion to the ith compartment. Compartments with identical ventilation–perfusion ratios x_i are generally lumped together.

After the following definitions, some results on equivalence to parallel ventilation and perfusion models are given.

1. Generalized Eigenvalues

Say as usual (Wilkinson, 1965) that g is an eigenvector of $A + \lambda B$ if either (1) there is a complex number μ such that $(A - \mu B)g = 0$, or (2) $Bg = 0$.

In case (1) we say that μ_i is an eigenvalue of $A + \lambda B$ associated with g_i. In case (2) we say that ∞ is an eigenvalue of $A + \lambda B$ associated with g_i.

2. Diagonable $A + \lambda B$

Call the system $A + \lambda B$ diagonable with extended real nonnegative eigenvalues if there are linearly independent eigenvectors $g_1, \ldots, g_n$ with associated eigenvalues $\mu_1, \ldots, \mu_n$ which are nonnegative or infinite. The following result holds for diagonable systems.

3. Theorem on Diagonable Systems

The following theorem is given and proved in Evans (1979a).

Theorem 1. Suppose that $A + \lambda B$ is diagonable with eigenvectors $g_1, \ldots, g_l$ having eigenvalues $\mu_1, \ldots, \mu_l \geq 0$ and eigenvectors $g_{l+1}, \ldots, g_n$ with eigenvalues equal to infinity. Then

$$R(\lambda) = \sum_{i=1}^{l} \frac{\lambda F_i}{\lambda + \mu_i}$$

where $F_1 + \cdots + F_l = 1$.

The diagonability condition does not result in complete equivalence to the parallel ventilation and perfusion models since diagonability alone does not ensure that $F_i \geq 0$ for $i = 1, \ldots, l$. Note that each eigenvector with eigenvalue $\mu_i \geq 0$ contributes to the above expression for $R(\lambda)$ just as a compartment with ventilation–perfusion ratio μ_i contributes to the retention–solubility relation for a parallel ventilation–perfusion lung model. An eigenvector with eigenvalue ∞ does not contributed to the expression and thus acts in a similar fashion to dead space (with infinite ventilation–perfusion ratio) in a parallel model.

Next it is seen that an assumption of symmetric transport between compartments does give complete equivalence to parallel models.

4. Symmetric Systems

Say that $A + \lambda B$ is symmetric if $A_{ij} = A_{ji}$ and $B_{ij} = B_{ji}$ for $1 \leq i, j \leq n$. In this case the following theorem proved in Evans (1979a) holds.

5. Theorem on Symmetric Systems

Theorem 2. If $A + \lambda B$ is symmetric, then the system is diagonable with extended nonnegative real eigenvalues, and $F_i \geq 0$ for $i = 1, \ldots, l$, where l and $F_1, \ldots, F_l$ are as in Theorem 1.

Applications are now given in the form of examples and counterexamples.

D. Dead Space and Series Ventilation

Let

$$
A = \begin{pmatrix}
\alpha\dot{V}_T & 0 & 0 & \cdots & 0 \\
0 & \alpha\dot{V}_T & -\alpha\dot{V}_1 & \cdots & -\alpha\dot{V}_n \\
0 & -\alpha\dot{V}_1 & \dot{V}_1 & & \\
\cdot & & & \cdot & \\
\cdot & & & & \cdot \\
\cdot & & & & \cdot \\
0 & -\alpha\dot{V}_n & & & \dot{V}_n
\end{pmatrix}
$$

$B = \mathrm{diag}(0, 0, \dot{Q}_1, \ldots, \dot{Q}_n)$, and $\mathbf{a} = A\mathbf{e}$, where $\dot{V}_T = \dot{V}_1 + \cdots + \dot{V}_n$. In this model the first two compartments together compromise the dead space. A fraction α of the total inspiratory and expiratory volume $\dot{V}_T$ goes to and from the first compartment with no communication between this and other compartments, and the same fraction α of the total ventilation $\dot{V}_i$ to and from the $(2 + i)$th compartment for $i = 1, \ldots, n$ goes to the second compartment and back. The first two compartments are unperfused and the remaining compartments are perfused in parallel.

Since this is a symmetric model there is an equivalent parallel ventilation and perfusion model by Theorem 2.

Parallel Equivalence for Series Ventilation

Let

$$
A = \begin{bmatrix}
\dot{V}_1 & -\dot{U}_1 & & & & \\
-\dot{U}_1 & & \cdot & & & \\
& \cdot & & \cdot & & \\
& & \cdot & & \cdot & \\
& & & \cdot & & -\dot{U}^{n-1} \\
& & & & -\dot{U}_{n-1} & \dot{V}_n
\end{bmatrix}
$$

$$B = \mathrm{diag}(\dot{Q}_1, \ldots, \dot{Q}_n), \qquad \mathbf{a} = A\mathbf{e}$$

where $\dot{V}_1 > \dot{U}_1$, $\dot{V}_i = \dot{U}_{i-1} + \dot{U}_{i+1}$ for $i = 2, \ldots, n - 1$, and $\dot{V}_n = \dot{U}_{n-1}$. Here the n compartments are symmetrically ventilated in series.

Again there is an equivalent parallel ventilation and perfusion model by Theorem 2.

E. Counterexamples with Nonequivalence to Parallel Models

1. Complex Eigenvalues

Let

$$A = \begin{pmatrix} 1 & 0 & 0 \\ -1 & 1 & 0 \\ 0 & -1 & 1 \end{pmatrix}, \quad B = \begin{pmatrix} 1 & -1 & 0 \\ 0 & 1 & -1 \\ 0 & 0 & 1 \end{pmatrix}$$

and

$$\mathbf{a} = A\mathbf{e}$$

Then

$$R(\lambda) = \frac{\lambda}{1 + \lambda + \lambda^2 + \lambda^3} = \frac{\frac{1}{2}}{\lambda + 1} - \frac{\frac{1}{2}(i + 1)}{\lambda + i} + \frac{\frac{1}{2}(i - 1)}{\lambda - i}$$

In this model blood flows in compartment 3, through compartment 2, and out compartment 1, while air flows in the opposite direction. There are complex eigenvalues i and $-i$ of $A + \lambda B$, where, of course, $i^2 = -1$. This model clearly has no parallel ventilation and perfusion equivalent.

2. Negative Fractional Perfusions

Let $B = \begin{pmatrix} 1/2 & 0 \\ 0 & 1/2 \end{pmatrix}$, $A = \begin{pmatrix} 1 & -1 \\ 0 & 1+\epsilon \end{pmatrix}$, and $\mathbf{a} = A\mathbf{e}$. Then

$$R(\lambda) = \frac{\lambda(1 + \epsilon)/2\epsilon}{2 + \lambda} - \frac{\lambda(1 - \epsilon)/2\epsilon}{2 + 2\epsilon + \lambda}$$

so that in the parallel equivalent interpretation one of the fractional perfusions is negative if $0 < \epsilon < 1$.

3. A Nondiagonable Model

Let $A = I$,

$$B = \begin{bmatrix} 1 & -1 & & & \\ & \cdot & \cdot & & \\ & & \cdot & \cdot & \\ & & & \cdot & -1 \\ & & & & 1 \end{bmatrix}$$

and $\mathbf{a} = A\mathbf{e}$, where I is the identity matrix. Then

$$R(\lambda) = \lambda^n/(1 + \lambda)^n$$

Here 1 is the only eigenvalue of $A + \lambda B$ and $(1, 0, \ldots, 0)$ is the only eigenvector, and so the system is not diagonable.

III. IMPAIRMENT OF INERT GAS EXCHANGE IN PARALLEL VENTILATION AND PERFUSION MODELS

In this section we give results from Colburn *et al.* (1974), where the effect of solubility on the impairment of gas exchange in nonhomogeneous parallel ventilation and perfusion lung models is studied. The ratio of the rate of transfer of an inhomogeneous lung model over the rate of transfer in a homogeneous model with the same total blood flow and ventilation is analyzed as a function of the blood–gas partition coefficient λ.

A. The Exchange Equations

As the equations of gas exchange in a single compartment we add to the usual balance equation for the inert gas under consideration

$$\dot{V}_{0i}P_i - \dot{V}_{i0}P_I = \lambda\dot{Q}_i(P_{\bar{v}} - P_i) \tag{6}$$

the equation

$$(1 - P_i)\dot{V}_{0i} = (1 - P_I)\dot{V}_{i0} \tag{7}$$

The second of these equations states that no net exchange of the remaining gases occurs. This assumption gives a good approximation in real lungs except in areas of very low ventilation–perfusion ratios. With this assumption the inert gas being studied is no longer taken as being present in trace amounts.

1. The Exchange Rate in the ith Compartment

Either side of (6) may be taken as the net exchange rate in the ith compartment. Solving for $\dot{V}_{i0}$ in (7) and substituting in (6), we obtain

$$\dot{V}_{0i}\left(\frac{P_i - P_I}{1 - P_I}\right) = \lambda\dot{Q}(P_{\bar{v}} - P_i) \tag{8}$$

On solving for P_i in (8) and substituting this value in the left-hand side of (8) we obtain for the net exchange rate in the ith compartment

$$\frac{\dot{V}_{0i}\lambda(P_{\bar{v}} - P_I)}{\lambda(1 - P_I) + \dot{V}_{0i}/\dot{Q}_i} \tag{9}$$

2. The Transfer Ratio $T(\lambda)$

On setting $\dot{V}_T = \dot{V}_{01} + \cdots + \dot{V}_{0n}$ and $\dot{Q}_T = \dot{Q}_1 + \cdots + \dot{Q}_n$ we have for fixed $P_{\bar{v}}$ and P_I that the ratio of the gas transfer rate of the n-compartmental model over the transfer rate of the homogeneous model with the same total (alveolar) ventilation and blood flow is

$$T(\lambda) \overset{\text{def}}{\equiv} \frac{\sum\limits_{i=1}^{n} \dot{V}_{0i}\lambda(P_{\bar{v}} - P_I)/[\lambda(1 - P_I) + \dot{V}_{0i}/\dot{Q}_i]}{\dot{V}_T\lambda(P_{\bar{v}} - P_I)/[\lambda(1 - P_I) + \dot{V}_T/\dot{Q}_T]}$$

$$= \sum_{i=1}^{n} \frac{\dot{V}_{0i}}{\dot{V}_T} \frac{\lambda(1 - P_I) + \dot{V}_T/\dot{Q}_T}{\lambda(1 - P_I) + \dot{V}_{0i}/\dot{Q}_i}$$

We are now ready to give the main result of this section, which is a theorem giving properties of the transfer ratio. In the statement of the theorem we let $T^{(0)}(\lambda) = T(\lambda)$, while for $m \geq 1$ we set $T^{(m)}(\lambda)$ equal to the mth derivative of T with respect to λ.

B. A Theorem on Impaired Gas Transfer

Theorem 3. For a fixed nonhomogeneous long model and fixed values of P_I, $P_{\bar{v}} \geq 0$, with $P_I \neq P_{\bar{v}}$, the following statements hold:

(1) $T(0) = 1$ and $T(\lambda) \to 1$ as $\lambda \to \infty$.
(2) There exist $0 < \lambda_1 < \lambda_2 < \cdots$ such that $T^{(m)}(\lambda_m) = 0$, $m \geq 1$.
(3) If $m \geq 1$ is an odd number then $T^{(m)}(\lambda) < 0$ for $0 \leq \lambda < \lambda_m$ and $T^{(m)}(\lambda) > 0$ for $\lambda_m < \lambda$.
(4) If $m \geq 2$ is an even number then $T^{(m)}(\lambda) > 0$ for $0 \leq \lambda \leq \lambda_m$ and $T^{(m)}(\lambda) < 0$ for $\lambda_m < \lambda$.

From the theorem we see that certain features of the transfer ratio are shared by all inhomogenous lung models. These are given next.

C. Significance: Qualitative Features of the Exchange Ratio

According to the above theorem, the first derivative of T is negative for $0 \leq \lambda < \lambda_1$ and is positive for $\lambda_1 < \lambda$. Thus T descends to a unique minimum at λ_1. Also the second derivative is positive before the unique inflection point λ_2 and is negative thereafter, so that T is convex before λ_2 and concave thereafter. We may therefore assert that the transfer of an inert gas is always impaired by inhomogeneity and that for a fixed inhomogeneous lung model there is a unique solubility at which the relative impairment is greatest.

IV. IMPAIRMENT OF GAS EXCHANGE IN INHOMOGENEOUS LUNG MODELS: NONLINEAR DISSOCIATION CURVES

We continue the analysis of the preceding section but consider gases with nonlinear dissociation curves. The results are taken from Evans *et al.* (1974).

A. The Exchange Equations

1. Nonlinear Dissociation Curves

Suppose now that volume of the gas of interest per unit volume of blood at a partial pressure P is given by a function $C(P)$. The exchange equations (6) and (7) become

$$\dot{V}_{0i}P_i - \dot{V}_{i0}P_I = \dot{Q}_i[C(P\bar{v}) - C(P)] \tag{10}$$

$$(1 - P_i)\dot{V}_{0i} = (1 - P_I)\dot{V}_{i0} \tag{11}$$

Again solving for $\dot{V}_{i0}$ in the second of these equations and substituting in the first, we have

$$\dot{V}_{0i}\left(\frac{P_i - P_I}{1 - P_I}\right) = \dot{Q}_i[C(P\bar{v}) - C(P_i)] \tag{12}$$

which implicitly defines P_i as a function of P_I, $P\bar{v}$, and $y_i \equiv^{\text{def}} \dot{Q}_i/\dot{V}_{0i}$. We denote this function for fixed P_I and $P\bar{v}$ as $P(y)$.

2. Homogeneous versus Nonhomogeneous Exchange

We assume that the content $C(P)$ is an increasing function of P and thus from (12) that P_i lies strictly between the minimum and the maximum of P_I and $P\bar{v}$ when $P_I \neq P\bar{v}$.

Setting $y_T \equiv^{\text{def}} \dot{Q}_T/\dot{V}_T$ we have that the net exchange for a homogeneous lung with alveolar ventilation $\dot{V}_T$ and perfusion $\dot{Q}_T$ is

$$\dot{V}_T\left(\frac{P(y_T) - P_I}{1 - P_I}\right) = \frac{\dot{V}_T P(y_T)}{1 - P_I} - \frac{\dot{V}_T P_I}{1 - P_I} \tag{13}$$

while the net exchange for the inhomogeneous lung is

$$\sum_{i=1}^{n} \dot{V}_{0i}\left(\frac{P(y_i) - P_I}{1 - P_I}\right) = \frac{\displaystyle\sum_{i=1}^{n} \dot{V}_{0i}P(y_i)}{1 - P_I} - \frac{\dot{V}_T P_I}{1 - P_I} \tag{14}$$

If $P\bar{v} > P_I$ this net exchange for both models is positive and the exchange is greater in the homogeneous lung if and only if

$$\dot{V}_T P(y_T) > \sum_{j=1}^{n} \dot{V}_{0i} P(y_i) \tag{15}$$

If $P_{\bar{v}} > P_I$ the net exchange is negative for both models and the magnitude of the exchange is greater in the homogeneous lung if and only if

$$\dot{V}_T P(y_T) < \sum_{i=1}^{n} \dot{V}_{0i} P(y_i) \tag{16}$$

3. Convexity Conditions on P(y)

We set $w_i = \dot{V}_{0i}/\dot{V}_T$ so that $w_i \geq 0$ for $i = 1, \ldots, n$ and $w_1 + \cdots + w_n = 1$. We note that

$$w_1 y_1 + \cdots + w_n y_n = \sum_{i=1}^{n} \frac{\dot{V}_{0i}}{\dot{V}_T} \frac{\dot{Q}_i}{\dot{V}_{0i}} = \dot{Q}_T/\dot{V}_T = y_T$$

and thus that (15) can be rewritten as

$$P(w_1 y_1 + \cdots + w_n y_n) > w_1 P(y_1) + \cdots + w_n P(y_n) \tag{17}$$

for $P_{\bar{v}} > P_I$, while (16) is just

$$P(w_1 y_1 + \cdots + w_n y_n) < w_1 P(y_1) + \cdots + w_n P(y_n) \tag{18}$$

for $P_{\bar{v}} < P_I$. These are simply the requirements that P is strictly convex in (17) and is strictly concave in (18).

4. The Second Derivative of P(y)

A function is strictly convex if and only if its second derivative is always nonnegative and never vanishes identically on any interval. A function is strictly concave if the negative of the function is strictly convex. Thus the second derivative of P with respect to y is of interest. From (12) it can be shown that

$$P'' = \frac{-\Delta C^3}{K^2(\Delta C + \Delta P C')} \left[2C' + \left(\frac{\Delta P \, \Delta C}{C + \Delta P C'} \right) C'' \right] \tag{19}$$

where prime denotes differentiation and where

$$K = 1/(1 - P_I), \qquad \Delta P = P(y) - P_I, \qquad \Delta C = C(P_{\bar{v}}) - C[P(y)]$$
$$C' = C'[P(y)], \qquad C'' = C''[P(y)]$$

If values of $P_{\bar{v}}$, and P_I, and y can be found so that (19) has a sign incompatible with (17) or (18) then a model can be constructed in which gas exchange is *enhanced* by inhomogeneity. We have the following theorem.

B. A Theorem Relating Convexity Conditions to Impaired Gas Transfer

Theorem 4. Theorem on convexity for $P_{\bar{v}} > P_I$ and concavity for $P_{\bar{v}} < P_I$ of $P(y)$.

(*1*) *The function $P(y)$ is strictly convex for $y > 0$ for all choices of $P_{\bar{v}} > P_I \geq 0$ if and only if $C(1/t)$, that is, the content plotted against the reciprocal of partial pressure, is convex for $t > 0$.*

(*2*) *The function $P(y)$ is strictly concave for $y > 0$ for all choices of $P_I > P_{\bar{v}} \geq 0$ if and only if $1/C(t)$, that is, the reciprocal of content plotted against the partial pressure, is convex for $t > 0$.*

C. Significance

When applied to the dissociation curves of O_2, CO_2, and CO, part (2) of the theorem shows that $P(y)$ is always strictly convex so that uptake of any of these gases is always impaired by inhomogeneity. In the same way part (1) shows that elimination of CO_2 is always impaired by inhomogeneity. The situation for elimination of O_2 and CO is more complex. There are regions where the convexity conditions are violated and models with enhanced elimination as a result of inhomogeneity are possible. This occurs only for mixed venous O_2 partial pressures in excess of 800 mm Hg or for CO partial pressures in excess of 51 mm Hg, conditions which greatly exceed those found under physiological circumstances.

V. INERT GAS ELIMINATION STUDIES WITHOUT MIXED VENOUS PARTIAL PRESSURES

We now give results from Evans (1979c), where the information present in an inert gas elimination study without measurement of mixed venous partial pressures is analyzed.

A. Retention and Excretion Related by the Fick Principle

We have defined the retention $R(\lambda)$ of an inert gas with blood–gas partition coefficient λ at steady state during intravenous test gas administration as $P_a/P_{\bar{v}}$. We now define as usual the excretion $E(\lambda)$ as $P_E/P_{\bar{v}}$. From the Fick principle of mass balance it follows that

$$\dot{Q}_T\lambda = \dot{Q}_T\lambda R(\lambda) + \dot{V}_T E(\lambda) \tag{20}$$

where $\dot{Q}_T$ is the total perfusion and $\dot{V}_T$ is the total alveolar or expiratory ventilation.

This gives

$$E(\lambda) = (\lambda/r)[1 - R(\lambda)] \tag{21}$$

where $r \equiv^{\mathrm{def}} \dot{V}_T/\dot{Q}_T$ is the ratio of total ventilation to total perfusion.

B. Elimination Divided by Retention of the E/R Function

1. The E/R Function S(λ) and Its Relation to R(λ)

If we now set

$$S(\lambda) = P_E/P_a \tag{22}$$

we have that $S(\lambda)$ is independent of $P_{\bar{v}}$ and is equal to $E(\lambda)/R(\lambda)$. We call $S(\lambda)$ the E/R *function of solubility* and note that

$$S(\lambda) = \lambda[1 - R(\lambda)]/rR(\lambda) \tag{23}$$

so that

$$R(\lambda) = \lambda/rS(\lambda) + \lambda \tag{24}$$

2. Retention of Parallel Ventilation and Perfusion Type with and without Shunt

Let us say that R is of PVP (parallel ventilation and perfusion) type if

$$R(\lambda) = \sum_{i=1}^{n} \lambda F_i/(\lambda + x_i) \tag{25}$$

where $0 \le x_1 < \cdots < x_n < \infty, F_1, \ldots, F_n > 0$, and $F_1 + \cdots + F_n = 1$. That is, the retention R is of PVP type if it represents the retention of $n \ge 1$ perfused compartments with fractional perfusions $F_1, \ldots, F_n$ at respective ventilation perfusion ratios of $x_1, \ldots, x_n$. If $x_1 = 0$ we say that R is *of PVP type with shunt*, otherwise we say that R is *of PVP type without shunt*. We treat the two cases separately.

C. Theorems Relating the E/R Function to the Retention

The following theorem deals with the form of $S(\lambda)$ and the relation between the parameters of $S(\lambda)$ and $R(\lambda)$ when $R(\lambda)$ is of PVP type.

Theorem 5. If R is of PVP type with shunt with fractional perfusions $F_1, \ldots, F_n > 0$ at ventilation–perfusion ratios $0 = x_1 < \cdots < x_n$ then

$$S(\lambda) = \sum_{j=1}^{n-1} \frac{\lambda L_j}{\lambda + b_j} \tag{26}$$

where $0 = x_1 < b_1 < x_2 < \cdots < b_{n-1} < x_n$ and

$$L_j = \frac{1}{r \sum_{i=2}^{n} F_i x_i / (x_i - b_j)^2} > 0 \tag{27}$$

for $j = 1, \ldots, n - 1$. The $b_1, \ldots, b_{n-1}$ are uniquely determined by the fact that

$$\sum_{i=2}^{n} \frac{F_i x_i}{x_i - b_j} = 1 \tag{28}$$

for $j = 1, \ldots, n - 1$. In addition $L_1 + \cdots + L_{n-1} \leq 1$.

If R is of PVP type without shunt with fractional perfusions $F_1, \ldots, F_n > 0$ at ventilation–perfusion ratios $0 < x_1 < \cdots < x_n$ then

$$S(\lambda) = \sum_{i=1}^{n} \frac{\lambda L_j}{\lambda + b_j} \tag{29}$$

where $0 = b_1 < x_1 < b_n < \cdots < b_n < x_n$ and

$$L_j = \frac{1}{r \sum_{i=1}^{n} F_i x_i / (x_i - b_j)^2} > 0 \tag{30}$$

for $j = 1, \ldots, n$. The $b_1, \ldots, b_n$ are uniquely determined by the fact that

$$\sum_{i=1}^{n} \frac{F_i x_i}{x_i - b_j} = 1 \tag{31}$$

for $j = 1, \ldots, n$. In addition, $L_1 + \cdots + L_n \leq 1$.

In both cases the sum of all the terms L_j is the fraction of the total ventilation $\dot{V}_T$ which comes from perfused compartments.

In light of the above theorem we may now give the following definition.

Definition: E/R of parallel ventilation and perfusion type with and without shunt. We say that an E/R function S is *of PVP type with shunt* if S is of the form given by (26) (with $0 < b_1$, $L_1, \ldots, L_{n-1} > 0$, and $L_1 + \cdots + L_{n-1} \leq 1$) and we say that S is *of PVP type without shunt* if S is of the form given by (29) (with $b_1 = 0$, $L_1, \ldots, L_n > 0$, and $L_1 + \cdots + L_n \leq 1$). We call the b_j terms appearing in (26) and (29) the (ventilation–perfusion) *barriers* and the L_j terms the *weights*. We call relation (26) or (29) the *E/R solubility relation*.

The following theorem, which is reciprocal to the one above, relates the parameters of $R(\lambda)$ to the parameters of $S(\lambda)$ when $S(\lambda)$ is of PVP type.

Theorem 6. If S of PVP type with shunt with weights $L_1, \ldots, L_{n-1} > 0$ at barriers $0 < b_1 < \cdots < b_{n-1}$ then

$$R(\lambda) = \sum_{i=1}^{n} \frac{\lambda F_i}{\lambda + x_i} \tag{32}$$

where $0 = x_1 < b_1 < \cdots < b_{n-1} < x_n$,

$$F_1 = \frac{1}{r \sum_{j=1}^{n-1} (L_j/b_j) + 1} > 0 \tag{33}$$

and

$$F_i = \frac{1}{r x_i \sum_{j=1}^{n-1} L_j/(b_j - x_i)^2} > 0 \tag{34}$$

for $i = 2, \ldots, n$. The $x_2, \ldots, x_n$ are uniquely determined by the fact that

$$\sum_{j=1}^{n-1} \frac{L_j}{b_j - x_i} = -\frac{1}{r} \tag{35}$$

for $i = 2, \ldots, n$. In addition $F_1 + \cdots + F_n = 1$.
   If S is of PVP type without shunt with weights $L_1, \ldots, L_n > 0$ at barriers $0 = b_1 < \cdots < b_n$ then

$$R(\lambda) = \sum_{i=1}^{n} \frac{\lambda F_i}{\lambda + x_i} \tag{36}$$

where $b_1 < x_1 < \cdots < b_n < x_n$,

$$F_i = \frac{1}{r_{x_i} \sum_{j=1}^{n} L_j/(b_j - x_i)^2} > 0 \tag{37}$$

for $i = 1, \ldots, n$. The $x_1, \ldots, x_n$ are uniquely determined by the fact that

$$\sum_{j=1}^{n} \frac{L_j}{b_j - x_i} = -\frac{1}{r}$$

for $i = 1, \ldots, n$ and $F_1 + \cdots + F_n = 1$.

D. Significance

These results show that in theory there is significant information in a steady state inert gas study without measurement of mixed venous partial pressures. Simple procedures detailed in Evans (1979c) give the distribution of fractional perfusions over the ventilation–perfusion $(\dot{V}_A/\dot{Q})$ scale as a function of $r = \dot{V}_T/\dot{Q}_T$ and the fractional shunt is expressed as a simple function of r, making it possible to comprehend all possible PVP models with a given E/R solubility relation.

VI. INSOLUBLE GAS WASH-OUT STUDIES

In this section we consider the wash-out of gases of negligible solubility (Lewis *et al.*, 1978). We first formally define the wash-out and the give general conditions for parallel equivalence (Evans, 1970). This is followed by the description of a compartmental model with dead space (Evans *et al.*, 1967).

A. The Open-Circuit Insoluble Gas Wash-Out

Suppose that an insoluble test gas is uniformly distributed at concentration C in the lung at full inspiration. If no further test gas is administered and if the expired gas is collected at each breath thereafter, we say that the sequence consisting of the amounts of test gas collected in each expiration constitutes an *open-circuit insoluble gas wash-out*. We label these amounts $C(k)$ for the kth expirate, calling the initial expirate the $k = 0$ expirate.

Assuming that the mixing processes in the lung are stationary from breath to breath, these processes may be described quite generally as follows.

B. Transfer Functions, Modeling Assumptions

1. The Transition Functions; Inspiration to Expiration

We represent the air spaces in inspiration by a set I of finite volume in Euclidean 3-space and represent the air spaces in expiration by a similar set E. For the test gas at concentration $f(x)$ in inspiration let

$$\int_I T_E(x, y)f(x)\,dV(x)$$

give the concentration at $y \in E$ on expiration, where dV denotes integration with respect to volume. Here $T_E(x, y)$ is the *transition density function* for expiration and must satisfy $T_E(x, y) \geq 0$ for all $x \in I$, $y \in E$, and $\int_E T_E(x, y) \, dV(y) \leq 1$ for all $x \in I$ since the amount of test substance cannot increase.

2. The Transition Function: Expiration to Inspiration

In a similar fashion let $T_I(x, y)$ for $x \in I$, $y \in E$, give the transition from expiration to inspiration. Again $T_I(x, y) \geq 0$ for all $x \in I$, $y \in E$, and in addition $\int_I T_I(x, y) \, dV(x) = 1$ for all $y \in E$ since no test substance is lost on inspiration.

Under mild regularity assumptions on $T_E(x, y)$ and $T_I(x, y)$, which are certainly satisfied in practice because of the smoothing effect of diffusion, we have the following theorem.

C. A Theorem on Insoluble Gas Wash-Out

Theorem 7. If respiration is symmetric in that $T_I(x, y) = T_E(x, y)$ for all $x \in I$, $y \in E$, and test gas is initially present at concentration C, then

$$C(k) = \sum_{i=1}^{\infty} A_i \lambda_i^k, \qquad \text{for} \quad k \geq 0$$

where $A_1, A_2, \ldots, \geq 0$ and $1 > \lambda_1 \geq \lambda_2 \geq \cdots \geq 0$ with

$$\sum_{i=1}^{\infty} \frac{A_i}{1 - \lambda_i} \leq C \int_I dV$$

and where $(\lambda_i)^0 = 1$ for $i \geq 1$.

D. Significance

The conditions of the theorem are met if convection in expiration is the reverse of that in inspiration. In a compartmental model the conditions are met if there is complete mixing in all compartments and if the compartments of the expiratory phase are assembled from fractions of the compartments of the inspiratory phase in a manner that is symmetric with the formation of the compartments of the inspiratory phase from fractions of the compartments of the expiratory phase. The conclusion of the theorem is that the output is equivalent to the output from a lung with parallel ventilation to compartments with inspiratory volume A_i and expiratory volume $\lambda_i A_i$ for $i = 1, 2, \ldots$.

E. Compartmental Model with Dead Space

We model the air spaces of the lung in a compartmental model as follows. Let D be the volume of the conducting airways (dead space) and let $V_1, \ldots, V_n$ be the volume of n functional compartments of the lung in full inspiration while $V'_1, \ldots, V'_n$ gives the volume of the same functional compartments in full expiration. Let T be the tidal volume so that

$$T = (V_1 - V'_1) + \cdots + (V_n - V'_n) \tag{38}$$

The Dynamics of Air Exchange in the Model

Let $g_0, \ldots, g_n$ give the concentration of a test gas in the conducting airways and the functional compartments at full inspiration. We then assume that at full expiration the conducting airways will contain an amount

$$\frac{D}{T} [(V_1 - V'_1)g_1 + \cdots + (V_n - V'_n)g_n] \tag{39}$$

of test substance while the output of test substance is

$$D_{g_0} + \frac{(T - D)}{T} [(V_1 - V'_1)g_1 + \cdots + (V_n - V'_n)g_n] \tag{40}$$

Assuming that no new test gas is inspired we assume that in the subsequent inspiration the conducting airways will contain no test gas and that the ith functional compartment will contain an amount $V'_i g_i$ of test substance which has remained in that compartment during expiration plus fraction $(V_i - V'_i)/T$ of the amount (39) left in the conducting airways during expiration. We add the following assumptions:

(1) $0 < D < T$.
(2) Any compartment with $V_i = V'_i$ has been removed from consideration.
(3) Compartments with the same ratio $\theta_i \equiv^{\text{def}} V'_i/V_i$ have been lumped together and $\theta_1 < \cdots < \theta_n$.
(4) The test gas has concentration 1 throughout the lung at the beginning of the wash-out test.

We then have the following theorem.

F. A Theorem on the Effect of the Dead Space

Theorem 8. The open-circuit insoluble gas wash-out has the form

$$C(k) = A_0 \lambda_0^k + \cdots + A_n \lambda_n^k$$

where $A_0, \ldots, A_n > 0$ and

$$0 = \lambda_0 \le \theta_1 < \lambda_1 < \theta_2 < \cdots < \theta_n < \lambda_n < 1$$

The following equations relate the model parameters D, $V_1, \ldots, V_n$, $V_1', \ldots, V_n'$ to the output parameters $A_0, \ldots, A_n$, $\lambda_0, \ldots, \lambda_n$, and suffice to determine one set of parameters when the other set is known.

$$T = (V_1 - V_1') + \cdots + (V_n - V_n') = A_0 + \cdots + A_n, \qquad D = A_0 \quad (41)$$

$$\frac{A_1(1 - \theta_i)}{\lambda_1 - \theta_i} + \cdots + \frac{A_n(1 - \theta_i)}{\lambda_n - \theta_i} - \frac{T(T - D)}{D} = 0, \qquad i = 1, \ldots, n \tag{42}$$

$$\frac{V_1(1 - \theta_1)^2}{\lambda_i - \theta_1} + \cdots + \frac{V_n(1 - \theta_n)^2}{\lambda_i - \theta_n} - \frac{T^2}{D} = 0, \; i = 1, \ldots, n \tag{43}$$

G. Significance

The theorem shows the effect of the conducting airway compartment in the model in slowing down the wash-out and in coupling the functional compartments.

VII. TRANSIENT INERT GAS TRANSFER

In the final section the transfer by the lungs of inert test gases in trace amounts under nonsteady state conditions is considered. This necessitates some consideration of the storage capacity of the lungs. The result in the compartmental formulation is a considerable increase in complexity for nonparallel models (Evans, 1979b).

A. Modeling Assumptions

1. The Assumption of Local Balance of Air Flow

We now add the assumption that the air flow into each compartment is equal to the air flow out. As we have seen previously for blood flow, the result is that $A\mathbf{e}$ is an n-vector giving the air flows to the n compartments from the outside while $\mathbf{e}^T A$ is a n-row vector giving the air flows to the outside.

2. Storage Capacity of the Lungs

We assign to each compartment an air volume V_i and a fluid volume F_i for $i = 1, \ldots, n$ and we set $V = \mathrm{diag}(V_1, \ldots, V_n)$ and $F = \mathrm{diag}(F_1, \ldots, F_n)$. We assume that if the partial pressures in the units at time t of a test gas with blood gas partition coefficient λ are given by $P(t) \equiv^{\mathrm{def}} [P_1(t), \ldots, P_n(t)]^{\mathsf{T}}$ then the amount of test gas in the compartments is $(V + \lambda F)P(t)$. Thus for simplicity λ serves as both the blood–gas partition coefficient and the tissue fluid–gas partition coefficient.

3. Transient Gas Exchange

If we combine the quantity

$$(V + \lambda F)P(t)$$

of test gas present at time t in the n compartments with the rate

$$P_I(t)A\mathbf{e} + P_{\bar{V}}(t)\lambda B\mathbf{e}$$

of inflow and the rate

$$(A + \lambda B)P(t)$$

of outflow of test substance, we obtain the ordinary differential equation

$$(V + \lambda F)\dot{P}(t) = -(A + \lambda B)P(t) + P_I(t)A\mathbf{e} + P_{\bar{V}}(t)\lambda B\mathbf{e} \quad (44)$$

Here $P_I(t)$ is the partial pressure in the inspired air and $P_{\bar{V}}(t)$ is the partial pressure in venous blood of the test gas at time t. The overdot on the P denote differentiation with respect to time.

To give a solution to (44) we set

$$M_\lambda \stackrel{\mathrm{def}}{=} (V + \lambda F)^{-1}(A + \lambda B)$$

and we have (Gantmacher, 1959)

$$
P(t) = \int_{-\infty}^{t} \exp[(s - t)M_\lambda]P_I(s)(\mathbf{v} + \lambda F)^{-1}A\mathbf{e}\, ds
$$

$$
+ \int_{-\infty}^{t} \exp[(s - t)M_\lambda]P_{\bar{V}}(s)(V + \lambda F)^{-1}B\mathbf{e}\, ds
$$

$$(45)$$

where $\exp(M) = \Sigma_{k=0}^{\infty} M^k/k!$ for any square matrix M.

4. The Output of the Transient Exchange Model

The expired air, which is a mixture of all the air leaving the compartments, has test substance at a partial pressure

$$e^T A P(t)/e^T A e \qquad (46)$$

while the arterial blood has test substance at a partial pressure

$$e^T B P(t)/e^T B e \qquad (47)$$

B. Transfer Functions

We now collect all terms that transfer the inputs P_I and $P_{\bar{V}}$ to the outputs P_E and P_a and set

$$T_E^I(\lambda,t) \overset{\text{def}}{=\!=\!=} e^T A \, \exp(-t M_\lambda)(V + \lambda F)^{-1} A e / e^T A e$$

$$T_a^I(\lambda,t) \overset{\text{def}}{=\!=\!=} e^T B \, \exp(-t M_\lambda)(V + \lambda F)^{-1} A e / e^T B e$$

$$(48)$$

$$T_E^V(\lambda,t) \overset{\text{def}}{=\!=\!=} e^T A \, \exp(-t M_\lambda)(V + \lambda F)^{-1} B e / e^T A e$$

$$T_a^V(\lambda,t) \overset{\text{def}}{=\!=\!=} e^T B \, \exp(-t M_\lambda)(V + \lambda F)^{-1} B e / e^T B e$$

for $t \geq 0$ and

$$T_E^I(\lambda,\, t) = T_a^I(\lambda,\, t) = T_E^V(\lambda,\, t) = T_a^V(\lambda,\, t) = 0$$

for $t < 0$.

The Outputs Expressed as Convolutions

We then have

$$P_E(t) = [T_E^I(\lambda,\, \cdot)*P_I](t) + [T_E^V(\lambda,\, \cdot)*P_{\bar{V}}](t)$$

$$P_a(t) = [T_a^I(\lambda,\, \cdot)*P_I](t) + [T_a^V(\lambda,\, \cdot)*P_{\bar{V}}](t)$$

$$(49)$$

where

$$f*g(t) \overset{\text{def}}{=\!=\!=} \int_{-\infty}^{\infty} f(t - s)g(s)\, ds = \int_{-\infty}^{\infty} f(s)g(t - s)\, ds$$

is the convolution of functions f and g evaluated at t.

C. Parallel Ventilation and Perfusion Models

If the off-diagonal terms of A (of B) are zero we say as before that ventilation (perfusion) is parallel. If both ventilation and perfusion are parallel the eigenvalues of M_λ are just the diagonal entries $\mu_{\lambda i} \overset{\text{def}}{=} (\dot{V}_i + \dot{Q}_i)/(V_i + \lambda F_i)$, where $B = \text{diag}(\dot{Q}_1, \ldots, \dot{Q}_n)$ and $A = \text{diag}(\dot{V}_1, \ldots, \dot{V}_n)$. We have at once that

$$T_E^I(\lambda, t) = \frac{1}{\dot{V}_T} \sum_{i=1}^{n} \frac{(\dot{V}_i)^2}{V_i + \lambda F_i} \exp(-t\mu_{\lambda i})$$

$$T_a^I(\lambda, t) = \frac{1}{\dot{Q}_T} \sum_{i=1}^{n} \frac{(\dot{V}_i \dot{Q}_i)}{V_i + \lambda F_i} \exp(-t\mu_{\lambda i})$$

$$T_E^V(\lambda, t) = \frac{1}{\dot{V}_T} \sum_{i=1}^{n} \frac{(\dot{V}_i \dot{Q}_i)}{V_i + \lambda F_i} \exp(-t\mu_{\lambda i})$$

(50)

$$T_a^V(\lambda, t) = \frac{1}{\dot{Q}_T} \sum_{i=1}^{n} \frac{(\dot{Q}_i)^2}{V_i + \lambda F_i} \exp(-t\mu_{\lambda i})$$

Three Ratios Used to Define a Parameter Space

If three ratios are defined for each compartment

$$r_1 = \text{perfusion/volume}$$

$$r_2 = \text{ventilation/volume}$$

$$r_3 = \text{fluid content/volume}$$

then the transfer functions may be expressed in terms of a distribution of lung volume in (r_1, r_2, r_3) space in the same manner that steady state models are described by a distribution of perfusion over ventilation–perfusion ratios. We have on using the superscript i on r_1, r_2, and r_3 to denote the ith compartment that

$$T_E^I(\lambda, t) = \frac{1}{\dot{V}_T} \sum_{i=1}^{n} V_i \frac{(r_2^i)^2}{1 + \lambda r_3^i} \exp\left(-t \frac{r_2^i + \lambda r_1^i}{1 + \lambda r_3^i}\right)$$

$$= \sum_{i=1}^{n} V_i G_E^I(r_1^i, r_2^i, r_3^i, t)$$

where

$$G_E^I(r_1, r_2, r_3, t) = \frac{(r_2)^2}{\dot{V}_T(1 + \lambda r_3)} \exp\left(-t \frac{r_2 + \lambda r_1}{1 + r_3}\right)$$

with similar expressions G_a^I, G_E^V, and G_a^V for the remaining transfer functions.

D. Test Description and Parameter Recovery

1. A Test Based on Transient Inert Gas Exchange

With this formulation we consider a test as follows:

(1) Administer test gases by mouth and in dissolved state by intravenous drip for $0 \leq t \leq T$.

(2) Measure $P_{\bar{v}}(t)$ and $P_I(t)$ for $0 \leq t \leq T$ for each gas. Include a correction for the conducting airways so that the $P_I(t)$ used is the inspiratory partial pressure to the functional units of the lungs.

(3) Measure $P_E(t)$ and $P_a(t)$ for $0 \leq t \leq T$.

Now given any distribution of volumes $V_1, \ldots, V_n$ at ratios $(r_1^1, r_2^1, r_3^1), \ldots, (r_1^n, r_2^n, r_3^n)$ we note that the dependence of the transfer functions on $V_1, \ldots, V_n$ is linear. Also for P_I and $P_{\bar{v}}$ fixed and known, the dependence of P_E and P_a on the transfer functions is linear from (50). Thus for P_I and $P_{\bar{v}}$ fixed the dependence of P_E and P_a on a distribution of volume over the (r_1, r_2, r_3) parameter space is linear. We may now ask for the distribution that gives an optimal approximation to the observed P_E and P_a. This formulation allows the use of a constrained linear least-squares approach similar to the treatment in Evans and Wagner (1977) and Lewis et al. (1978).

2. Parameter Determination

It is assumed that given any sum of exponential decay factors for $t \geq 0$ of the form $\sum_{i=1}^{k} a_i e - \alpha_i t$ where $0 < \alpha_1 < \alpha_2 < \cdots < \alpha_k$ and $a_1, \ldots, a_k \geq 0$ the decay rates $\alpha_1, \ldots, \alpha_k$ and the coefficients $a_1, \ldots, a_k$ can be recovered. For each distinct α in $\mu_{\lambda 1}, \ldots, \mu_{\lambda n}$ let J_α be the set of $1 \leq i \leq n$ with $\mu_{\lambda i} = \alpha$. Then set

$$a_\alpha = \sum_{i \in J_\alpha} \frac{(\dot{V}_i)^2}{V_i + \lambda F_i}, \qquad b_\alpha = \sum_{i \in J_\alpha} \frac{(\dot{Q}_i)^2}{V_i + \lambda F_i}, \qquad c_\alpha = \sum_{i \in J_\alpha} \frac{(\dot{V}_i \dot{Q}_i)}{V_i + \lambda F_i} \quad (51)$$

Under the above assumptions a_α, b_α, and c_α can be determined from a transient inert gas study. We observe that

$$(a_\alpha + \lambda c_\alpha)/\alpha = \sum_{i \in J_\alpha} \dot{V}_i$$

$$(c_\alpha + \lambda b_\alpha)/\alpha = \sum_{i \in J_\alpha} \dot{Q}_i \qquad (52)$$

$$(a_\alpha + 2\lambda c_\alpha + \lambda^2 b_\alpha)/\alpha^2 = \sum_{i \in J_\alpha} (V_i + \lambda F_i)$$

Thus the total ventilation, perfusion, and storage capacity are known for each characteristic decay rate or wash-out rate α.

In addition as a measure of the dispersion over different ventilation–perfusion ratios we have

$$\left(\frac{a_\alpha}{\alpha}\right)\left(\frac{b_\alpha}{\alpha}\right) - \left(\frac{c_\alpha}{\alpha}\right)^2 = \sum_{\substack{i<j \\ i,j \in J_\alpha}} \frac{(\dot{V}_i/\dot{Q}_i - \dot{V}_j/\dot{Q}_j)^2}{(\dot{V}_i/\dot{Q}_i + \lambda)(\dot{V}_j/\dot{Q}_j + \lambda)} \qquad (53)$$

So that $a_\alpha b_\alpha = c_\alpha^2$ if and only if all units with index i in J_α have the same ratio of ventilation to perfusion, which is then $(\Sigma_{i \in J_\alpha} \dot{V}_i)/(\Sigma_{i \in J_\alpha} \dot{Q}_i)$.

3. Lung Volume and Fluid Content

By summing the storage capacity over all distinct α in $\mu_{\lambda 1}, \ldots, \mu_{\lambda n}$ we obtain

$$\sum_{i=1}^{n} V_i + \lambda \sum_{i=1}^{n} F_i \tag{54}$$

so that in theory knowledge of the transfer functions for $\lambda_1 \neq \lambda_2$ results in a determination of lung volume and fluid content.

E. Models with No Parallel Ventilation and Perfusion Equivalence

If we assume that the matrices A and B are symmetric there is for a fixed blood gas partition coefficient λ a strong similarity to the behavior of some parallel ventilation and perfusion model in transient inert gas elimination. The following two examples with symmetric A and B, however, do not have an equivalent parallel ventilation and perfusion model for λ not fixed.

Example 1. Let $A = \begin{pmatrix} 6 & -4 \\ -4 & 12 \end{pmatrix}$, $B = \begin{pmatrix} 1 & 0 \\ 0 & 1 \end{pmatrix}$, and $V = F = \begin{pmatrix} 1 & 0 \\ 0 & 4 \end{pmatrix}$. This model has parallel blood flow and has a fluid content equal to the air volume of each of the two compartments.

Example 2. Let A and V be as above and set $B = F = \begin{pmatrix} 1 & 0 \\ 0 & 1 \end{pmatrix}$. This model has parallel blood flow with a fluid content equal to the blood flow.

It is a fact that if $V^{-1}F$, $V^{-1}A$, and $V^{-1}B$ all commute, then there is a parallel ventilation and perfusion model with equivalent transient inert gas exchange.

REFERENCES

Cantor, D. G., and Evans, J. W. (1970). A correction for the effect of the dead space in pulmonary gas washout studies. *Bull. Math. Biophys.* **32,** 215–218.

Colburn, W. E., Evans, J. W., and West, J. B. (1974). Analysis of the effect of solubility on gas exchange in nonhomogeneous lungs. *J. Appl. Physiol.* **37,** 547–551.

Evans, J. W. (1970). The gas washout determination under a symmetry assumption. *Bull. Math. Biophys.* **32,** 59–63.

Evans, J. W. (1979a). On steady state inert gas exchange. *Math. Biosci.* **46,** 209–222.

Evans, J. W. (1979b). On transient inert gas exchange. *Math. Biosci.* **46,** 233–250.

Evans, J. W. (1979c). Inert gas elimination studies without mixed venous partial pressures. *Math. Biosci.* **46,** 223–232.

Evans, J. W., and Wagner, P. D. (1977). Limits on $\dot{V}_A/\dot{Q}$ distributions from analysis of experimental inert gas elimination. *J. Appl. Physiol.* **42,** 889–898.

Evans, J. W., Cantor, D. G., and Norman, J. R. (1967). The dead space in a compartmental lung model. *Bull. Math. Biophys.* **29,** 711–718.

Evans, J. W., Wagner, P. D., and West, J. B. (1974). Conditions for reduction of pulmonary gas transfer by ventilation–perfusion inequality. *J. Appl. Physiol.* **36,** 533–537.

Farhi, L. E. (1967). Elimination of inert gas by the lung. *Respir. Physiol.* **3,** 1–11.

Farhi, L. E., and Yokoyama, T. (1967). Effects of ventilation–perfusion inequality on elimination of inert gases. *Respir. Physiol.* **3,** 12–20.

Gantmacher, F. R. (1959). "The Theory of Matrices." *Chelsea,* Bronx, New York.

Jaliwala, S. A., Mates, R. E., and Klocke, F. J. (1975). An efficient optimization technique for recovering ventilation–perfusion distributions from inert gas data. Effects of random experimental error. *J. Clin. Invest.* **55,** 188–192.

Lewis, S. M., Evans, J. W., and Jalowayski, A. E. (1978). Continuous distributions of specific ventilation recovered from inert gas washout. *J. Appl. Physiol.* **44,** 416–423.

Nye, R. E. (1970). Influence of cyclical pattern of ventilatory flow on pulmonary gas exchange. *Respir. Physiol.* **10,** 321–337.

Olszowka, A. J. (1975). Can $\dot{V}_A/\dot{Q}$ distributions in the lung be recovered from inert gas retention data. *Respir. Physiol.* **25,** 191–198.

Wagner, P. D., and Evans, J. W. (1977). Conditions for equivalence of gas exchange in series and parallel models of the lungs. *Respir. Physiol.* **31,** 117–138.

Wagner, P. D., Laravuso, R. B., Uhl, R. R., and West, J. B. (1974a). Continuous distributions of ventilation–perfusion ratios in normal subjects breathing air and 100% O_2. *J. Clin. Invest.* **54,** 54–68.

Wagner, P. D., Naumann, P. F., and Laravuso, R. B. (1974b). Simultaneous measurement of eight foreign gases in blood by gas chromatography. *J. Appl. Physiol.* **36,** 600–605.

Wagner, P. D., Saltzman, H. A., and West, J. B. (1974c). Measurement of continuous distributions of ventilation–perfusion ratios: Theory. *J. Appl. Physiol.* **36,** 588–599.

Wagner, P. D., Dantzker, D. R., Iacovoni, V. E., Schillaci, R. F., and West, J. B. (1975). Distributions of ventilation–perfusion ratios in asthma. *Am. Rev. Respir. Dis.* **111,** 940. (Abstr.)

Wagner, P. D., Dantzker, D. R., Dueck, R., Clausen, J. L., and West, J. B. (1977). Ventilation–perfusion inequality in chronic obstructive pulmonary disease. *J. Clin. Invest.* **59,** 203–216.

Wagner, P. D., Dantzker, D. R., Iacovoni, V. E., Tomkin, W. C., and West, J. B. (1978). Ventilation–perfusion inequality in asymptomatic asthma. *Am. Rev. Respir. Dis.* **118,** 511–524.

Wilkinson, J. H. (1965). "The Algebraic Eigenvalue Problem." Oxford Univ. Press, London and New York.

Index